PRACTICAL
VETERINARY
ULTRASOUND

PRACTICAL VETERINARY ULTRASOUND

Robert E. Cartee, D.V.M., M.S.

Barbara A. Selcer, D.V.M., M.S.

Judith A. Hudson, D.V.M., M.S., Ph.D.

Susan T. Finn-Bodner, D.V.M., M.S.

Mary B. Mahaffey, D.V.M., M.S.

Pamela L. Johnson, B.S.

Ken W. Marich, B.S., M.B.A.

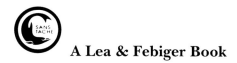

A Lea & Febiger Book

Williams & Wilkins

PHILADELPHIA • BALTIMORE • HONG KONG
LONDON • MUNICH • SYDNEY • TOKYO

A WAVERLY COMPANY
1995

Executive Editor: Carroll C. Cann
Developmental Editor: Susan Hunsberger
Production Coordinator: Marette D. Magargle
Project Editor: Robert D. Magee

Copyright © 1995
Williams & Wilkins
Rose Tree Corporate Center
1400 North Providence Road
Building II, Suite 5025
Media, PA 19063-2043 USA

Accurate indications, adverse reactions, and dosage schedules for drugs are provided in this book, but it is possible they may change. The reader is urged to review the package information data of the manufacturers of the medications mentioned.

Printed in the United States of America

Library of Congress Cataloging in Publication Data

Practical veterinary ultrasound / Robert E. Cartee . . . [et al.].
    p. cm.
  "A Lea & Febiger book."
  Includes index.
  ISBN 0-683-01483-8
  1. Veterinary ultrasonography.   I. Cartee, Robert E.
SF772.58.P74   1995
636.089'607543—dc20   94-44192
                       CIP

The Publishers have made every effort to trace the copyright holders for borrowed material. If they have inadvertently overlooked any, they will be pleased to make the necessary arrangements at the first opportunity.

95 96 97 98 99
1 2 3 4 5 6 7 8 9 10

PREFACE

The purpose of this book is to help the practicing veterinarian and the veterinary student to understand and use diagnostic ultrasound in the evaluation of small animal diseases. Basic physics and instrumentation are hopefully covered in a concise, practical way so that they may be applied to new situations that may arise for the veterinarian. Because ultrasound images represent somewhat unfamiliar planes of section through the body, Chapter 3 is devoted to cross-sectional anatomy, and provides a representative section of the major body regions in three planes (transverse, sagittal and frontal).

In many cases (e.g., cardiac), the best way to learn normal and abnormal sonographic appearances is by viewing a videotape. In these instances, we provide a verbal description to augment the still photos.

The normal and abnormal descriptions provided are the culmination of 100 years of study by many veterinary and nonveterinary sonographers. Their observations and those of the authors have been analyzed, compared, and compiled to facilitate today's sonographic studies. Many of the early observations were found inaccurate. The reader of this text is encouraged to add to the validation of our observations and to expand the knowledge base by exploring new frontiers of use. Sonographic imaging is not in its infancy; it is still maturing and is a long way from being complete. We hope that readers will use this information as an aid to diagnosis and, more importantly, to the expansion of our understanding.

ACKNOWLEDGMENT

I would like to acknowledge the patience, expertise, and untiring efforts of Mrs. Debbie Allgood in the preparation of this book.

CONTRIBUTORS

Robert E. Cartee, B.A., B.S., D.V.M., M.S.
Associate Professor
Departments of Anatomy/Histology and Radiology
CVM, Auburn University
Department of Anatomy/Histology
College of Veterinary Medicine
Auburn University, Alabama

Barbara A. Selcer, D.V.M.
Associate Professor and Diplomate A.C.V.R.
Department of Anatomy and Radiology
College of Veterinary Medicine
University of Georgia
Athens, Georgia

Judith A. Hudson, D.V.M., Ph.D.
Assistant Professor and Diplomate A.C.V.R.
Department of Radiology
Auburn University College of Veterinary Medicine
Auburn, Alabama

Susan T. Finn-Bodner, D.V.M., M.S.
Diplomate A.C.V.R.
Assistant Professor Radiology
Auburn University College of Veterinary Medicine
Auburn, Alabama

Mary B. Mahaffey, D.V.M., M.S.
Diplomate A.C.V.R.
Associate Professor Radiology
University of Georgia College of Veterinary Medicine
Athens, Georgia

Pamela L. Johnson, D.V.M.
Auburn University College of Veterinary Medicine
Auburn, Alabama

Kenneth W. Marich, B.S., M.B.A.
Adjunct Instructor, Auburn University, Alabama
Vice-President, Focus Surgery, California

CONTENTS

THE PHYSICS OF ULTRASOUND

Robert E. Cartee

DEFINITION AND PRODUCTION

Ultrasound is nothing more than sound at a frequency or tone that is higher than most humans can hear. That level or frequency is usually about 20,000 cycles per second or 20 kilohertz (kHz). Diagnostic medical ultrasound is usually produced at frequencies in millions of cycles per second, called megahertz (mHz). Ultrasound at this frequency is produced by materials called piezoelectric crystals, which have the ability to transfer electrical energy into mechanical ultrasound waves and to reconvert mechanical ultrasound waves into electrical energy. Staggering the electrical stimulation of these crystals can make them both transmitters and receivers of ultrasound. Deliberately constructing a piezoelectric material to a certain thickness and encasing it in a damping medium can make it produce ultrasound of a main or predominant tone or frequency. The crystal will also be able to receive ultrasound waves of that frequency or others when it is "listening."[1,2]

CHARACTERISTICS

Ultrasound emitted from a crystal has three basic properties. One, which has already been mentioned, is a certain frequency measured in megahertz that depends on the prescribed thickness and damping of the crystal. The frequency is analogous to the pitch or tone of audible sound and has a great bearing on the resolution and penetration capabilities of the ultrasound. The second property is the intensity or loudness of the ultrasound, which is measured in a relative value system of decibels like that used to measure audible sound. Intensity can also be measured in watts per centimeter squared, referring to its concentration at a particular depth. The intensity is determined by the signal that is stimulating the crystal but is altered by the medium through which the ultrasound passes. The third property of ultrasound is that it passes through a medium (the body in this case) at a certain speed or velocity. Although this velocity may vary slightly within soft tissues and varies greatly between hard and soft tissues, it is generally accepted to be a constant 1540 meters (m) per second in a mammalian body. This assumption of constant speed is one of the prime determinants of the operation of all ultrasound equipment. After production, a portion of the intensity is reflected back toward the crystal from somewhere in the body while another portion may travel deeper into the body to be reflected back at some later time or greater depth. As a result of the varying times that ultrasound returns to the crystal, an electronic picture created by the echoes can be

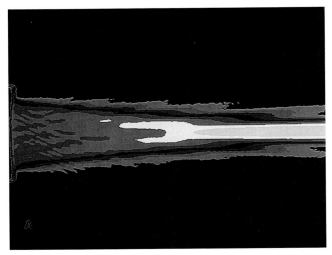

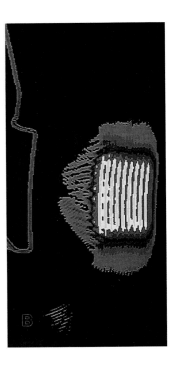

Figure 1–1

A, A Schlieren image of a beam of ultrasound. Note the various colors of different amplitudes (intensity) along the beam. In a narrow focal zone, the intensity is highest (orange). **B,** A Schlieren image of a pulse of ultrasound shows the individual wavelets contained in the pulse (alternating bands of color).

recreated on a screen. On the screen, one parameter always equals distance from the crystal, or depth into the body. The relative brightness of the images represents the relative intensity or loudness of the returning echoes (Fig. 1–1).[1,2]

ATTENUATION

Attenuation is a term used to indicate what happens to the intensity of the ultrasound after it enters the body. Neither the frequency nor the velocity changes appreciably; therefore, the variable characteristic, the one used to construct visual images, is the intensity or loudness. On the basis of this fact, attenuation can be described as consisting of five main occurrences. The intensity can be *reflected* at various levels and depths, to be reconstructed electronically into the image. To be reflected at various levels, it must also be *transmitted* to those levels. In this process, some of the intensity may be changed into some unavailable form or may be redirected so that it does not return to the crystal. *Absorption, scatter,* and *refraction* are terms used to describe other forms of attenuation.[1,2]

Different acoustic impedances of adjacent biologic materials determine the amount of reflected intensity of the ultrasound at a particular interface. The term "acoustic impedance" describes the relationship between the density and the stiffness of a particular substance. The differences in impedance of adjacent materials determine the reflectivity and transmissibility of the intensity of the ultrasound. If the impedance difference is great, the intensity of the reflection will be great. If the impedance of adjacent materials is equal, no reflection of the ultrasound occurs and the ultrasound is totally transmitted. This concept can become complex because of the laws governing the direction of reflection relative to the direction of incidence based on the stiffness/density determination of propagation speed. For the purpose of this discussion, however, it is possible that the direction of the ultrasound wave front can be altered by a curved surface and a variable propagation speed.[1–3]

An ultrasound wave front with a certain tone (frequency) and a certain loudness is produced by the crystal. As the wave front enters the body, some of the loudness is reflected back to the crystal, some goes deeper, and some is lost. The loudness of the echo depends on the differences in density and stiffness of adjacent biologic materials and how much loudness remains at that point. In most cases, the deeper into the body a reflector lies, the less loud the echo, unless little loss has occurred superficial to the reflector. What has been reflected is no longer available for deeper reflection, and what has been absorbed is also not available.[1-3]

RESOLUTION

The two resolutions of ultrasound imaging are axial and lateral. The axial, or longitudinal, is related to frequencies and refers to how close two reflectors can be on an axis parallel to the direction of travel of the ultrasound wave front and still be seen as two reflectors. Major components of this determination are the frequency of the crystal and the frequency at which it is stimulated. Usually, the higher the frequency, the better the axial resolution and the more detailed the image can be.[1-3]

Lateral resolution refers to how close two reflectors can be perpendicular to the direction of travel of the ultrasound wave front and still be seen as separate reflections. This resolution is directly related to the width of the crystal and the distance of the reflectors from it. If the reflectors are both within the wave front of one crystal, they will be seen as one reflector. If the reflectors are outside the crystal's wave front and in another crystal's wave front, or if a crystal can be moved back and forth, the two reflectors may be distinguished as separate. Ultrasound wave fronts, like light beams, tend to converge and then diverge; therefore, in some zones, lateral resolution may be better or worse than in others. Methods used to arrange the crystals to produce concentric rings of wave fronts may improve the lateral resolution; these techniques are discussed in a subsequent section. The level of attenuation is directly related to the frequency: the higher the frequency, the greater the attenuation per centimeter of tissue. Therefore, a trade-off exists between axial resolution and the ability to penetrate deeply. Lower frequencies produce better capabilities of penetration before the intensity diminishes, but the axial resolution is not as good. Conversely, higher frequencies produce better resolution but lose loudness sooner. In this case, reducing the amount of initial loudness lost by using a contrast medium with homogenous acoustic impedance allows more penetration.[1-3]

Sonographic resolution may be summarized as follows:

1. The brightness of the image produced is proportional to the loudness of the echo, which is directly related to differences in the densities or stiffness of the adjacent tissue and in the depth from which the echoes came.
2. The detail of the image is proportional to stimulation frequency, crystal frequency, width of the crystal, and depth from which the echo came.
3. Usually, higher frequencies are associated with better resolution but less penetration, and lower frequencies are associated with more penetration but less resolution.

MODES OF DISPLAY

Modes of display refer to how the electronic signal generated by the returning echo striking the crystal is presented for interpretation. Of the many modes of display, the simplest is an A mode display, which is a vertical deflection of a beam of electrons that is tracing out a straight line across an oscilloscope screen. The height of the deflection corresponds to the loudness of the returning echo, and the space between the deflections corresponds to depth or time between echoes. Because the height corresponds to loudness and loudness or intensity is not an electronic term, the height corresponds to the amplitude of the signal and therefore A mode stands for amplitude mode. This mode of display is used with high-frequency transducer crystals in measuring distances in the eye.[4] It has been used in veterinary medicine for the detection of pregnancy in pigs and sheep.[5,6]

The mode used most commonly today is the B mode. In this case, the loudness of the echo is displayed by correspondingly bright spots on a screen. Progressively more sophisticated methods of displaying the relative brightness have been developed based on relative echo intensities. The "B" in B mode stands for brightness. The display of different levels of brightness is called a gray scale display. The ability through computerization of the signal position to update the location of the echo from microsecond to microsecond ("real-time" ultrasound) has enabled visualization of movement within the entire field of view. Before the availability of real-time imaging, the entire field of view was frozen on the screen until erased and replaced by another, the static B mode display.[1–3]

The ability to select a specific portion of a real-time image and/or to look only at the patterns described by motion within a specific area has been called M or "motion" mode. M mode is used especially in cardiac evaluation and has become synonymous with echocardiography. Most systems now use both B mode real-time gray scale displays and M mode displays.[1–3]

DOPPLER ULTRASONOGRAPHY

The frequencies produced from reflectors do not necessarily remain the same as that being produced by the crystal. If the reflector is moving and the crystal is made capable of receiving and recording the echo frequency from that reflector, then it is possible to display the direction and amount of the frequency shift or change produced. Knowing the frequency of the originally produced ultrasound, the angle at which the wave front is striking the moving reflector, and the "constant" propagation speed of ultrasound creates a formula that allows the calculation of the amount of change and direction of change in frequency. Manipulation of the *Doppler shift formula* also allows calculation of the velocity of and direction in which the reflector is moving. This information may be displayed in the form of a profile similar to an A mode intensity display, a histogram, an audible pulsed display, or a colored image over a B mode intensity display. Doppler ultrasonography is used primarily to detect blood flow in vessels and in the heart. Through mathematical comparisons of differing flow velocities during stages of the cardiac cycle, many useful indices and values may be studied.[7]

ARTIFACTS

With a concept of the basic physics of ultrasonographic imaging comes the awareness of the possibilities of errors in the display, called "imaging artifacts." Some of these errors are easy to recognize and are even helpful in diagnostic procedures. Three examples are *acoustic shadowing, reverberation,* and *enhancement.*

Acoustic shadowing occurs when the intensity of the reflection is so great that there is little or no intensity remaining to be transmitted, producing a shadow deep to the reflection (Fig. 1–2). This shadowing indicates that the reflection is different in acoustic impedance and is likely to be bony, metallic, or a large bubble of gas. (One is stiff or dense and the other is elastic. Therefore, the acoustic impedance is different from biologic materials, but each in its own separate way.)

Reverberation occurs when the wave front is scattered and delayed in returning to the crystal but the intensity is still great (Fig. 1–3). This type of artifact may indicate a big acoustic impedance difference and many small or irregular reflectors (air within lung alveoli). Reverberation is useful in that it may help to determine the nature of the reflector (e.g., little gas bubbles or an irregular surface). Some examples of deep reverberation artifacts are called "comet tail" and "ring down" artifacts.

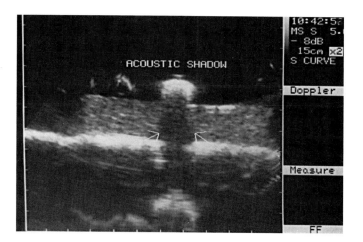

Figure 1–2

An acoustic shadow (arrows) produced by a stronger reflective interface.

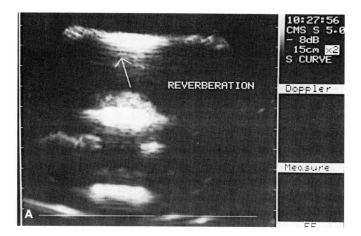

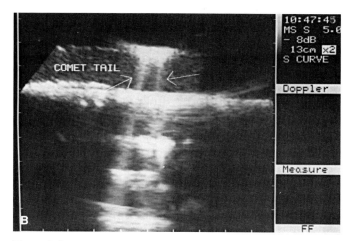

Figure 1–3

A, A reverberation artifact is produced by two strongly reflective interfaces in close proximity (i.e., surface of air close to surface of probe). Note the repetitive echogenic lines (arrow). **B,** Comet tail artifact, parallel white lines (arrows), caused by deep reverberation.

Enhancement occurs when there is little or no attenuation of the intensity so that all reflections deep to the nonattenuating area appear more intense than normal (Fig. 1–4). This phenomenon is noted most commonly deep to cystic structures such as the gallbladder or the urinary bladder. When enhancement occurs, the fair assumption is that the nonattenuating area is homogeneous in its acoustic impedance.

Other less useful types of artifacts are *mirror image, slice thickness*, and *refraction*. Mirror image artifacts occur as a result of repetitive or delayed wave front reflections that duplicate an area displayed previously. A common example is duplication of liver parenchyma echoes so that they arrive later at the crystal and the liver appears to be superficial *and* deep to the diaphragm, creating the illusion of a diaphragmatic hernia (Fig. 1–5). Slice thickness artifacts occur because the ultrasound beam has a finite thickness. If a portion of the thickness includes both the wall and the lumen of a fluid-filled structure, both will

Figure 1–4

Enhancement artifact (arrows) created by more proximal, weakly attenuating materials such as homogeneous fluids.

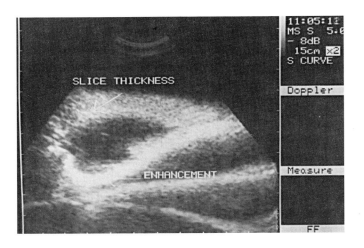

Figure 1–5

Mirror image artifact created by a deeply placed, strongly reflective interface and a more proximal reflective interface resulting in a repetitive path before arriving at the probe surface. Note the appearance of two objects, one on each side of the diaphragm (arrows).

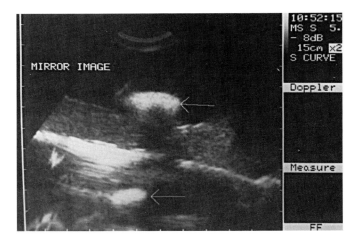

be displayed simultaneously and the appearance will be that of material (wall) within the fluid. This artifact is noted most often when scanning the gallbladder (Fig. 1–6). Refraction artifacts occur when propagation speeds vary and cause a wave front that is striking an acoustic impedance interface at a non-90° angle to be bent away or toward a 90° incidence. Echoes returning from deeper structures in the path of the refracted wave front are displayed improperly on the screen because ultrasound equipment assumes that all echoes come back at 90° (Fig. 1–7). Refraction may also lead to acoustic shadowing at the borders of curved structures if the propagation speed within the curved structure is greater than that of the material around it.[1]

Figure 1–6

Slice thickness artifact (arrow) created by inclusion of the wall of the organ in the same beam thickness as the lumen. Note the appearance of a material within the lumen that is really the wall of the gallbladder and adjacent lumen.

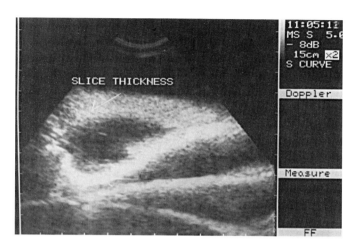

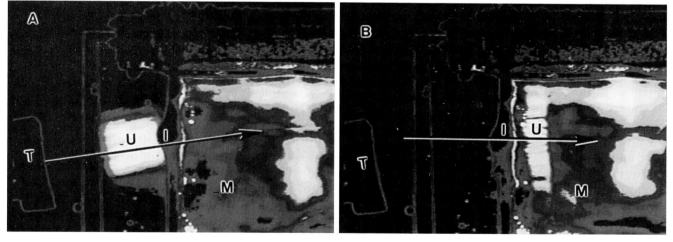

Figure 1–7

A, A black and white image of a Schlieren image shows a bundle of ultrasound (U) approaching an interface (I) between a water bath and a higher density material (M). The arrow indicates the angle of inclination that the ultrasound would follow without refraction occurring. T, transducer. **B,** Because the medium (M) density is higher than that of the water and the propagation velocity is less than that of water, the bundle of ultrasound (U) is refracted in the direction of the arrows, which could lead to artifacts on the returning echoes from deeper layers.

REFERENCES

1. Kremkau F: *Diagnostic Ultrasound.* New York, Grune & Stratton, 1989.
2. Powis RL: Ultrasound physics for the fun of it. Unirad Corp., 1978.
3. Ginther OJ: Ultrasonic imaging and reproductive events in the mare. Equiservices, 4343 Garfoot Road, Gross Plains, WI, 1986.
4. Schiffer SP, et al: Biometric study of the canine eye, using A mode ultrasonography. Am J Vet Res *43*:826, 1982.
5. Cartee RE, Powe TA, Ayer RL: Ultrasonographic detection of pregnancy in sows. Mod Vet Pract Jan:23, 1985.
6. Meredith MJ, Medani MUK: The detection of pregnancy in sheep by A mode ultrasound. Br Vet J *136*:325, 1980.
7. Kremkare FW: *Doppler Ultrasound.* New York, Grune & Stratton, 1990.

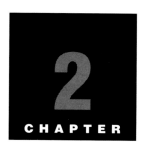

CHAPTER 2

INSTRUMENTS AND THEIR OPERATION

Robert E. Cartee

PROBES

The transducer or probe is the most important part of the instrumentation in diagnostic sonography. Choosing the appropriate type and frequency of transducer is essential to the value of the examination. In many studies, several frequencies and types are used. Higher frequency probes improve the axial resolution but the image usually appears enlarged. Lower frequency probes have less axial resolution and more penetration. Switching from a high to a low frequency probe may also create differences in size and echogenicity. Low frequency images usually appear more echogenic and require adjustment of gain controls.

Type and Selection (Fig. 2–1)

Ultrasound transducers or probes are categorized by the arrangement of the piezoelectric material/crystals, and by the firing sequence or method of electrical stimulation of the crystals. In a *linear array* probe, the material/crystal is arranged in a straight line. In an *annular array* probe, the material/crystal is arranged in concentric rings. A *sector* probe refers to the fact that there may be only one or two crystals, but these crystals are in motion while being stimulated. This motion allows the duplication of the image of a linear array while minimizing the size of the probe surface. Reducing the size facilitates access to smaller windows for viewing structures that a longer linear array probe might not be able to reach. Concentric rings of crystals (annular arrays) purportedly improve the lateral resolution of the ultrasound beam by creating overlapping areas within the same image field. By varying the number and overlapping the crystals stimulated in a linear array probe, a *phased linear array* probe is created. The resulting image is smoother and lateral resolution is improved. Altering the direction of the electrical stimulus from one end of the probe to the other and back produces a *steered linear array*. Again, this technique improves lateral resolution.

Lenses have been used to create focal zones of various depths. When a lens is used, the probe is designated as "focused." Focusing may also be accomplished by altering the timing of the electrical stimulus to the crystals. If this process is done and a lens is also used, the probe is then double focused.

Current advances in both probe design and receiver processing have enabled the pro-

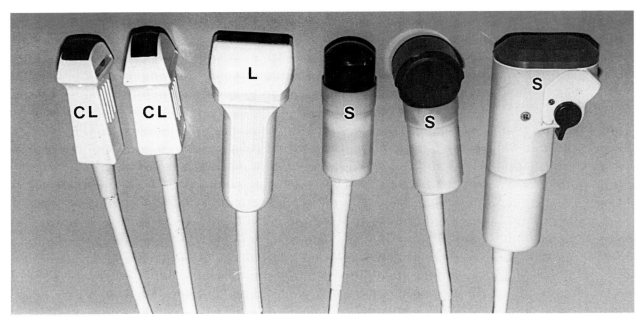

Figure 2–1

Examples of different kinds of ultrasound transducers (probes). Note the flat surface of the linear array (L). S, sector (mechanical); CL, curved linear; A, annular.

duction of curved or convex linear arrays or curved phased arrays. Both of these designs result in the superior image field of the linear array with fewer artifacts, as well as in a smaller active portion of the probe surface for easier access to body structures (e.g., heart).

Probes are also categorized according to their particular usage. Endovaginal probes are designed specifically for scanning the genital structures from within the vagina. Transrectal probes, used from within the rectum, have been used primarily for veterinary pregnancy examinations and for human prostate studies. Other terms such as "intraoperative," "near field," and "small parts" are used to describe probes with specific application for determining vascular supply during surgery, in the examination of the eye, and for evaluation of the thyroid gland, respectively. Probes are also designated according to the frequency of ultrasound produced. These frequencies vary from 2.25 megahertz (mHz) for use in studies of the abdomen to 50 mHz for some dermatologic applications.

Care and Cleaning

All types of probe require care and maintenance. Piezoelectric crystals should never be heated to extreme temperatures, such as in an autoclave. Overheating can result in permanent damage. Dropping or striking the probe surface against hard objects should be avoided because chipping and scratching of the soft material that covers the crystals tend to create areas of discontinuity in which air may collect and create acoustic shadows. Dropping may also result in damage to the piezoelectric material.

Probes should be wiped clean of the contact gel as soon as possible. Washing the probe with cold water and wiping it dry with a soft towel keeps the probe from accumulating harmful dried particles of gel. Although it makes a good contact medium, especially in horses, mineral oil is hard to remove and may be corrosive to the soft probe coverings.

Immersion of the entire probe in water or other liquids should be avoided. Tiny leaks in the cable may cause electrical shorting, which could result in electrical shock and certainly damage to the probe. Limited immersion of the probe surface in fluids is acceptable and, in many cases, is preferred to create a better image.

Doppler Probes

Doppler probes are of two basic types. A continuous wave Doppler probe requires the presence of two crystals, one that sends and the other that receives the returning echoes. These probes effectively record the flow of blood in vessels but they are not discriminatory as to the position of the vessel, so the exact depth of the vessel is difficult to determine. Pulsed Doppler probes have one crystal that acts as both transmitter and receiver. These probes are not as effective at picking up flow in any vessel in the path of the beam, but they are discriminating as to the exact depth of the vessel that is detected. Doppler signals received by these probes can be processed into audible signals, a spectral analysis display, and a color signal indicative of direction and velocity of flow.

GAIN CONTROLS

Ultrasound instruments have various complexities of gain controls. Gain refers to amplification of the electrical signal generated by the returning echoes. The intensity of the echo is the main determinant of the level of brightness of the image. The purpose of the gain control is to adjust the amplitude to create more contrast at some particular area of the image. Typically, near field echoes are brighter than those from the far field. Adjustment of the near field gain control may increase or decrease this brightness for a better image. Overall gain controls allow improvement of a poor contrast image in both the near and far fields. Gain controls are usually inoperable after the image is frozen. On some equipment, gain amplifications may be present in the form of preset curves. In addition to manual adjustment of gain, present curve options may be chosen in advance or during the scanning process, and may allow enhancement of the gray levels after freezing.

POWER

Power controls determine the intensity of the ultrasound being produced. Increasing the output power may help penetration and also will appear to have the same effect on the image as increasing gain. The quantitation of these controls is somewhat variable. Some manufacturers display power as absolute decibels of intensity, whereas others ascribe a value that is electronically relative to that instrument (e.g., -0 = maximum power and -14 = minimum power; Diasonics, Inc., Milpitas, CA). Images can be vastly improved by balancing the power and gain controls. Manipulating these two controls can compensate for deficiencies in penetration in order to improve resolution.

Other controls include depth of field, temporal (time) processing, reject, orientation, annotation, left-right invert, polarity, pointers, format, biopsy controls, pulsed Doppler cursors, M mode cursors, configuration controls, and, finally, measurement controls. Not all of these control options are available on every ultrasound machine. Usually, the more options available, the more expensive the equipment. The following is a brief listing of these controls and their practical function (Fig. 2–2).

1. *Depth of field*: Allows an increase or reduction in the size of the image to enable visualization of a structure that might be out of an image field. An additional option connected with this area is a *zoom* control that allows magnification of the image.
2. *Temporal processing*: Not usually available, but this gain control option processes the image based on time of echo arrival.

Figure 2–2

Example of an ultrasound machine. P, printer; C, color monitor; B, black and white monitor; K, keyboard controls; M, camera.

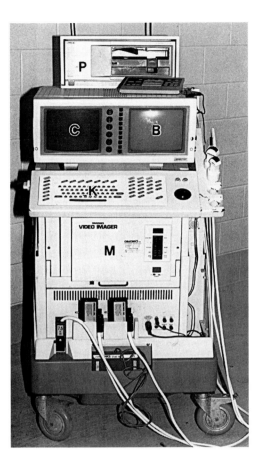

3. *Reject*: Another gain control option that allows the operator to reject near field echoes of high intensity.

4. *Orientation*: Allows documentation of the plane in which the probe is oriented relative to the body (e.g., transverse, sagittal, etc.).

5. *Annotation*: Available on many but not all systems, this control allows predesignation of body parts scanned (e.g., left kidney, spleen, etc.).

6. *Left-right invert*: Allows reversal of the left and right sides of the image if needed in order to align the image with the probe orientation on the body. This control enables the operator to maintain probe contact.

7. *Polarity*: Determines if echoes appear white or black. This control is not found on newer systems because most operators are accustomed to images in which echoes are white. Older systems may have this option.

8. *Pointers*: Allows the use of arrows or tracing cursors to designate specific areas or structures.

9. *Format*: Allows the use of split screen images or a combination of split screen images for accurate comparison of structures or for more accurate measurement of structures that are larger than the normal image field.

10. *Biopsy cursors*: Designed to be used with an external biopsy guide, this control allows the operator to align the needle in a guide and to know that, on the screen, the needle will be found at some depth within two cursor lines.

11. *Pulsed Doppler cursor*: Allows accurate placement of a sample volume box for determining the flow of blood within a vessel. The display of flow is in the form of a spectral analysis and usually includes an audible sound presentation.

12. *M mode cursor.* Allows the placement of a cursor line and box over the heart to determine the limits of the M mode display of the contractile motions of the heart.
13. *Configuration controls.* Allows the adjustment of a previously configured annotation, image size, or echo density.
14. *Measurement.* Allows for multiple measurement parameters depending on the level of sophistication of the equipment. From a simple cursor separation distance measurement to M mode measurements of the heart and subsequent computer calculations of cardiac output, this control has many functions.

As the level of technology increases, the capacity for image improvement and quantitation also increases. Many pieces of equipment now require only software upgrades in order to improve the capacities.

The methods of recording images vary from Polaroid cameras attached to the face of the monitor to complex cameras using radiographic film with black and white or color printers. Most instruments also have the capability of recording the real-time images using a video cassette recorder.

3

CHAPTER

ANATOMIC PLANES

Robert E. Cartee

Three basic anatomic planes are used in describing the relations between adjacent abdominal structures: (1) transverse, (2) sagittal (or longitudinal), and (3) frontal (or coronal) (Fig. 3–1**A–C**). The following series of figures illustrates the thoracic and abdominal structures in these planes. Presentation of structures in all possible oblique planes was not feasible. The figures do not necessarily represent sequential sections but are representative of the anatomy within areas commonly assessed sonographically. Well-accepted labels for anatomic areas of the abdomen are used in the discussion of the location of each section (Fig. 3–1**D**).

Because modern ultrasound probes are not large enough to cover the entire width, length, or thickness of the body, the sonographic image of a particular area may include only part of the section. At the beginning of each section unit (transverse, sagittal, or frontal) is another perpendicular template plane with red lines illustrating the approximate level of each of the subsections. Each number of a subsection corresponds to a plane illustrated on the template or between the planes of that template. To facilitate the use of this chapter, a list of the anatomic structures and their regions are presented in Table 3–1.

ATLAS OF PLANES

Transverse (Figs. 3–2 to 3–7)

The transverse section number corresponds to that level or to some point between the numbered red lines. For example, level 26 on the template indicates that the cranial pole of the left kidney and the dorsal spleen should appear in transverse section on the cross section numbered 26. The caudal pole of the left kidney and the ventral tip of the spleen occur on the template at section 30. Sections 1 through 10 include the cervical region and do not appear on the template. The transverse planes of the atlas include representative sections that feature organs usually visualized during an examination of the thorax or abdomen. These sections are as follows from cranial to caudal: sections 15, 18, 24, 36, and 39.

Sagittal (Figs. 3–8 to 3–13)

The red lines on the *frontal* section template represent the levels through which sagittal sections were cut. These sections are labeled by number and with an "M" or "L" to indicate medial and lateral sides. They are presented here from left to right as follows: 4M, 5M, 8M, 13L, and 16M.

Frontal (Figs. 3–14 to 3–19)

The red lines on the *sagittal* template represent the planes of frontal sections. The "V" and "D" represent the dorsal and ventral sides of that particular section. The representative frontal sections presented are as follows: 6V, 7D, 8V, 10V, and 12V.

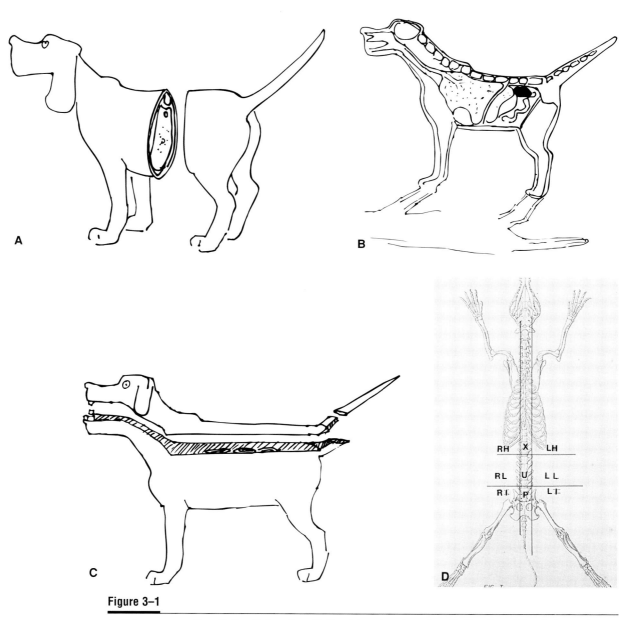

Figure 3–1

A, Transverse section. **B,** Sagittal section. **C,** Frontal or dorsal section. **D,** Drawing of the abdomen (ventral view) indicating the regions used to describe the location of abdominal and thoracic organs. RH, right hypochondriac; LH, left hypochondriac; RL and LL, right and left lateral; RI and LI, right and left inguinal; X, xiphoid; U, umbilical; P, pubic.

TABLE 3–1
Anatomic Structures and Their Regions

Organ	Region	Other Landmarks
Thorax Heart	3rd rib to caudal border of 6th rib; long axis is 45° from ventral plane	
Abdomen Esophagus	Left hypochondriac	Ventral or slightly cranial to last thoracic vertebra. Thickness—6 mm
Stomach (fundus) (empty) (1) Stomach (fundus) (full) (2,3)	1. Left hypochondriac 2. Left and right lateral 3. Right hypochondriac, xiphoid umbilical	1. Caudal to last rib 2. Caudal to costal arch 3. Caudally through a transverse plane through umbilicus
Stomach (body)	Xiphoid and left hypochondriac, umbilical	
Stomach (pylorus)	Right xiphoid and right hypochondriac Right lateral or umbilical	
Duodenum	Dorsal right hypochondriac opposite 9th intercostal space goes to tuber coxae level	
Cecum	Right lateral region ventral to right transverse process of L1–L4	
Descending colon	Left lateral, left inguinal region	
Liver	Right and left hypochondriac xiphoid region; 6th to 12th interconstal space	
Gallbladder	Right hypochondriac—6th rib to costal arch when full (5 cm long by 1.5 cm wide)	
Pancreas (right lobe)	Right hypochondriac, right lateral, dorsal to duodenum	9th intercostal space to 4th lumbar vertebrae (1–3 cm in width, 1 cm thick) 15 cm long
Pancreas (body)	Right xiphoid region, ventral to portal vein	
Pancreas (left lobe)	Left hypochondriac and left lateral regions	End at cranial pole of left kidney and middle portion of spleen
Spleen	Left hypochondriac	Cranial to cranial pole of left kidney
Left kidney	Left lateral	Adrenal gland and pancreas craniomedial
Right kidney	Right hypochondriac	Adrenal gland and liver medial and cranial
Left adrenal	Left lateral	Cranial pole of left kidney. Aorta, caudal vena cava, medially.
Right adrenal	Right hypochondriac	Right kidney hilus. Caudal vena cave medially.
Portal vein	Xiphoid—right umbilical region	1.2 cm in diameter
Bladder	Pubic, umbilical	
Prostate	Pubic—pelvis	Bladder cranially—size = LWTH = 2.2 × 2.2 × 1.7 for 30–50 lb. dog
Left ovary	Left lateral	1–3 cm from caudal pole of left kidney
Right ovary	Right lateral	10 cm from caudal pole of right kidney
Uterus	Right and left lateral inguinal and pubic and pelvic cavity	
Medial iliac lymph nodes	Left lateral or inguinal	Adjacent to aortic bifurcation
Peripheral Thyroid gland	Cervical	Larynx cranially; esophagus, trachea medially; carotid artery laterally; 5 cm × 1.5 cm × 0.5 cm (dog)

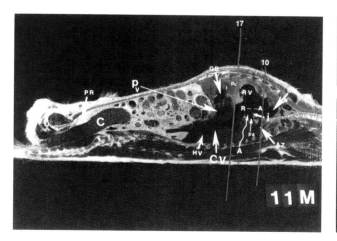

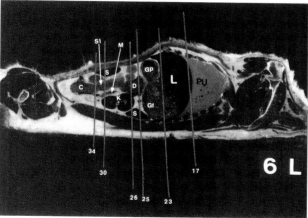

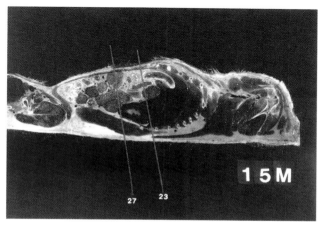

Figure 3–2

The red lines indicate the planes of transverse section through the body.

Figure 3–3

E, esophagus; A, aorta; VA, azygos vein; b, right bronchus; PU, lung; pa, pulmonary artery; pv, pulmonary vein; CV, caudal vena cava; RV, right ventricle; rw, right ventricular wall; s, septum of heart; LV, left ventricle; lw = left ventricle wall; SS, sternum.

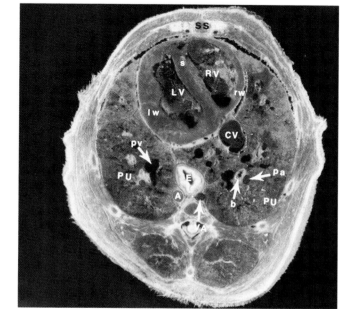

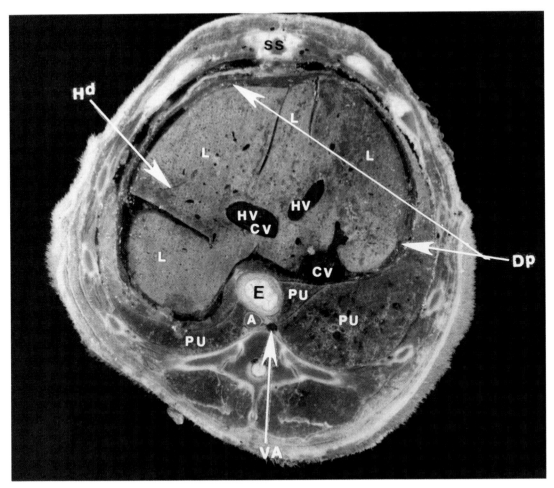

Figure 3–4

E, esophagus; A, aorta; L, liver; CV, caudal vena cava; HV, hepatic vein; PU, lung; VA, azygos vein; DP, diaphragm; Hd, hepatic duct; SS, sternum.

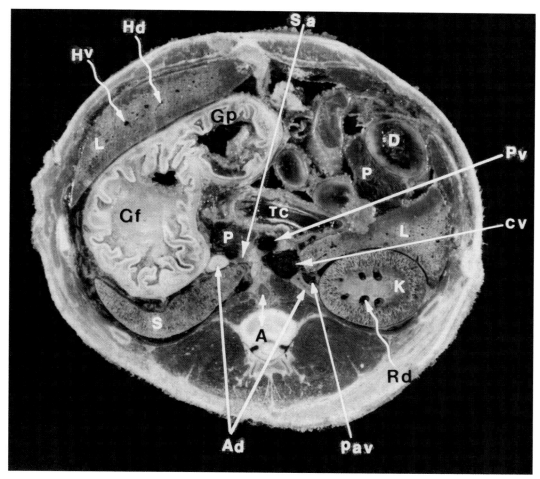

Figure 3–5

A, aorta; S, spleen; Ad, adrenal gland; cv, caudal vena cava; K, right kidney; Rd, renal diverticulum; L, liver; Pv, portal vein; P, pancreas; D, duodenum; TC, transverse colon; Sa, splenic artery; Gf, fundus of stomach; Gp, pylorus of stomach; Hv, hepatic vein; Hd, hepatic duct; pav, phrenicoabdominal vein.

Figure 3–6

B, bladder; Ut, ureter; C, colon.

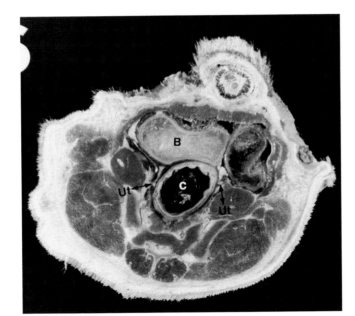

Figure 3–7

P, prostate; R, rectum; U, urethra.

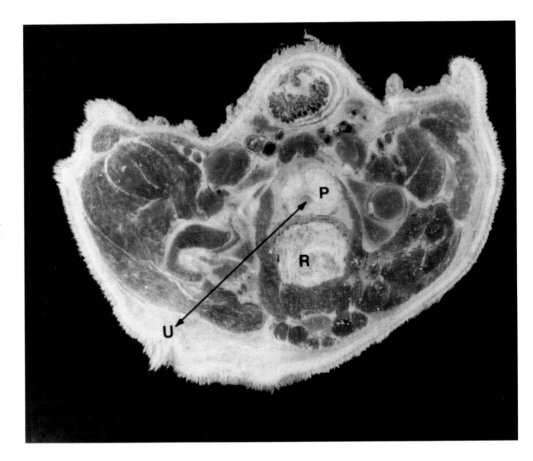

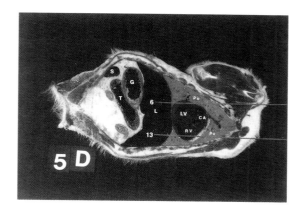
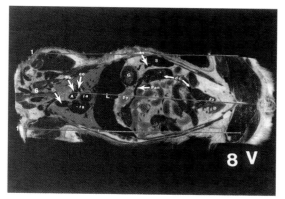
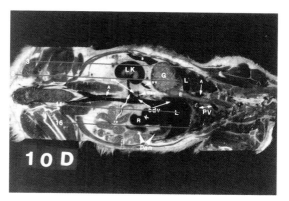

Figure 3–8

The red lines indicate the planes of sagittal sections through the body.

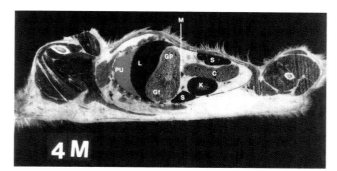

Figure 3–9

The medial side of sagittal section number 4. Gp, pyloric region of stomach; Gf, gastric fundus; M, mesenteric vessel; L, liver; PU, lung; S, spleen; K, left kidney; C, colon.

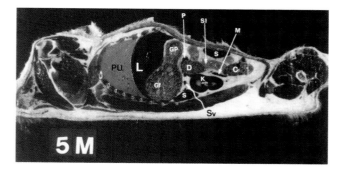

Figure 3–10

Medial side of sagittal section 5. PU, lung; L, liver; Gf, gastric fundus; Gp, gastric pylorus; P, pancreas; D, duodenum; S, spleen; K, left kidney; SI, small intestine; M, mesenteric veins; C, colon; Sv, splenic vessel.

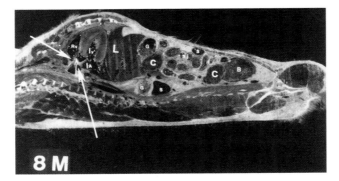

Figure 3–11

Medial side of sagittal section 8. Rv, right ventricle; Iv, left ventricle; Ia, left atrium; A, aorta; arrows, pulmonary arteries; L, liver; G, stomach; C, colon; si, small intestine; B, urinary bladder; S, spleen.

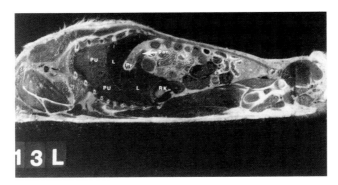

Figure 3–12

Lateral side of sagittal section 13. PU, lung; L, liver; PY, pylorus; pan, pancreas; RK, kidney.

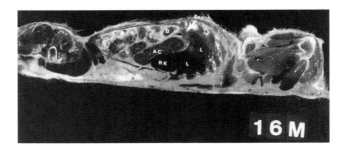

Figure 3–13

Medial side of sagittal section 16. pan, pancreas; D, duodenum; L, liver; AC, ascending colon; RK, right kidney.

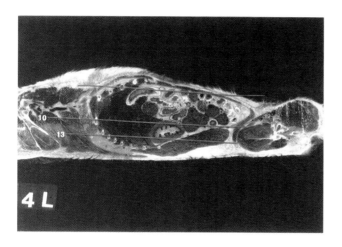

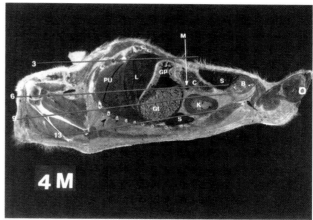

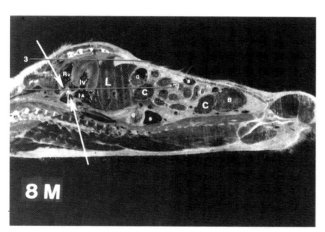

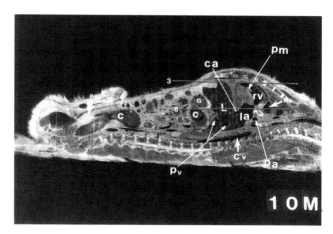

Figure 3–14

The red lines indicate the planes of frontal section through the body.

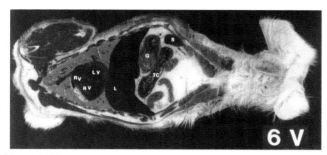

Figure 3–15

The ventral side of frontal section 6. RV, right ventricle; LV, left ventricle; L, liver; G, stomach; TC, transverse colon; S, spleen.

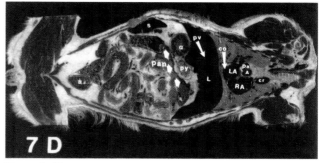

Figure 3–16

The dorsal side of frontal section 7. Pa, pulmonary artery; A, aorta; LA, left atrium; RA, right atrium; cr, cranial vena cava; co, coronary vessel; pv, portal vein; G, stomach fundus; py, pylorus; pan, pancreas; S, spleen; B, urinary bladder.

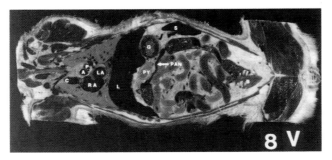

Figure 3-17

The ventral side of frontal section 8. C, cranial vena cava (thorax); A, aorta; P, pulmonary trunk; RA, right atrium; LA, left atrium; L, liver; G, stomach; PY, pylorus; PAN, pancreas; B, urinary bladder; S, spleen.

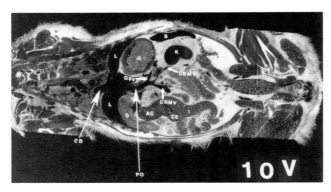

Figure 3-18

The ventral side of frontal section 10. CD, caudal vena cava; L, liver; GSV, gastrosplenic vein; G, stomach; D, duodenum; PO, portal vein; S, spleen, K, left kidney; CDMV, caudal mesenteric vein; CRMV, cranial mesenteric vein; AC, ascending colon; CE, cecum; I, ileum.

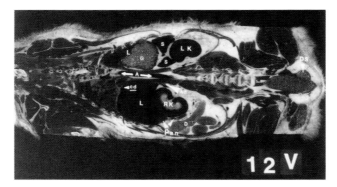

Figure 3-19

The ventral side of frontal section 12. L, liver; G, stomach; A, aorta; cd, caudal vena cava; pan, pancreas; D, duodenum; RK, right kidney; Ad, right adrenal gland; S, spleen; LK, left kidney; PS, paranal sinus.

THE NERVOUS SYSTEM

Judith A. Hudson

Judith A. Hudson

THE BRAIN

Indications

Neurosonography is not a new technique in veterinary medicine. A mode sonography was used in 1972 to detect experimentally created intracranial lesions in dogs.[1] Real-time B mode examination is now easily performed in selected animals. The most common indications for sonographic examination of the brain are to determine the size of the lateral ventricles in cases of possible hydrocephalus, to evaluate the extent of neoplasia, to guide biopsy of brain lesions, and to determine vascularity of brain lesions. The appearance of hemorrhage in the brain has been described.[2] In a research environment, Doppler ultrasound is being used to characterize the vascular system of young dogs.[3] Although most reports cite studies in dogs, B mode evaluation of the brain of cats has also been reported.[4]

Pediatric sonography has become an important specialty in human medicine. Premature infants can be examined for intraventricular or intraparenchymal hemorrhage, and periventricular leukomalacia. Subsequent hydrocephalus or cerebral atrophy can also be evaluated sonographically.[5] Peri-intraventricular hemorrhage has been shown to occur naturally in puppies,[6] although a connection between these conditions and hydrocephalus has not been demonstrated in dogs. Thorough serial examination of the brain of neonatal puppies may reveal such a connection or shed light on some other etiology.

Scanning and Biopsy Techniques

Sonographic examination of the brain is limited, to some extent, by the thick osseous skull. Sonography of the brain of most puppies less than 3 to 4 weeks of age can be accomplished through the bregmatic fontanelle or "soft spot" in the middle of the top of the skull. Some toy or small breed dogs have a fontanelle that persists into adult life. Adult dogs with closed sutures can be examined after a craniotomy, the size of which can vary from a 1-cm burr hole to a large defect made to allow dissection of the brain lesion (usually a neoplasm). Low frequency probes have also been used with some success to evaluate dilated lateral ventricles using the thinnest part of the temporal bone (Fig. 4-1). The foramen magnum has been used successfully in children to examine the posterior fossa.[7] This window can be used also in dogs, but the sonographic anatomy of this area has yet to be described.

Figure 4-1

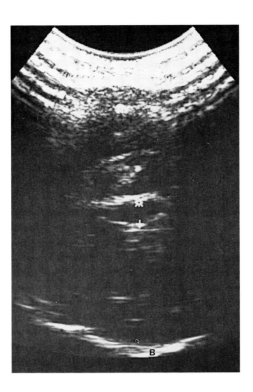

Sagittal sonogram of the brain of a 6-month-old Pekingese imaged through the temporal bone with a 5.0-mHz probe. The rostral aspect is to the left. Calipers indicate the roof (*) and floor (+) of the left lateral ventricle. The black area between the calipers is cerebrospinal fluid in the lateral ventricle. B, bony floor of the cranial vault.

High frequency probes are preferred for most applications. Excellent results have been obtained with both 10- and 7.5-mHz probes. An increase in frequency results in better resolution but less penetration, however, so the 10-mHz probe is best for very small animals. The frequency associated with a probe actually refers to its operating or resonance frequency, but the probe produces pulses that contain a spectrum or "bandwidth" of frequencies. Some sophisticated ultrasound machines can be set to "listen" for frequencies other than the operating frequency. With such a machine, a 7.5-mHz probe could be used to produce images closer to those that could be obtained with a 10-mHz probe.

Probes are prepared for intraoperative use according to several methods. Many probes can be gas sterilized, but draping the probe with a sterilized cover is usually easier and does not require removal of the probe from clinical service. It is possible to place the probe in a sterile surgical glove[8] or condom and to cover the connecting cord with sterile bandaging material. Alternatively, the probe can be wrapped in gas-sterilized plastic wrap.[9]

The brain is scanned using a windshield wiper technique, examining structures in transverse images from rostral to caudal and back again. The probe is then rotated 180° and swept from side to side to obtain images that are oblique to the sagittal plane (Fig. 4-2).[10,11]

If one or both lateral ventricles appear enlarged, the height of the lateral ventricle is measured between the floor and the roof of the lateral ventricle.[12] In one series of dogs, the mean height of normal lateral ventricles, measured at or immediately caudal to the level of the interthalamic adhesion, was 0.15 mm (0.04 to 0.35 mm).[12] Ratios also have been used to evaluate lateral ventricular size.[12,13] Cerebral mantle thickness is the distance between the roof of the lateral ventricle and the dorsal surface of the brain (the brain parenchyma dorsal to the lateral ventricle). The ventricle-mantle ratio is a ratio of the height of the lateral ventricle to the cerebral mantle thickness. The ventricle-hemisphere ratio is a ratio of the height of the lateral ventricle to the hemispheric width. Hemispheric width is measured in transverse scans from the center of the third ventricle to the lateral aspect of the brain. Normal ratios in a group of normal dogs were 0.08

(range: 0.05 to 0.18) and 0.07 (range: 0.04 to 0.17) for the ventricle-mantle ratio and the ventricle-hemisphere ratio, respectively. Another useful ratio is the percent of brain occupied by the dorsoventral dimension of the lateral ventricle. The percentage in a group of normal dogs was 0.14%.[13] Depending on the ultrasound machine and connected peripheral equipment, images can be recorded on videocassette tape, photographic paper, Polaroid film, or radiographic film.

Doppler sonography can measure blood flow velocity in cerebral arteries of dogs (Fig. 4–3).[3,14] Because the proximal portion of the basal cerebral arteries does not vary much in diameter, Doppler variables give insight into changes in cerebral blood flow and can provide prognostic information. In man, suggested applications include cases of perinatal asphyxia, patent ductus arteriosus (which can cause secondary changes in cerebral blood flow), and hydrocephalus; determination of brain death; and evaluation of drug effects on cerebral blood flow.[15] Blood flow information also can be obtained by color coding amplitude information to create an "ultrasonic angiogram" (Fig. 4–4). Use of these technologies in larger veterinary centers should add to the knowledge base regarding pathophysiology of disease and effects of drug therapy in the brain of dogs.

Normal Findings

Several rules of thumb may aid in the interpretation of sonograms. Cerebrospinal fluid (CSF) in the ventricular system is anechoic. The choroid plexus is hyperechoic. The appearance of the lateral and third ventricles varies depending on the relative amounts of CSF or choroid plexus. Pulsations can be seen in the choroid plexus of the third and especially the lateral ventricles. These pulsations can be followed in serial sections to aid in identification of the ventricles. The brain is smoother and the gyri less obvious in

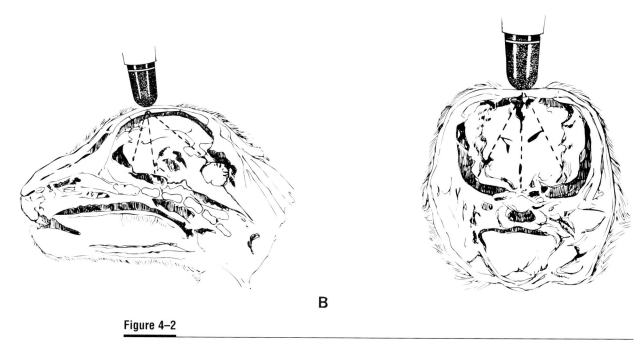

A   B

Figure 4–2

Diagrams of the head of a dog showing probe placement to obtain transverse **(A)** and sagittal **(B)** images. Dotted lines represent transverse and sagittal imaging planes, respectively. (From Hudson JA, et al: Ultrasonographic examination of the normal canine neonatal brain. Vet Radiol 32:50, 1991.)

Figure 4–3

Sagittal color flow Doppler scan of the brain of a 13-day-old dog. The rostral aspect of the brain is to the left. M, middle cerebral artery; R, rostral cerebral artery; C, callosal artery in the callosal sulcus. Branches of the callosal artery course dorsally. A typical Doppler spectral waveform of the middle cerebral artery is shown.

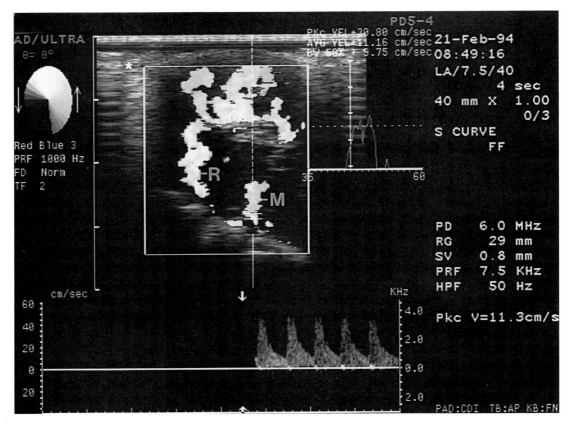

Figure 4–4

Sagittal "ultrasonic angiogram" created by color coding amplitude information. Compare to the color flow Doppler image in Figure 4–3. R, rostral cerebral artery; C, callosal artery in the callosal sulcus with branches coursing dorsally; T, thalamus.

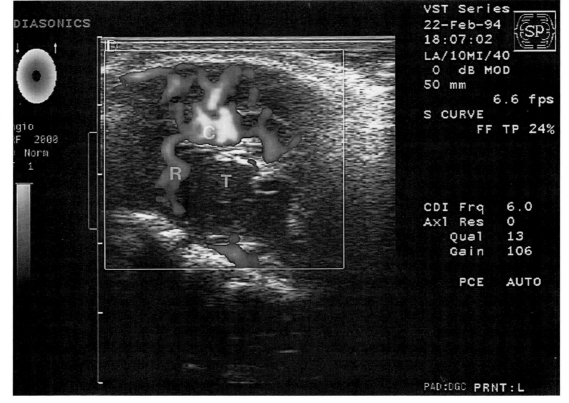

neonatal animals than in adult animals. The hippocampus is better visualized in adult animals. The lateral ventricles in day-old puppies are usually slit-like.[10,11] Occasionally, one or both lateral ventricles are large at birth but decrease in size within the next few days. True hydrocephalus in neonatal animals manifests as a progressive increase in lateral ventricular size.

Transverse Images

The falx cerebri, splenial sulci, and callosal sulci form a readily recognizable landmark in transverse images. Together, they comprise a hyperechoic umbrella-like structure. The falx cerebri forms the hyperechoic stem of the umbrella. The splenial sulcus curves laterally and ventrally to each side from the falx cerebri, thereby forming the "roof" of the umbrella. The small callosal sulci form a T-shaped handle.[10,11]

In rostral images (Fig. 4–5), normal lateral ventricles appear as anechoic slit-like areas medial to the respective head of the caudate nucleus. The superficial aspect of the head of the caudate nucleus is hyperechoic. More caudally (Fig. 4–6), the fornix is visible between the lateral ventricles. The deep portion of the falx cerebri appears as a hyperechoic area superficial to the fornix. The callosal sulci extend laterally and may contribute to the echogenicity of this structure. The area of the lateral ventricles has mixed echogenicity because CSF appears anechoic whereas choroid plexus is hyperechoic. In some normal neonates, only three hyperechoic amorphous areas are seen, indicating the site of the lateral ventricles and the midline fornix and deep portion of the falx cerebri. The pyriform lobe is located ventrally, separated from the diencephalon by a hyperechoic line.[10,11]

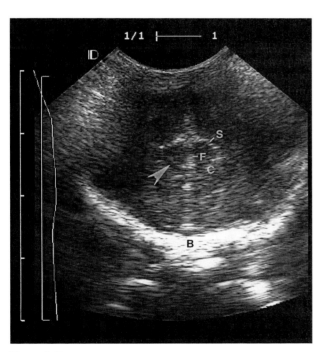

Figure 4–5

Rostral transverse sonogram of the brain of an 11-day-old dog. Cerebrospinal fluid causes a normal lateral ventricle to appear as an anechoic slit-like area medial to the respective head of the caudate nucleus. The superficial aspect of the head of caudate nucleus is hyperechoic. Arrowhead, right lateral ventricle; C, left caudate nucleus; F, falx cerebri; S, splenial sulcus; B, bony floor of the cranial vault.

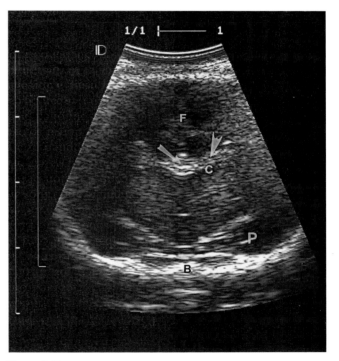

Figure 4–6

Transverse sonogram at the level of the rostral fornix of the brain of an 11-day-old dog. Note the hyperechoic line between the diencephalon and the pyriform lobe. Arrowhead, area of the left lateral ventricle; C, left caudate nucleus; arrow, fornix; P, left pyriform lobe; F, falx cerebri; B, bony floor of the cranial vault. The deep portion of the falx cerebri is a hyperechoic area superficial to the fornix. The callosal sulci extend laterally and may contribute to the echogenicity of this area.

As the probe is angled to allow visualization of more caudal structures (Fig. 4–7), the dorsal portion of the hippocampus appears as a hypoechoic structure medial to the lateral ventricles. Choroid plexus in the dorsal portion of the lateral ventricles causes the lateral ventricles to appear hyperechoic. In some images at this level, the ventral portion of the hippocampus is medial to the hyperechoic choroid plexus in the ventral portion of the lateral ventricles. In these scans, the third ventricle is seen deep to the dorsal portion of the hippocampus. The angle of some scanning planes may be such that the mesencephalon or midbrain may be seen ventral to diencephalic structures (see Fig. 4–7). Only a thin membrane lies between the third ventricle and the subarachnoid space. Because both choroid plexus in the third ventricle and the subarachnoid space are hyperechoic, the division between the two is indistinguishable.[10,11]

In caudal images, with the probe held vertically, the midbrain appears as a dome-shaped hypoechoic structure outlined dorsally and laterally by interfaces between CSF, vessels, and trabeculae in the subarachnoid space. The choroid plexus and occasionally the CSF are seen laterally in the lateral ventricles. Again, pulsations in the lateral ventricles can be followed caudally to help identify the lateral ventricles.[10,11]

In the most caudal images (Fig. 4–8), the vermis of the cerebellum is seen as a stack of horizontal hyperechoic lines. The cerebellar hemispheres are hypoechoic and are located laterally. The membranous tentorium does not present a barrier to ultrasound, but the osseous tentorium interferes with visualization of more caudal structures in the adult. In the adult, this structure resembled an upside-down "V".[10,11]

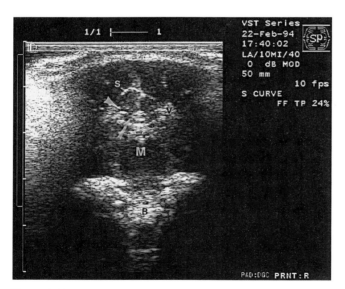

Figure 4–7

Transverse sonogram of the brain, caudal to the interthalamic adhesion, in an 11-day-old dog. The scanning plane of this image is such that the diencephalon is seen dorsally and the mesencephalon appears ventrally. The subarachnoid space (S), rather than the third ventricle (V), is visible. Arrow, dorsal portion of the hippocampus; arrowhead, cerebrospinal fluid in the dorsal portion of the right lateral ventricle; open arrow, subarachnoid space (S); M, mesencephalon; B, bony floor of the cranial vault.

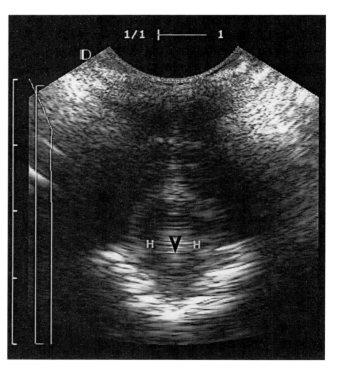

Figure 4–8

Transverse sonogram of the brain of an 11-day-old dog at the level of the vermis of the cerebellum (V). H, cerebellar hemisphere in the adult. The membranous tentorium does not present a barrier to ultrasound, but the osseous tentorium interferes with visualization of more caudal structures.

Sagittal Images

Images that are oblique to the sagittal plane have been loosely referred to as parasagittal images in the ultrasound literature. In such images, the lateral ventricle appears as a C-shaped structure. As with transverse images, CSF causes some portions of the lateral ventricles to appear anechoic, whereas the choroid plexus causes other portions to appear hyperechoic. The lateral ventricle surrounds the thalamus on each side. The thalamus is hypoechoic but the borders are outlined by the hyperechoic choroid plexus in the respective lateral ventricle. Rostral to the thalamus, the caudate nucleus is of variable echogenicity. Most of this dorsally curved structure is hypoechoic, but the superficial portion may be hyperechoic, particularly in adult dogs. The splenial sulcus is an undulating hyperechoic line curved caudally. The hypoechoic cingulate gyrus appears deep to this sulcus. In adult dogs, the callosal sulcus is often visualized as a second hyperechoic line. A third line representing the interface between brain parenchyma and CSF in the lateral ventricle is seen when sufficient CSF is present. In newborn dogs, a hyperechoic clump of choroid plexus in the region of the thalamocaudate groove should not be mistaken for hyperechoic hemorrhage.[10,11]

The third ventricle is occasionally identified in midline sagittal images (Fig. 4–9) but, usually the thickness of the ultrasound beam causes portions of the lateral ventricles to be included in these images (slice thickness artifact). The interthalamic adhesion is present in these images.[10,11]

Abnormal Findings

Hydrocephalus

Although a relationship between the presence of a persistent fontanelle and lateral ventricular enlargement has been suggested,[13] the presence of a fontanelle in an adult dog should not be taken as evidence of hydrocephalus. In three separate studies, 29 of 73 dogs examined through a persistent fontanelle had normal sonographic findings. Because similar breed dogs without persistent fontanelles cannot be readily examined, the incidence of dilated lateral ventricles in these dogs in not known. The percentage of hydrocephalic dogs may be independent of the presence of a persistent fontanelle. It is equally important to realize that many dogs with dilated lateral ventricles display minimal or no clinical signs, and that lateral ventricular size does not correlate with severity of clinical signs in dogs that are neurologically abnormal.[12,13]

Hydrocephalus implies enlargement of all or part of the ventricular system associated with hypoplasia or atrophy of surrounding nervous tissue.[12,13,16,17] In one series of dogs, a lateral ventricle was considered enlarged if the lateral ventricular height at the level of the interthalamic adhesion exceeded 3.5 mm (Fig. 4–10).[12] Ventricle-mantle ratios above 0.25 and ventricle-hemisphere ratios above 0.19 also were used as criteria to determine lateral ventricular dilatation.[12] In another study, enlargement was considered moderate if the percent of brain occupied by the dorsoventral dimension of the lateral ventricle was 15 to 25%. Severe dilatation was indicated by a percentage greater than 25%.[13]

Biopsy

Brain biopsy can be guided by computed tomography, magnetic resonance imaging, or ultrasound. Ultrasound-guided biopsy allows real-time examination of the vascular system if the ultrasound machine has Doppler capability. Sonography provides a lower cost alternative and may be more readily available in some areas.

A pseudobiopsy technique has been described for biopsy of brain lesions in dogs.[2] A biopsy guide was handmade using metallic bands designed for use in automotive work and a protractor. Procedures were performed using sterile surgical technique with the ultrasound probe prepared as described previously. A midline burr-hole large enough to accommodate the ultrasound probe was made in the skull using a pneumatic perforator. A second hole was made in the target area for biopsy. The brain was examined thor-

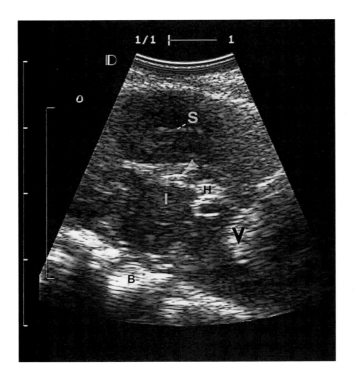

Figure 4-9

Sonogram of the brain of an 11-day-old dog, slightly oblique to the midsagittal plane. The rostral aspect of the brain is to the left. Arrowhead, choroid plexus in the lateral ventricle; H, hippocampus; I, interthalamic adhesion; V, vermis; S, splenial sulcus; B, bony floor of the cranial vault.

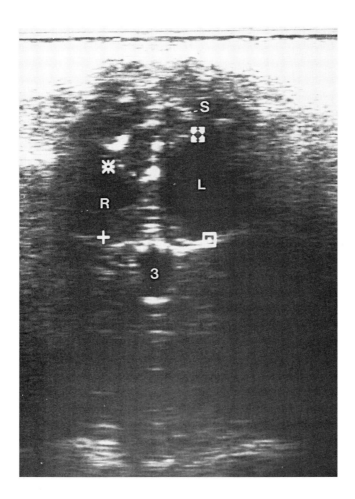

Figure 4-10

Transverse sonogram of the brain of a Chihuahua puppy with hydrocephalus. Calipers measure the height of the lateral ventricle and the thickness of the cerebral mantle on each side. Both lateral ventricles and the third ventricle are dilated. R, right lateral ventricle; L, left lateral ventricle; 3, third ventricle; S, splenial sulcus.

oughly using a 7.5-mHz intraoperative probe. The biopsy guide was attached to the probe and the probe was placed in a holder to minimize operator error. After a site was chosen for biopsy, an electronic pointer was placed on the monitor screen to indicate the chosen site. The probe and biopsy guide were removed from the holder and placed in a saline bath. The biopsy needle was placed into the guide hole of the biopsy guide. A 16-gauge Menghini needle, with the tip roughened to increase echogenicity, was used. The angle of the biopsy needle was adjusted until the needle path intersected the pointer mark on the ultrasound monitor. The probe and biopsy guide were then returned to the holder apparatus, being careful not to disturb the needle angle. The dura was elevated and incised where the needle was to enter the brain. The brain was imaged as the needle was passed through the guide hole. When the needle tip was in the lesion, a 3-ml syringe was attached to the needle hub and the plunger was withdrawn 1 ml. A core of tissue was obtained by rotating the needle tip around its long axis. After biopsy, imaging continued for 30 minutes to monitor for hemorrhage. Routine surgical closure followed. Hemorrhage tended to be minor and unassociated with neurologic dysfunction.[2]

Neoplasia

Most neoplasms described in human studies were hyperechoic. Although peritumoral edema is also hyperechoic, edges of tumor can usually be detected better with sonography than with computed tomography.[18] Limited experience with intraoperative examination of brain neoplasms in dogs suggests that these tumors also are likely to be hyperechoic (Figs. 4–11 and 4–12). Ultrasound can be used to evaluate the brain for evidence of remaining neoplasia after resection of a brain neoplasm (see Fig. 4–12**B**). Doppler ultrasound can be used, if available, to help the surgeon avoid large blood vessels. If a skull defect is present after surgery, the defect can be used to provide a window for postoperative re-examination (Fig. 4–13).

Figure 4–11

Intraoperative sonogram of the brain of a 7-year-old Shar-Pei with a nonresectable brain stem mass. Injection of an experimental compound was performed under ultrasound guidance. Calipers measure the diameter of the hyperechoic mass. M, mass; S, sulcus; B, bony floor of the cranial vault.

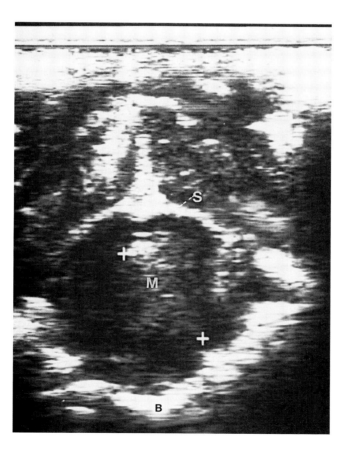

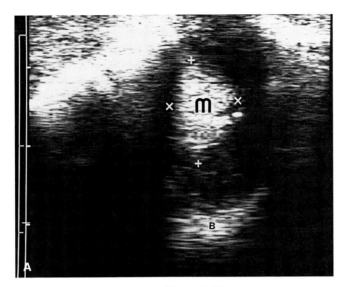
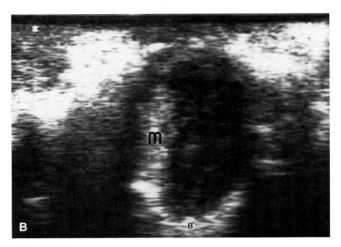

Figure 4–12

A, Intraoperative transverse sonogram of the brain of 9-year-old mixed breed dog with an astrocytoma that extended rostrally into the brain from the cerebellopontine angle. Note that the astrocytoma is hyperechoic. Calipers measure the diameter of the astrocytoma. M, mass; B, bony floor of the cranial vault. **B,** Intraoperative transverse sonogram after resection of the neoplasm. Only a small echogenic mass remains. Doppler sonography showed that the remaining tissue was highly vascular. M, remaining portion of the meningioma; B, bony floor of the cranial vault.

Figure 4–13

Parasagittal sonogram of the brain of a 14-year-old mixed breed dog with a meningioma. Treatment consisted of surgical debulking followed by radiation therapy. Sonography was performed after regression of the mass through the defect created during craniectomy. Calipers measure the mass (M). T, thalamus; V, dilated right lateral ventricle; triangular arrowheads, margins of the dilated right lateral ventricle.

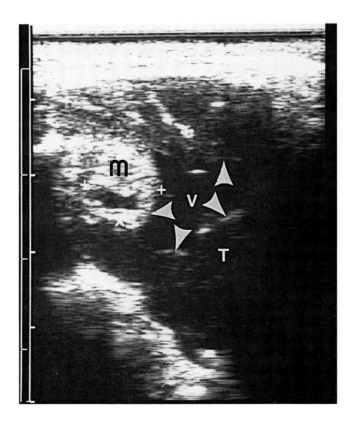

Intraoperative Sonography

Biopsy and ultrasound-guided resection of neoplasia are two examples of the use of intra-operative sonography. Complete recovery occurred in a lamb with neurologic deficits after ultrasound was used to locate and guide surgical removal of a Coenurus cerebralis cyst. Skull trephination and sonography were necessary in this case because skull soften-ing was not present to enable localization and removal of the cyst.[19] Other applications in man include imaging and drainage of cysts or abscesses, guidance of intraventricular catheters into the ventricles, evaluation of hemorrhage, and intraoperative monitoring of arteriovenous lesions. Abscesses have a center with variable echogenicity. Hemorrhage is initially hypoechoic but rapidly becomes hyperechoic. One advantage of ultrasound over stereotaxic localization for drainage of lesions is that displacement of the lesion by the needle can be seen during the procedure.[18] Clinical applications of ultrasound in vet-erinary medicine grow in number as students learn and begin to apply this relatively new technology.

Congenital Anomalies

Congenital brain lesions investigated using ultrasound in babies are numerous, but include absence of the corpus callosum, cerebellar hypoplasia, holoprosencephaly, Dandy-Walker syndrome, and meningocele.[5] These lesions also occur in dogs.[20] Sonographic evaluation of the brain of neonatal dogs or dogs with persistent fontanelles should allow premortem diagnosis.

THE SPINAL CORD

Indications

As with the brain, the inaccessibility of the spinal cord has delayed the routine use of sonography as a method by which to examine the spinal cord of small animals. The spinal cord of human neonates has been examined noninvasively using sonography[21,22], and intraoperative sonography has been used in older children and adults for evaluation of spinal cord trauma[23] and the diagnosis of intramedullary and extramedullary lesions. Indications for its application include neoplasia, cysts, hematomas, hemorrhage, myelo-malacia, syringomyelia, intervertebral disk herniation, gunshot wounds, arachnoiditis, and epidural scar tissue.[24,25] The strength of spinal cord pulsations imaged using a 7.5-mHz probe was used to predict outcome after decompressive surgery of cervical spinal cords in man.[26] Intraoperative gray-scale and color flow Doppler imaging and Doppler spectral analysis of normal and experimentally traumatized spinal cords of dogs have been described.[27–30] The spinal cord of some of these dogs was assessed through the intact skin postoperatively after laminectomy (Fig. 4–14). The invasiveness of spinal neo-plasms (like brain neoplasms) can be evaluated sonographically. Indications for its use should increase with more experience in imaging the spinal cord and improved instru-mentation.

Scanning and Biopsy Techniques

Optimal examination of the spinal cord requires a dorsal or dorsolateral laminectomy. A 7.5- or 10-mHz probe is required to provide sufficient resolution. In one study of the effi-cacy of a drug for treatment of spinal cord trauma, a 7.5-mHz linear array probe with an axial resolution of 0.45 mm and a lateral resolution of 0.4 mm was used with a triplex ultrasound machine.[a] This relatively large, rectangular probe allowed only sagittal images to be obtained through a dorsolateral laminectomy made in the vertical lamina of L2.[28] When this probe was used with a long dorsolateral laminectomy, transverse images were obtained.[29] The use of smaller probes also allows transverse images to be obtained.

a Spectra Ultrasound Machine. Diasonics, Milpitas, CA

Postoperatively, the spinal cord can be evaluated through the intact skin using the laminectomy site as a window. Also, portions of the spinal cord can be visualized by scanning between vertebrae from a dorsal approach, through intervertebral foramina from a lateral approach, or through the abdomen and intervertebral disks from a ventral approach without the need to perform a laminectomy. One can gain experience looking at the lumbar spinal cord by scanning dorsally between the vertebrae during routine abdominal sonography. Examination of the human cervical spinal cord using an ultrasound probe placed in the esophagus has been reported.[31] Data such as sagittal and tranverse diameters and ratios are recorded.

The central region of the spinal cord of dogs (and man) is supplied by a central or centrifugal arterial system arising from the ventral (anterior) spinal artery.[32] The peripheral region is supplied by a peripheral or centripetal system supplied by the single ventral and paired dorsal spinal arteries. The area between these regions, referred to as a border zone, is supplied by both the central and the peripheral systems.[33,34] Branches of the central arteries can be easily examined with Doppler sonography ventrolateral to the central canal using a dorsolateral laminectomy. When the probe is held at 30 to 45° from a perpendicular to the spinal cord, the Doppler signal is as parallel as possible to the vessel examined. Such a position maximizes the Doppler signal so that Doppler waveforms can be obtained and analyzed.

Normal Findings

Sonograms of the spinal cord of the dog[27,28,35] are similar in many ways to those described for man.[24,25,31] In sagittal images (Fig. 4–15), the dura mater and adjacent thin arachnoid appear as a linear horizontal echo. The subarachnoid space, when apparent, is anechoic because of the presence of CSF. The pia mater forms a second hyperechoic linear echo on the surface of the spinal cord. The spinal cord parenchyma has variable echogenicity with no distinction between gray and white matter. The central canal appears as one or two hyperechoic lines located centrally. Fat and connective tissue in the ventral epidural space appear as lobular echoes. Surrounding bone has a bright hyperechoic surface but it absorbs sound, causing distal acoustic shadowing.[27,28]

Figure 4–14

Sagittal sonogram of a canine spinal cord made through the intact skin and musculature 48 hours after laminectomy. Calipers on the pial surfaces measure spinal cord diameter. C, central canal; L, laminectomy site.

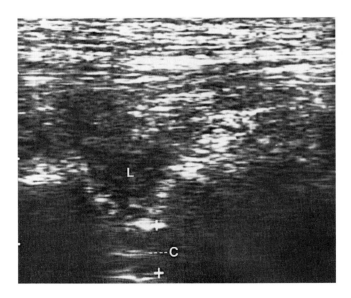

If the probe is sufficiently small or the laminectomy is large enough, the probe can be rotated 180° to obtain transverse images. The central canal will appear as a circular echogenicity surrounded by a relatively hypoechoic spinal cord parenchyma.[35]

Not all structures are visible in all scans. In one report describing a dorsolateral approach, the dura mater was seen both superficial and deep to the spinal cord, but the dorsal and ventral subarachnoid spaces were well defined only 58% and 71% of the time, respectively.[28] The spinal cord parenchyma was uniformly hypoechoic in 27%, contained subtle low level echoes in 23%, was hypoechoic with clusters of defined echogenic foci in 37%, and had well-delineated linear echoes in 13%. Differences in parenchymal appearance were believed to result from differences in vascularity in the dogs.[28]

Although a detailed description is beyond the scope of this book, a few comments about color flow Doppler imaging and Doppler spectral analysis of the spinal cord are made because these techniques will be more available as technology improves. Arterial waveforms of spinal arteries show high end-diastolic blood flow typical of intraparenchymal arteries in other low resistance organs such as the brain and kidney.[36] The mean and standard deviation of the peak systolic velocity for central arterial branches was 5.78 ± 2.5 cm/sec (range: 2.3 to 14.3 cm/sec) in one report.[30]

Abnormal Findings

Trauma

The spinal cord is hyperechoic after trauma,[29] possibly because of hemorrhage (Fig. 4–16). An initial increase in vascularity seen with color flow Doppler imaging in 11 of 34 dogs was usually followed by a decrease 30 minutes after trauma. Peak systolic velocity, minimum diastolic velocity, and mean velocity also decreased after trauma.[30] Some preliminary evidence shows that higher peak systolic velocities after trauma suggest a better prognosis.

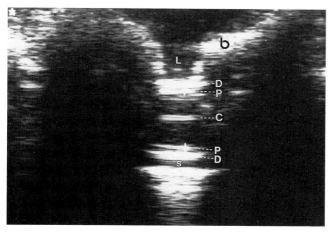

Figure 4–15

Sagittal sonogram of a normal canine spinal cord. The central canal (C) appears as two hyperechoic lines located centrally. Calipers measure the diameter of the spinal cord from the superficial pial layer to the deep pial layer. Acoustic shadowing is seen deep to the bony vertebral column. D, dura mater and adjacent thin arachnoid; P, pia mater; S, subarachnoid space; L, laminectomy site; b, vertebral bone.

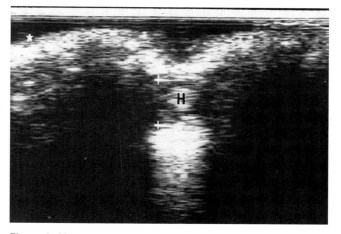

Figure 4–16

Sagittal sonogram of the spinal cord after trauma. Calipers on the pial surfaces measure spinal cord diameter. The hyperechoic area represents hemorrhage (H). Compare to the image of the normal spinal cord in Figure 4–15.

Disk Disease

The use of sonography to assess complete removal of herniated disk material in a dog has been described. After initial surgery, hyperechoic disk material was seen compressing the spinal cord ventrally. Subsequent removal was confirmed sonographically. M mode imaging, which consistently shows oscillations ("pulsations") of the spinal cord in normal dogs, only showed oscillations in this dog after compression was relieved by complete removal of disk material. The dog recovered. In another dog that remained paralyzed after spinal cord trauma, oscillations could not be demonstrated.[35] Similar findings have been reported in human studies in which the presence of oscillations suggested a better prognosis, but this technique is not a reliable prognostic tool. In other cases, oscillations correlated poorly to neurologic status.[26] Also, oscillations can occur because of extrinsic anterior (ventral) compression cranial or caudal to the examined area. Such oscillations may reflect increased pulsations in the anterior (ventral) spinal artery rather than normal dural motion.[24,25] Doppler sonography may prove useful for providing a more reliable evaluation of spinal cord vascularity as the technique becomes more available.

Congenital Anomaly

Sonography has been used in man to determine the best sites to cannulate for drainage of syringomyelia. With this technique, it is possible to demonstrate that all cystic areas in a syrinx may not be interconnected and that multiple areas may require cannulation.[24,25] Arteriovenous malformations usually appear as multiple, cystic masses, although echogenic masses have been reported. Doppler sonography may aid in resection.[24,25] Caudal displacement of the spinal cord associated with meningocele and extramedullary intradural lipoma (tethered cord syndrome) was investigated in a Manx cat with sonography and computed tomography. The meningocele was a hypoechoic tract containing the lipoma that appeared as a hyperechoic mass.[37]

Neoplasia

Intramedullary spinal neoplasms in man usually are more hyperechoic than the normal spinal cord.[24] Also noted is expansion of the cord with disruption or loss of the central canal echo complex. Intraoperative sonography can be used to select sites for biopsy and to determine extent of tumor. Because edema can result in a diffusely expanded, echogenic spinal cord, both edema and neoplasia should be considered when the lesion is diffuse. Drugs to decrease edema and re-examination might be of benefit in these cases. The extent of extramedullary neoplasia and the degree of involvement of the spinal cord can be determined sonographically. Limited numbers of canine studies show that spinal neoplasia in dogs is also hyperechoic and that sonography has similar applications in animals.

THE PERIPHERAL NERVES

Indications

Improved technology has provided sufficient resolution to allow examination of peripheral nerves. Some potential uses include determination of the extent of injury after trauma, evaluation of nerve healing to determine whether transected nerve endings have rejoined, examination for neuroma formation, and investigation of the involvement of nerves in neoplasia, granulomas, or other lesions.[38]

Scanning and Biopsy Techniques

The small size of peripheral nerves dictates the use of a high frequency probe such as a 10- or 7.5-mHz probe. Size also makes transverse images difficult to obtain, except at the proximal areas of the largest nerves. Examination of nerves is further complicated by the similarity of nerves to the surrounding tissues and their changing course. Nerves are readily recognizable in some areas, but in others, their identification is not as easy because of the linear appearance of muscle and tendon fibers and vessels. Although some nerves can be followed for many centimeters, tracking becomes difficult as the nerve dives between muscle planes. A thorough knowledge of anatomy is necessary to prevent confusing the nerve with other structures. In areas in which a nerve is usually accompanied by a vein and artery, color flow Doppler imaging, if available, can be used to find adjacent vessels and thus, isolate the nerve.

A nerve is usually identified by its hyperechoic surfaces and location (Fig. 4–17). Once a nerve is identified, the probe should be rotated slowly to maximize its dimensions in the sagittal planes. The nerve is then slowly followed proximally and distally, moving the probe as necessary to keep the dimensions as large as possible.

Care is needed to avoid compression of tissues during scanning. Compression causes collapse of vessels, making their identification and that of the accompanying nerves more difficult. Also, muscle should be evaluated during scanning. Compressed muscle appears more hyperechoic than normal muscle.

Normal Findings

In sagittal images (see Fig. 4–17), sciatic, tibial, and peroneal nerves have hyperechoic near and deep surfaces. The internal area has multiple linear echo densities. Although vessels have a similar appearance, they are more anechoic, can be compressed, and have less distinct borders (JA Hudson, JE Steiss, unpublished research).

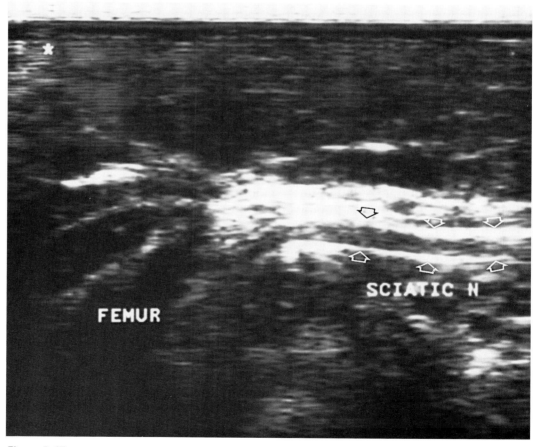

Figure 4–17

Sagittal sonogram of a normal sciatic nerve of a dog. Note the hyperechoic near and far surfaces (arrows).

Figure 4–18

Sagittal sonogram of a sciatic nerve that was severed inadvertently during closed reduction and repair of a femoral fracture using an intramedullary pin. This scan was obtained approximately 1 week later, before surgical amputation of the limb. The near and far surfaces (open arrows) of the nerve are visualized less clearly than those of the normal nerve in Figure 4–17. The distal end of the proximal segment of the nerve is "flared" (solid arrows) because of pathologic swelling. Wallerian degeneration of the nerve distal to the injury causes poor visualization of the distal segment.

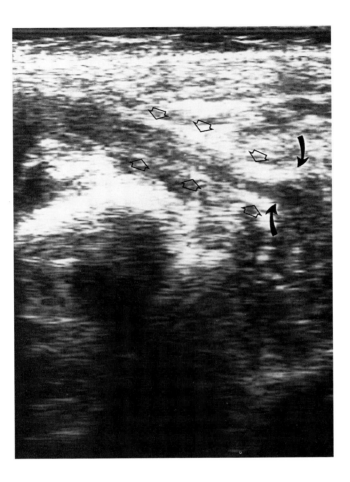

Abnormal Findings

Transection

When transection is suspected (Fig. 4–18), a normal section of the nerve should be identified. The nerve is then followed to the potential area of transection to determine whether or not the nerve is intact. Preferably, examination of the nerve begins proximal to the lesion. Unless transection is recent, the distal nerve will have undergone Wallerian degeneration and will be difficult to identify. Comparison of the affected nerve with the nerve in the normal opposite limb is beneficial to avoid misinterpretation of normal findings. Nerves can be difficult to follow where they change course, appearing as though they have been transected.

Wallerian Degeneration

The nerve distal to an area of transection appears slightly smaller than normal. The borders are less hyperechoic and have become slightly irregular. Confusion with blood vessels or muscle or tendon fibers is more likely to occur.

Other Considerations

Surrounding muscle should be examined for evidence of lesions or atrophy. As noted previously, care is needed to avoid compression of muscle tissue, which would result in artificially increased echogenicity.

REFERENCES

1. Smith CW, Marshall AE, Knecht CD: Detection of artificially produced intracranial midline shifts of the brain in the dog with A-mode echoencephalography. Am J Vet Res *33*:2423, 1972.

2. Thomas, WB, Sorjonen DC, Hudson JA: Ultrasound-guided brain biopsy in dogs. Am J Vet Res *54*:1942, 1992.

3. Hudson JA, et al: Color flow Doppler imaging and Doppler spectral analysis of the brain of neonatal dogs. Vet Radiol Ultrasound, Submitted for publication.

4. Wolfson B, et al: Ultrasound evaluation of kittens with experimental hydrocephalus and ventriculoperitoneal shunts (abstract). J Ultrasound Med *7*:S39, 1988.

5. Fawer CL, Calame A: *Ultrasound.* In *Imaging Techniques of the Central Nervous System of Neonates.* Edited by J Haddad, D Christmann, J Messer. Berlin: Springer, 1991.

6. Ment LR, et al: Beagle puppy model of intraventricular hemorrhage. J Neurosurg *57*:219, 1982.

7. Sudakoff GS, Montazemi M, Rifkin MD: The foramen magnum: The underutilized acoustic window to the posterior fossa. J Ultrasound Med *12*:205, 1993.

8. Mittelstaedt CA, et al: The intraoperative uses of real-time ultrasound. Radiographics *4*:267, 1984.

9. Laing FC, et al: Plastic wrap for US transducer sterility or sanitization. Radiology *160*:846, 1986.

10. Hudson JA, et al: Ultrasonographic anatomy of the canine brain. Vet Radiol *30*:13, 1989.

11. Hudson JA, et al: Ultrasonographic examination of the normal canine neonatal brain. Vet Radiol *32*:50, 1991.

12. Hudson JA, et al: Ultrasonographic diagnosis of canine hydrocephalus. Vet Radiol *31*:50, 1990.

13. Spaulding KA, Sharp NJH: Ultrasonographic imaging of the lateral cerebral ventricles in the dog. Vet Radiol *31*:59, 1990.

14. Koons AH, et al: Cerebral blood flow measurements in the newborn dog. Biol Neonate *63*:120, 1993.

15. Messer J: *Cerebral Doppler in the neonate.* In *Imaging Techniques of the Central Nervous System of Neonates.* Edited by J Haddad, D Christmann, J Messer. Berlin: Springer, 1991, pp. 107–115.

16. Rivers WJ, Walter PA: Hydrocephalus in the dog: Utility of ultrasonography as an alternate diagnostic imaging technique. J Am Anim Hosp Assoc *28*:333, 1992.

17. Chrisman CL: *Problems in Small Animal Neurology,* 2nd Ed. Philadelphia: Lea & Febiger, 1991, pp. 136–138.

18. Chandler WF: *Use of ultrasound imaging during intracranial operations.* In *Ultrasound in Neurosurgery.* Edited by JM Rubin, WF Chandler. New York: Raven Press, 1990, pp. 67–106.

19. Doherty ML, McAllister H, Healy A: Ultrasound as an aid to Coenurus cerebralis cyst localization in a lamb. Vet Rec *124*:591, 1989.

20. Jubb KVF, Huxtable CR: *Malformations of the central nervous system.* In *Pathology of Domestic Animals.* 4th Ed. Edited by KVF Jubb, PC Kennedy, NC Palmer. New York: Academic Press, pp. 270–292.

21. Leadman M, et al: Ultrasound diagnosis of neonatal spinal epidural hemorrhage. JCU *16*:440, 1988.

22. Kawahara H, et al: Normal development of the spinal cord in neonates and infants seen on ultrasonography. Neuroradiology *29*:50, 1987.

23. Eismont FJ, et al: The role of intraoperative ultrasonography in the treatment of thoracic and lumbar spine fractures. Spine *9*:782, 1984.

24. Rubin JM, et al: Spinal ultrasonography. Intraoperative and pediatric applications. Radiol Clin North Am *26*:1, 1988.

25. Rubin JM: *Ultrasonography in spinal cord surgery.* In *Ultrasound in Neurosurgery.* Edited by JM Rubin, WF Chandler. New York: Raven Press, 1990.

26. Yamaoka K: Significance of intraoperative ultrasonography in anterior spinal operation. Spine *14*:1192, 1989

27. Cartee RE, Hudson JA, Finn-Bodner ST: Ultrasonography/Echocardiography. Vet Clin North Am Small Anim Pract, January/February, 1993.

28. Finn-Bodner ST, et al: Sonographic appearance of the normal canine spinal cord. Vet Radiol Ultrasound, In press.

29. Hudson JA, et al: Grey-scale and color flow Doppler imaging of the normal and traumatized spinal cord of dogs. Presented at the Annual Meeting of the American College of Veterinary Radiology, Orlando, August, 1992.

30. Hudson JA, et al: Doppler spectral analysis of the normal and traumatized spinal cord of dogs. Presented at the Annual Meeting of the American College of Veterinary Radiology, Orlando, August, 1992.

31. Mügge A, et al: Ultrasound imaging of the spinal cord via the esophagus in conscious patients: Initial experience. JCU *19*:187, 1991.

32. de Lahunta A, Alexander JW: Ischemic myelopathy secondary to presumed fibrocartilaginous embolism in nine dogs. J Am Anim Hosp Assoc *12*:37, 1976.

33. Hukuda S, Wilson CB: Experimental cervical myelopathy: Effects of compression and ischemia on the canine cervical cord. J Neurosurg *37:*631, 1972.

34. Gillilan LA: *Blood supply to the central nervous system.* In *Correlative Anatomy of the Nervous System.* Edited by EC Crosby, T Humphrey, EW Lauer. New York: Macmillan, 1962, pp. 550–564.

35. Nakayama M: Intraoperative spinal ultrasonography in dogs: Normal findings and case-history reports. Vet Radiol Ultrasound *34:*264, 1993.

36. Strandness DE: *Duplex Scanning in Vascular Disorders.* New York: Raven Press, 1990, pp. 53, 57–60.

37. Plummer SB, et al: Tethered spinal cord and an intradural lipoma associated with a meningocele in a Manx-type cat. J Am Vet Med Assoc *203:*1159, 1993.

38. Swaim SF: *Peripheral nerve surgery. Nerve degeneration.* In *Veterinary Neurology.* Edited by JE Oliver, BF Hoerlein, IG Mayhew. Philadelphia: WB Saunders, 1987, pp. 495–496.

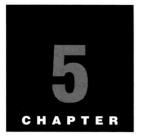

THE EYE

Barbara A. Selcer

Although there are few reports in the veterinary literature on the use of two-dimensional real-time sonographic imaging of the eye, ocular sonography can provide important diagnostic information that is not readily available using other diagnostic techniques.[1–10] The eye is ideally suited to sonographic examination because of its fluid-like content and the presence of several internal reflective surfaces. Sonography is indicated when evaluation of internal ocular structures is necessary, but corneal opacity, hyphema, or vitreolar opacity hinder conventional examination. Retrobulbar abnormalities, which may be difficult to detect radiographically, frequently can be identified sonographically, and ocular foreign bodies are best localized using this technique. Thus, ocular ultrasound can be an important diagnostic tool.

TECHNIQUE

Ocular sonography is easily performed in conscious patients. In fact, sedation should be avoided if possible to decrease the likelihood of membrana nictitans prolapse. A topical ophthalmic anesthetic is administered before scanning. Direct corneal contact scanning, in which the transducer head is placed directly on the corneal surface, is the technique of choice for visualization of the lens, vitreous, choroid/retina/scleral surface, and retrobulbar tissues. The use of a water bath offset may enhance visualization of the anterior chamber. With either technique, sterile acoustic coupling gel should be applied to the cornea to facilitate transducer-eye contact. After the examination, eye wash is used to flush the eyes to decrease potential irritation from the gel.

High-frequency, 7.5- to 10-mHz transducers are recommended for ocular sonography. Sector scanners provide small transducer-head surface area and are therefore preferable to larger linear array transducers. Scans should be made in at least two scan planes, i.e., the coronal (horizontal) and sagittal (vertical) planes. Oblique sagittal images may be required to see some lesions.

ANATOMY

Normal ocular sonographic anatomy can depict the cornea, anterior chamber, lens, iris, ciliary body, vitreous, posterior wall of the globe, retrobulbar tissues, and optic nerve (Fig. 5–1). The choroid, retina, and posterior sclera are tightly adherent and are seen as a single structure. The posterior chamber is not well visualized sonographically. The

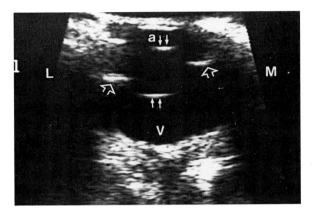

Figure 5–1

Dorsal (coronal) plane sonogram of a normal canine eye. The normal lens is sonolucent bounded anteriorly and posteriorly by thin echogenic lines (solid arrows). The anterior chamber (a) is small and sonolucent. The vitreous chamber (V) is larger and also sonolucent. Often, the iris and ciliary body are identified by short echogenic lines on either side of the lens (open arrows). L, lateral; M, medial.

optic nerve, iris, and ciliary body are not always visible in all scan planes. The cornea is usually identified as an echogenic curvilinear structure in the extreme near field. Just deep to the cornea is the anterior chamber, which is usually small and sonolucent. The caudal boundary of the anterior chamber is formed by the anterior surface of the lens. The lens itself is sonolucent but it is bounded anteriorly and posteriorly by short, thin echogenic lines. Deep to the lens lies the large sonolucent vitreous chamber. In some sections, the iris and ciliary body may be identified as thin echogenic lines on either side of the lens. The posterior wall of the globe comprises the sclera, choroid, and retina, which form an echogenic line somewhat thicker than the individual boundary lines of the lens. The retrobulbar tissues are usually echogenic because of their fat content. Frequently, sonolucent bands that represent extraocular muscles are visible in the retrobulbar tissue. The optic nerve can also be identified in some scans as a relatively hypoechoic linear band surrounded by echogenic fat. The optic disk can appear as a slightly thickened echogenic area in the posterior globe.

OCULAR SONOGRAPHIC ABNORMALITIES

Abnormalities of the cornea usually are not evaluated sonographically. Hyphema in the anterior chamber, on the other hand, can be identified when the normal anechoic nature of the anterior chamber becomes echogenic.[11] After trauma, the anterior chamber may collapse and the cornea will lie adjacent to the iris.[11] Another possible cause of increased anterior chamber echogenicity is hypopyon (Fig. 5–2), in which inflammatory cells are present within the chamber.[11]

The iris and ciliary body can be evaluated sonographically. In people, benign nevi (clusters of dense melanophore concentration) are reportedly seen as small nodular echogenic foci involving the iris.[11] A similar appearance might be expected in animals, but it has not yet been confirmed. Malignant melanoma of the iris and ciliary body has been reported in the veterinary literature.[4] Similar to lesions in people, iris/ciliary body melanoma appears sonographically as a large echogenic mass originating at the plane of the iris and ciliary body and extending into the anterior chamber and the vitreous chamber (Figs. 5–3 and 5–4).[4,11] Associated lens subluxation may be seen.[4]

Cataracts usually are identified clinically. Sonographic examination of the eye before cataract removal may be necessary to rule out retinal detachment or disease within the vitreous. The most common sonographic finding associated with cataract formation is thickening of the anterior and posterior lens surface (Figs. 5–5 to 5–7). In addition, a larger surface area is seen along the margin of the lens. Sonography may also identify lens luxation into the anterior chamber or vitreous (Fig. 5–8).[2,11]

Hemorrhage within the vitreous chamber may be identified sonographically. Small-volume acute hemorrhage is difficult to identify;[11] however, as clots form, variably sized amorphous echogenic heterogenous masses can develop. Blood clots are indistinguishable from other lesions that may produce vitreolar echogenic masses (Figs. 5–9 and 5–10). Other irregular, nonhemorrhagic mass-like echogenic lesions within the vitreous reported in the veterinary literature include fungal granuloma,[4] purulent panophthalmitis,[4] and proteinaceous inflammatory reaction associated with a penetrating foreign body.[4] Small "floating" echogenic specks seen within the vitreous in some patients possibly represent asteroid hyalosis (Fig. 5–11), calcium and fatty acid foci that do not impair vision.[11,13]

Sonographic ocular examination is frequently used to identify retinal detachment.[2,4–6,8,11] Detachments can occur along the entire surface of the retina or focally. Sonographically, thin echogenic lines are seen within the vitreous either freely movable (viewed in real time) or attached at the optic disk or ora serrata. They may also be associated with an echogenic mass or blood clot within the vitreous.[4,11] Severe detachment of the retina with points of attachment at the optic disk or ora serrata is seen as echogenic lines in a characteristic "V" shape (Figs. 5–7 and 5–12).[2,4,11] Small focal detachments may be difficult to recognize. Sonographically similar lesions include choroidal detachment and vitreous hemorrhage.[4]

The choroidal lesion most often detected sonographically is melanoma.[11] Choroidal melanomas vary in size and shape and can protrude into the vitreous.[11] Small melanomas are usually uniform and moderately echogenic, whereas larger tumors may appear heterogeneous.[11] Retinal detachment is commonly associated with these tumors.[11] Metastatic neoplasia of the choroid can be difficult to distinguish from choroidal melanoma on two-dimensional real-time sonograms.[11]

Some penetrating foreign bodies can be identified sonographically.[4,11] Metallic foreign bodies are usually highly echogenic, with possible reverberation artifact or acoustic shadowing seen posteriorly (Fig. 5–13).[2,11] Sonographic localization of the foreign body within the globe is often superior to radiographic localization.

Figure 5–2

Sagittal sonogram of the eye of a horse with hypopyon related to a corneal lesion. Diffuse medium level echoes are seen within the anterior chamber (A). The lens (L) and vitreous (v) remain sonolucent.

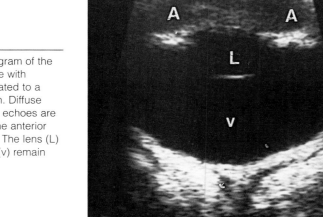

Sonography is an important method of examining the retrobulbar and periorbital soft tissues. Exophthalmos is a common indication for ocular sonography. Although magnetic resonance and CT imaging may produce slightly superior periorbital images, sonography is usually more readily available and is considerably less expensive. The etiology of retrobulbar masses ranges from neoplastic to inflammatory.[1,4,8,9] In a series of cases in which ultrasound was used to confirm the presence of retrobulbar disease, Morgan found neoplasia as a frequent cause.[9]

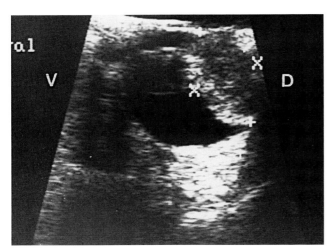

Figure 5–3

Sagittal sonogram of the eye of a dog with an iris/ciliary body melanoma. A large, medium level echogenic mass (X—X) is seen dorsally protruding into both the anterior chamber and the vitreous chamber. The lens is displaced ventrally. D, dorsal; V, ventral.

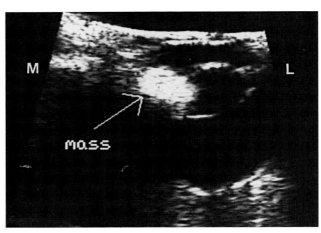

Figure 5–4

Dorsal (coronal) sonogram of the eye of a dog with an undiagnosed iris/ciliary body mass. The mass is highly echogenic. Compare to the mass in Figure 4–3. M, medial; L, lateral.

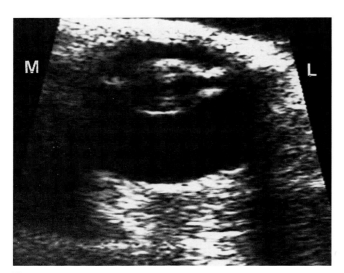

Figure 5–5

Dorsal (coronal) sonogram of the eye of a dog with a mature cataract. The anterior and posterior lens surfaces are thickened and more echogenic. No vitreal or retinal abnormalities are present. M, medial; L, lateral.

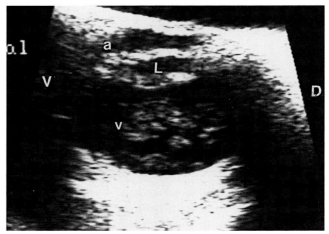

Figure 5–6

Sagittal sonogram of an eye of a dog with a hypermature cataract and vitreal echoes consistent with a diagnosis of lens-induced uveitis. The anterior and posterior lens surfaces are thick and hyperechoic. The lens diameter is reduced. Medium level echoes are present within the vitreous chamber and may be related to hemorrhage or an inflammatory response. V, ventral; D, dorsal; a, anterior chamber; L, lens; v, vitreous chamber.

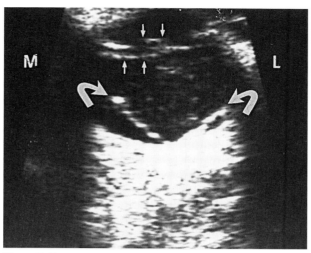

Figure 5–7

Dorsal (coronal) sonogram of an eye in a dog with a hypermature cataract and retinal detachment. The lens (straight arrows) is collapsed. Hypoechoic foci are present within the vitreous chamber, and the retina (linear echogenic lines [curved arrows]) is detached in a characteristic "V" shape. M, medial; L, lateral.

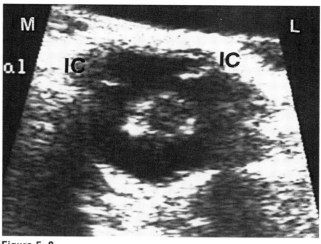

Figure 5–8

Dorsal (coronal) plane sonogram of the eye in a dog with a cataract and a posterior lens luxation. The lens is displaced into the vitreous chamber. Short linear echoes (IC) represent the plane of the iris/ciliary body. M, medial; L, lateral.

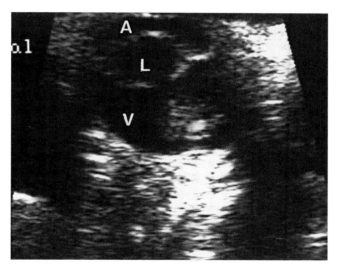

Figure 5–9

Sagittal plane sonogram of the eye in a dog with a focal vitreolar mass. Note the thickening of the anterior and posterior lens surfaces (cataract). An irregular, medium level echogenic mass with a hyperechoic central focus is present within the vitreous chamber (v). A, anterior chamber; L, lens.

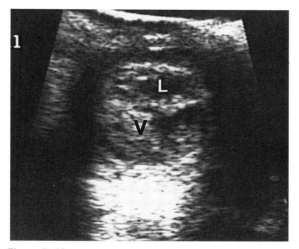

Figure 5–10

Dorsal (coronal) plane sonogram of the eye of a dog with severe amorphous vitreolar echoes. The vitreous chamber is almost filled with a medium level echogenic mass. The lens surfaces are thickened and echogenic (cataract). The etiology of the lesion was not determined. L, lens; V, vitreous chamber.

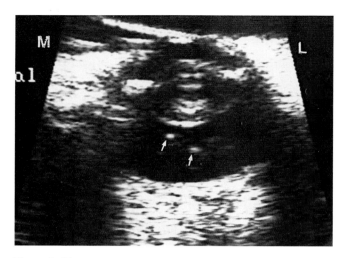

Figure 5–11

Dorsal (coronal) plane sonogram of the eye of a dog with a cataract and small floating echogenic foci presumed to be asteroid hyalosis (small arrows) within the vitreous chamber. M, medial; L, lateral.

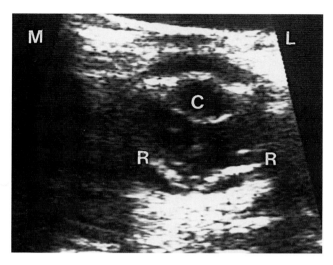

Figure 5–12

Dorsal (coronal) plane sonogram of the eye of a dog with a cataract (C) and detached retina. Linear "V"-shaped echogenic lines (R) seen within the posterior vitreous chamber attached to the optic disk represent the retinal detachment. M, medial; L, lateral.

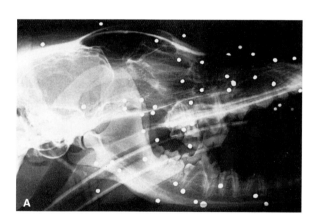

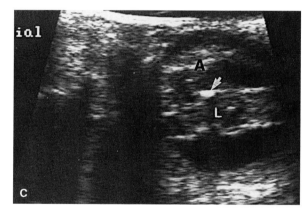

Figure 5–13

A and **B,** Lateral and ventrodorsal skull radiographs of a dog with a gunshot injury to the head. Numerous metallic shot pellets are present over the plane of the eyes. Sonography **(C)** was useful in localizing a pellet within the globe of the eye. **C,** Dorsal (coronal) oblique sonogram reveals a highly echogenic focus (arrow) in the anterior lens capsule. Note the posterior shadowing deep to the pellet. Increased medium level echoes are present in the anterior chamber (A) and within the lens (L).

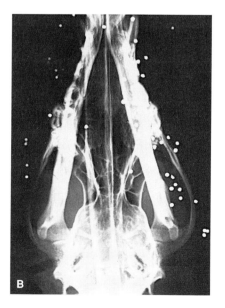

The sonographic appearance of the following tumor types has been described in the veterinary literature: lymphosarcoma (highly echogenic mass),[9] lymphoblastic lymphoma (diffuse increased echogenicity initially, followed 2 weeks later by a hypoechoic mass with deformation of the posterior globe),[8] chondrosarcoma (echogenic mass deforming the shape of the globe),[9] osteosarcoma (echogenic mass deforming the shape of the globe),[9] and optic nerve meningioma (medium level echogenic mass deforming the shape of the globe).[1] Inflammatory conditions such as retrobulbar abscesses (Fig. 5–14) appear sonographically as discreet hypoechoic to anechoic masses with slight deformation of the globe.[8,9]

Other retrobulbar abnormalities that may be detected sonographically include periorbital cysts (Fig. 5–15),[4] retrobulbar cellulitis,[9] salivary gland adenitis,[11] retrobulbar foreign bodies,[11] and extraocular muscle hypertrophy associated with hyperthyroidism.[11] The latter has not yet been reported in the veterinary literature.

Ocular ultrasound can play a significant role in the diagnosis of ocular and retrobulbar disease not readily identified by routine or conventional ophthalmic examination, especially when corneal opacity or cataracts preclude visualization of the vitreous chamber and retina.

Figure 5–14

Oblique sonogram of the eye and retrobulbar tissues of a dog with a retrobulbar abscess. Only a small section of the lateral globe is seen (G). A large mixed echogenic mass (abscess) (A) is in the periorbital soft tissues. The mass is predominantly hypoechoic with hyperechoic margins. The abscess has displaced the globe and has distorted the normal landmarks. Caud, caudal.

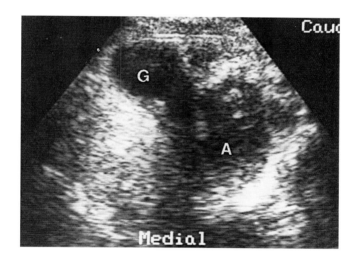

Figure 5–15

Oblique sonogram of the periorbital soft tissues of a dog with a lacrimal cyst adenoma. The globe of the eye is not seen in this scan. Multiple anechoic cystic structures are present (C). Note the posterior enhancement and the large, linear transducer artifact (A).

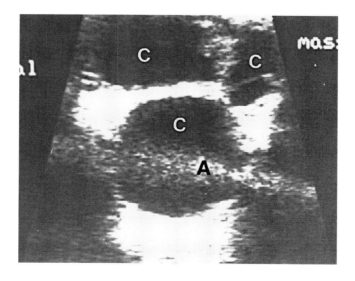

REFERENCES

1. Abrams K, Toal RL: What is your diagnosis? J Am Vet Med Assoc *196:*951, 1990.
2. Barr F: Diagnostic Ultrasound in the Dog and Cat. Oxford: Blackwell Scientific, 1990, pp. 159–168.
3. Cottrill NB, Banks WJ, Pechman RD: Ultrasonographic and biometric evaluation of the eye and orbit of dogs. Am J Vet Res *50:*898, 1989.
4. Dziezyc J, Hager DA, Millichamp NJ: Two-dimensional real-time ocular ultrasonography in the diagnosis of ocular lesions in dogs. J Am Anim Hosp Assoc *23:*501, 1987.
5. Dziezyc J, Hager DA: Ocular ultrasonography in veterinary medicine. Semin Vet Med Surg (Small Anim) *3:*1, 1988.
6. Eisenberg HM: Ultrasonography of the eye and orbit. Vet Clin North Am *15:*1263, 1985.
7. Hager DA, Dziezyc J, Millichamp NJ: Two-dimensional real-time ocular ultrasonography in the dog; technique and normal anatomy. Vet Radiol *28:*60, 1987.
8. Miller WW, Cartee RE: B-scan ultrasonography for the detection of space-occupying ocular masses. J Am Vet Med Assoc *187:*66, 1985.
9. Morgan RV: Ultrasonography of retrobulbar diseases of the dog and cat. J Am Anim Hosp Assoc *25:*393, 1989.
10. Rogers M, et al: Evaluation of the extirpated equine eye using B-mode ultrasonography. Vet Radiol *27:*24, 1986.
11. Munk PL, et al: Sonography of the eye. AJR Am J Roentgenol *157:*1079, 1991.

THE GLANDS AND LYMPH NODES

Robert E. Cartee and Mary B. Mahaffey

SALIVARY GLAND—*R. E. Cartee*

The use of ultrasound in the diagnosis of salivary gland diseases in man is well documented. In one report, sonography had a sensitivity of 100% in the detection of salivary masses, but only 59% in the detection of sialoadenitis.[1] Salivary masses appeared hypoechoic and either sharply marginated (benign) or irregular (malignant); sialoadenitis was seen as enlarged, inhomogeneous hypoechoic areas.[1] In another report, a cavernous hemangioma detected sonographically in the submandibular gland appeared hyperechoic to echo-free.[2] Gritzmann reported that sonographic detection of salivary calculi was 95% specific in a group of human patients.[3] The author also indicated that sonography can be used to detect diseases and acute inflammation of the salivary gland. Abscesses were hypoechoic and acute inflammation appeared as inhomogeneous areas.[3] Hematomas and cysts were echo-free, and the latter often accompanied chronic inflammatory or autoimmune disease. Calculi were reported to be echogenic with acoustic shadowing. The normal salivary gland was usually more echogenic than the surrounding tissue.[3]

Zbaren and Ducommon reported that sonography is superior to sialography in the assessment of salivary gland disease.[4] They also indicated that sonography is an effective tool in the detection of lesions in the gland parenchyma and also in both intra- and extraductal ectasia.[4] Other authors stated that sonography was as sensitive as magnetic resonance imaging (MRI) in detecting lesions of the parotid salivary gland.[5] Diederich and colleagues stated that sonography is the method of choice in evaluating salivary glands in children.[6]

The sonographic appearance of a normal mandibular salivary gland in the dog is shown in Figure 6–1. The mandibular salivary gland lies at the caudal edge of the mandible and the probe may be applied in either a rostral-to-caudal or a dorsal-to-ventral orientation. The use of a standoff pad may be desirable and a frequency of 7 to 10 mHz is preferred. Wisner and colleagues reported that the canine mandibular salivary gland appears as a low echo intensity oval structure with a hyperechoic margin. Thin linear streaks of high intensity echoes occur internally. The parotid salivary gland may be scanned in either orientation just ventral to the base of the ear. Because of its thickness, the parotid salivary gland is difficult to image, and is seen as a poorly marginated, low intensity-echo structure.[7]

The incidence of salivary gland disease in dogs and cats is low. Salivary mucocele is the most common finding.[8] Other conditions that do occur are rupture, inflammation, dilation, necrosis, fistula, foreign bodies, autoimmune tissue, calculi, and neoplasia.[9]

Figure 6–1

Sonogram of the normal mandibular salivary glands of the dog.

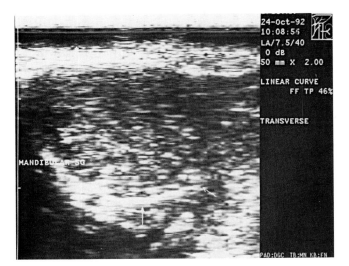

There have been few reports on the use of sonography in the diagnosis of salivary gland disease in animals; however, MRI has been used to evaluate the salivary glands of laboratory dogs after ductal ligation.[10]

THE THYROID AND PARATHYROID GLANDS—*R. E. Cartee*

The use of sonography in the diagnosis of diseases and in the calculation of volume changes of the human thyroid gland has been extensively reported.[11–23] Decreased echogenicity is associated with thyroiditis, hyperthyroidism, and abscesses.[12–15,20] Normal volumes were determined for adults, children, and fetuses, and change in volume was related to iodism and hypothyroidism.[11,16,19,21,23] Changes in vascularity of both the thyroid and parathyroid glands as noted by color Doppler analysis were investigated and found to be of little value.[18,22]

Sonographic imaging of the thyroid and parathyroid glands of animals is not as well documented. In 1991, Wisner et al. described the normal appearance of the thyroid and parathyroid glands of the dog. They reported that the thyroid gland was well marginated and homogeneous in echotexture (Fig. 6–2A), and was found by first locating the common carotid artery. The gland was ventral and medial to the artery in the craniocervical region. The parathyroid gland could not be identified.[24] In a later study, the parathyroid glands were located using a 10-mHz probe. Abnormal parathyroid glands were found to be hypoechoic compared to the thyroid gland.[25]

In a study in cats, the thyroid gland was found adjacent to the trachea slightly caudal to the cricoid cartilage. Sonographically, it was hypoechoic and well marginated (Fig. 6–2B). The parathyroids could not be discriminated sonographically.[26] In cats, measurements of size using B mode sonography appear to be inaccurate and unreliable at this time.[26]

THE PANCREAS—*M. B. Mahaffey*

Ultrasound has become a useful tool in the evaluation of the canine pancreas. Unfortunately, the normal pancreas is difficult to image because it is small, is similar in echogenicity to surrounding mesenteric fat, lacks distinct sonographic margins, and, most importantly, is in close proximity to gas-containing gastrointestinal structures.[27,28] Identifiable, adjacent anatomic landmarks are therefore used when scanning the pancreatic region.

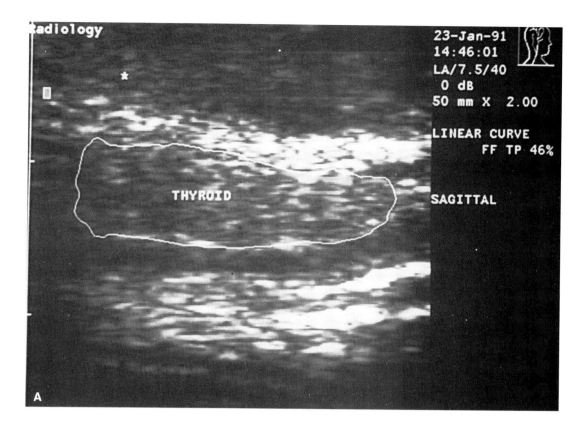

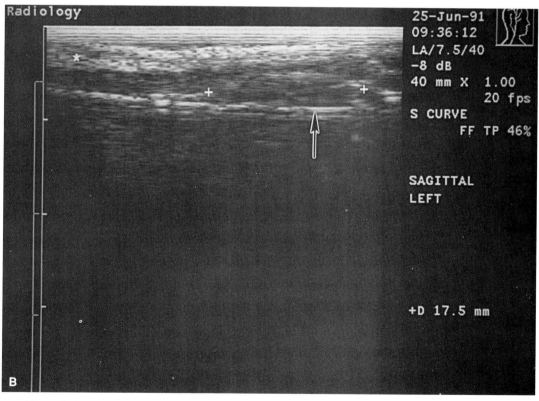

Figure 6–2

Sonogram of the normal canine (**A**) and feline (**B**, arrow) thyroid glands.

The pancreas is composed of right and left lobes joined together by the body. The right lobe is long and slender, and is located in the mesoduodenum dorsomedial to the descending duodenum and ventromedial to the right kidney. The left lobe is shorter and wider than the right lobe, and is located between the stomach and transverse colon, with its distal tip adjacent to the spleen and cranioventral surface of the left kidney.[29] The body lies ventral to the portal vein and unites the two lobes at the caudal surface of the pylorus. The portal vein courses dorsal to the body of the pancreas (Fig. 6–3).

Scanning Procedure

The dog is placed in dorsal recumbency[30,31] or in lateral recumbency (left side down to scan the right lobe and right side down to scan the left lobe).[32] Longitudinal and transverse scan planes are used. A systematic method to scan the pancreatic area is important. Patients are scanned after fasting so the amount of gas within the stomach is minimized.[30,32]

The transducer with the highest frequency that allows adequate depth penetration should be selected. In cats and small to medium-sized dogs, a 7.5-mHz transducer provides sufficient depth penetration and resolution to evaluate the pancreas. In larger dogs, a 5.0-mHz probe may be necessary to obtain adequate depth penetration, but much of the fine detail of the pancreas is lost. Therefore, a 7.5-mHz transducer should be used as much as possible.

The major landmarks used to find the right pancreatic lobe are the descending duodenum and the right kidney. Using a longitudinal scan plane, the stomach is found by scanning the ventral abdomen. While still in the longitudinal plane, the probe is shifted to the right until the pylorus and proximal duodenum are located. These structures are seen in cross section and have a round "bulls-eye" appearance. As the probe is moved slightly more to the right and caudally, the duodenum is seen in its long axis (see Fig. 6–4A). This section of bowel appears straighter than other adjacent small intestine. The area dorsal to the descending duodenum from the right kidney laterally to the portal vein and caudal vena cava medially should also be scanned. Occasionally, the pancreati-

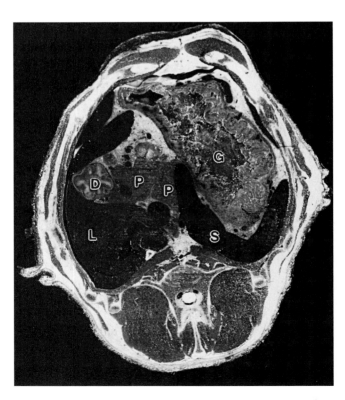

Figure 6–3

Section of abdomen showing the position of the normal pancreas (P). D, duodenum; G, stomach; L, liver; S, spleen.

coduodenal vein, which lies within the pancreas and runs parallel to the duodenum, can be identified, but only when a 7.5-mHz transducer is used.[32] Following the duodenum caudally to its caudal flexure ensure the entire area containing the right lobe is imaged.

Another approach to the right pancreatic lobe is to locate the cranial pole of the right kidney and, with the probe in a longitudinal plane, move the probe medially until the descending duodenum is found. After scanning in the longitudinal plane, the probe is rotated in order to scan the area in the transverse plane.

In deep-chested dogs or in dogs with abdominal pain that disallows applying adequate pressure to the ventral abdomen, the pancreatic area can be scanned by placing the probe on the right lateral side of the patient at the 11th or 12th intercostal space. The area medial and ventral to the right kidney is scanned until the duodenum is found. It is more difficult to evaluate the pancreas using the right lateral approach because the ribs block much of the scanning area, and if the patient is lying on its left side, bowel gas often blocks the sound. The distal portion of the right lobe can be scanned by placing the probe caudal to the 13th rib. The problem of overlying bowel gas occasionally can be overcome by placing the patient on its right side so that fluid may fill the duodenum and displace the gas. The probe is positioned between the table and the patient. The right kidney is located in the longitudinal plane, and then the probe is pulled ventrally until the duodenum comes into view.[32] Any free peritoneal fluid present will flow to the dependent right side and improve visualization of the pancreatic region. In some practices, a table with a slot or hole is used for cardiac scanning from the dependent side. Such a table, if present, would be helpful in this instance.

In the cat, the right lobe of the pancreas is visualized from the left side using the spleen as a window.[32] The probe is placed just behind the ribs and the area is scanned until the spleen is identified. Pressure is placed on the probe so the right kidney comes into view in the far field. Pressure on the probe is then decreased so that the right pancreatic lobe region between the right kidney and the portal vein can be viewed.

The left lobe of the pancreas is more difficult to see because gas, often present in the stomach, transverse colon, and small intestine adjacent to the pancreas, blocks the sound waves. Even so, the area caudal to the greater curvature of the stomach and cranial to the transverse colon should be scanned from the pylorus laterally with the patient in dorsal or right lateral recumbency. Because the tip of the left lobe may contact the spleen and left kidney, lateral movement of the probe should continue until these structures are identified. If the patient is in right lateral recumbency, the area between the spleen, left kidney, and stomach is visualized by placing the probe on the left side behind the ribs. The splenic vein can also be used as a landmark to find the left pancreatic lobe because the lobe is located just caudal to the vessel.[31,32] The branches that exit the spleen medially form the large splenic vein.[32]

The Normal Pancreas

As stated previously, the normal pancreas is seldom seen as a distinct structure sonographically because it is small, its echogenicity is similar to that of the adjacent mesenteric fat, and the presence of overlying bowel gas.[27] When seen, the pancreas has indistinct margins (Fig. 6–4) and is somewhat hypoechoic; its echogenicity is slightly greater than that of the liver[30,32] and less than that of the spleen.[32] The normal pancreas is more likely to be identified in puppies, thin dogs, and dogs with peritoneal fluid.[32] Saline infusion into the peritoneal space improves visualization of the normal pancreas,[33] but this technique is rarely used in clinical practice. Filling the stomach with fluid to provide an acoustical window is of little benefit.[30] In people, as in dogs, the normal pancreas is hypoechoic or isoechoic when compared to the liver. The echogenicity may increase to that of the surrounding fat, however, when fatty infiltration occurs, making the pancreas difficult to identify.[34–36] Some causes of pancreatic fatty infiltration in man include aging, obesity, chronic pancreatitis, steroid therapy, obstruction of the pancreatic duct, and diabetes mellitus.[36,37] Perhaps fatty infiltration of the pancreas occurs in dogs and cats and is one of the reasons the normal pancreas is difficult to identify as a distinct structure.

Pancreatitis

Pancreatitis can be difficult to diagnose accurately. Patient history, clinicopathologic results, and radiographic findings are used to arrive at the diagnosis as no one test is pathognomonic. Sonography has become a valuable tool in identifying pancreatitis in man,[38] and within the last few years, it has become an important adjunct in evaluating dogs and cats with suspected pancreatitis.[28,30–32,39–44]

In mild pancreatitis, the pancreas may appear as a distinct hypoechoic structure surrounded by hyperechoic mesenteric fat[28,32] (Fig. 6–5). Occasionally, small hypoechoic foci (approximately 2 to 3 mm in diameter) are found in the area of the pancreas (Fig. 6–6). Hypoechoic to anechoic finger-like projections may extend from the duodenal wall into the pancreas (Fig. 6–7). More severe pancreatitis is associated with irregularly shaped areas of increased and decreased echogenicity in the pancreatic area (Fig. 6–8). The affected pancreas may appear as a mass displacing the duodenum ventrally (Fig. 6–9).[31] Hypoechoic and anechoic areas are probably caused by pancreatic necrosis and hemorrhage,[30,32] as was shown in experimentally induced acute pancreatitis in dogs.[45] Hyperechoic areas may represent fibrosis.[28] A less common finding in dogs with pancreatitis is dilation of the pancreatic duct.[41] Other findings in dogs with pancreatitis include peripancreatic fluid; a gas- or fluid-filled, thick-walled duodenum with ileus[30,32,39]; cyst formation (Fig. 6–10); and dilation of the common bile duct and gallbladder because of obstruction.[32,39,43]

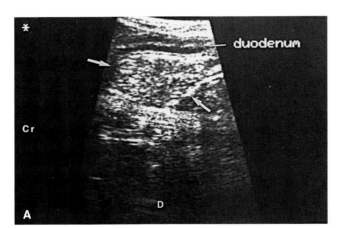
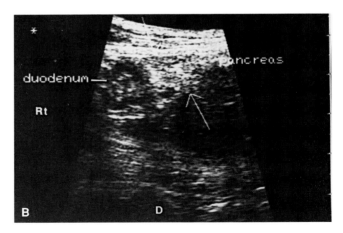

Figure 6–4

Sagittal **(A)** and transverse **(B)** scans of the right pancreatic region of two normal dogs. The pancreas (arrows) lies in the area dorsal and medial to the duodenum. It is not seen as a distinct structure because it is small and its echogenicity is similar to that of the surrounding mesenteric fat. A 7.5-mHz transducer was used. Cr, cranial; Rt, right; D, dorsal.

Figure 6–5

Transverse scan of the right lobe of the pancreas of a dog with mild pancreatitis using a 7.5-mHz transducer. The pancreas (arrow), located just medial to the duodenum, appears as a triangular hypoechoic structure surrounded by echogenic mesenteric fat. Rt, right; D, dorsal.

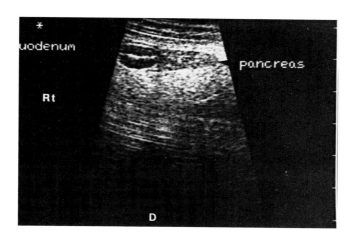

Figure 6–6

Sagittal scan of the right pancreatic region of a dog with pancreatitis using a 7.5-mHz transducer. Note the ill-defined, hypoechoic foci (arrows) in the area of the right pancreatic lobe. Cr, cranial; D, dorsal.

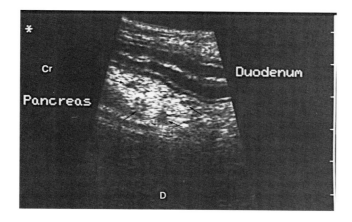

Figure 6–7

Sagittal scan of the right pancreatic region of a dog with pancreatitis using a 7.5-mHz transducer. Hypoechoic to anechoic finger-like projections extend from the duodenal wall into the adjacent pancreatic tissue that is increased in echogenicity. Cr, cranial; D, dorsal.

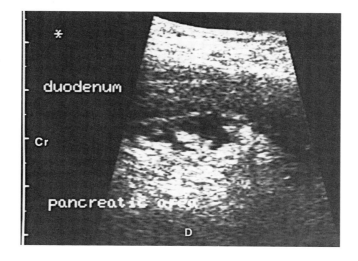

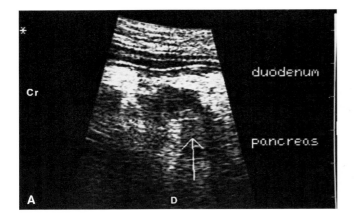

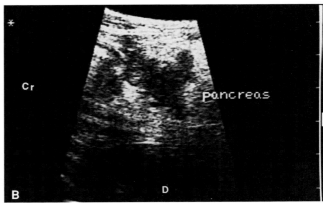

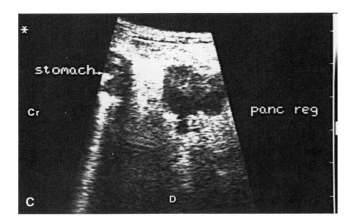

Figure 6–8

Sagittal scans of the region of the right pancreatic lobe **(A** and **B)** and left pancreatic lobe **(C)** of dogs with pancreatitis. Irregularly shaped areas of increased and decreased echogenicity in the pancreatic region are common findings in dogs with moderate to severe pancreatitis. A 7.5-mHz transducer was used. Cr, cranial; D, dorsal; panc reg, pancreatic region.

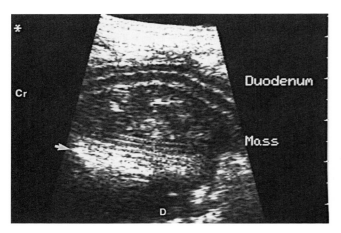

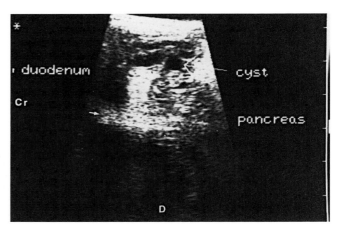

Figure 6–9

Sagittal scan of the region of the right pancreatic lobe of a dog with pancreatitis. The pancreas appears as a hypoechoic mass displacing the duodenum ventrally. The bright area (arrow) is a probe artifact. A 7.5-mHz transducer was used. Cr, cranial; D, dorsal.

Figure 6–10

Sagittal scan of the right pancreatic area of a dog with diabetes mellitus secondary to pancreatitis. An anechoic focus (cyst) measuring approximately 4 mm in diameter was found in the pancreas adjacent to the duodenum. It may have been a small pseudocyst. Surgery was not performed. The horizontal white band (small arrow) is a probe artifact. A 7.5-mHz transducer was used. Cr, cranial; D, dorsal.

Pancreatic pseudocysts and abscesses (Fig. 6–11) are possible sequelae to pancreatitis in dogs.[42–44] A pseudocyst is a collection of fluid within the pancreas resulting from disruption of a pancreatic duct.[46,47] Pseudocysts resolve spontaneously or require surgical removal.[42,44] They can measure from 6 to 10 cm in diameter. Sonographically, they appear as mostly anechoic masses with acoustic enhancement and may contain low-level internal echoes. These findings suggest a fluid-filled mass containing cellular debris.[42,44] The appearance of pancreatic abscesses is often similar to that of pseudocysts, so it may not be possible to differentiate between the two entities sonographically.[43]

Pancreatitis is uncommon in the cat. In one reported case, the sonographic findings were more subtle than those in dogs. The pancreas was seen as a well-defined, sharply marginated, hypoechoic structure. Peritoneal effusion was also present.[32]

Pancreatic Neoplasia

Neoplasms of the pancreas are uncommon. Carcinomas of the exocrine pancreas are rare, but when they occur, they tend to invade the wall of the duodenum and metastasize readily to regional lymph nodes, liver, and, occasionally, the peritoneum.[48] Functional islet cell tumors may be suspected in dogs with persistent hypoglycemia. These tumors may be benign or malignant and occur as single or multiple nodules within the pancreas (Fig. 6–12). Spread of malignant tumors may be to local lymph nodes and the liver.[48]

Sonographically, either type of tumor may appear as a discrete hypoechoic nodule in the region of the pancreas.[27,32,49] The pancreatic tissue itself may not be identified. In that instance, an enlarged lymph node must also be ruled out. If a nodule is found in the pancreas, one should look for involvement of regional lymph nodes and the liver. In a report of three dogs with insulinomas, discrete hypoechoic nodules were found in two dogs and multiple hypoechoic nodules were found throughout the pancreas in a third. Insulinomas are too small to be detected with ultrasound, so a normal pancreatic sonogram does not rule out the presence of a tumor.[32] Sonographic examination is recommended nonetheless as metastasis may be detected even if the primary tumor is not.

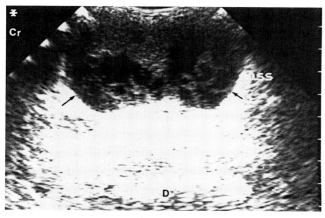

Figure 6–11

Sagittal scan of the left pancreatic region of a dog with chronic vomiting and a palpable abdominal mass. Note the mixed hypoechoic and anechoic mass (arrows), approximately 8 cm in diameter, in the region of the left lobe of the pancreas. A pancreatic abscess was found at surgery. A 5-mHz probe was used. Cr, cranial; D, dorsal.

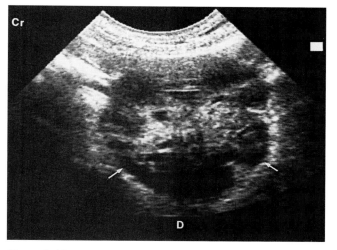

Figure 6–12

Sagittal scan of a dog with a pancreatic acinar tumor reveals a distinctly marginated, mixed echogenic mass (arrows) measuring 7 cm in diameter in the region of the left pancreatic lobe. A 5-mHz probe was used. Cr, cranial; D, dorsal.

THE ADRENAL GLAND

Sonographic examination of the adrenal gland is a routine procedure in both human and veterinary medicine.

Both longitudinal and transverse scanning planes are effective in imaging the adrenal glands in man.[50-52] The transverse scans are less diagnostic than those in the sagittal plane.[52] Location of the adrenal by transgastric and cava-suprarenal line positions has also been described.[53,54]

In man, the adrenal cortex is described as hypoechoic and the medulla as hyperechoic.[55,56] In one report, the hyperechoic area was called suprarenal fat.[57] In two other reports, it was difficult to distinguish adrenal from renal tissue.[58,59]

Several studies of sonographic size and volume determinations have been conducted in man.[60-63] Calculations of human fetal adrenal gland area, circumference, and length showed variable correlation with abnormal fetuses. The area of the adrenal correlated with high maternal estrogen levels.[61] Area measurements demonstrated shrinkage of the adrenal gland between the neonatal and early antenatal periods.[62] In vitro studies of volume determinations of the adrenal gland using water displacement are reported to be an accurate method of measurement.[63]

A similar appearance of the adrenal gland has been described in dogs.[64,65] In both dogs and cats, the adrenals are hypoechoic triangular structures with a hyperechoic border. The left adrenal lies craniomedial to the cranial pole of the left kidney and lateral to the aorta. The phrenicoabdominal artery and vein may be identified passing through the adrenal (Fig. 6–13). The right adrenal lies medial to the right kidney and caudate process of the caudate lobe of the liver (Fig. 6–14). No studies of sonographic size and volume have been done in dogs and only one has been reported in cats.[66]

The single feline study showed good correlation between sonographic measurements of length and thickness and physical measurements of these parameters; averages of 10 mm and 3.9 mm, respectively, were reported.[66] Estimation of the extent of change in the

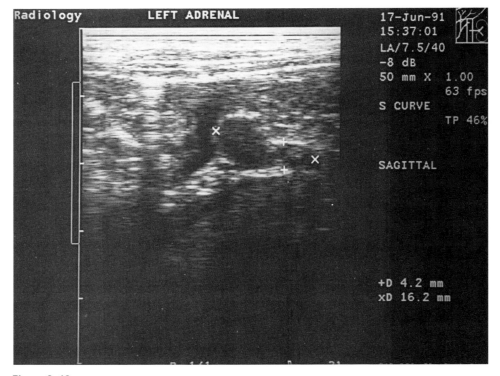

Figure 6–13

The left adrenal gland of a cat (x—x) is medial to the left kidney. A 7.5-mHz transducer was used.

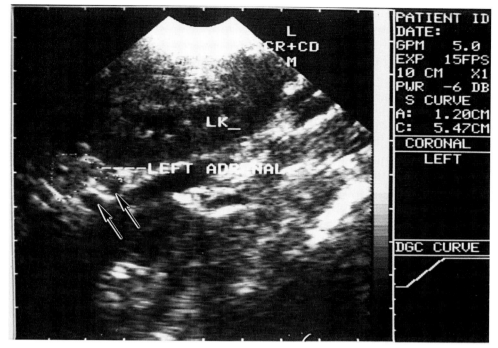

Figure 6–14

Left adrenal gland of a dog. The phrenicoabdominal artery/vein complex (arrows) is adjacent to the adrenal. LK, left kidney. A 7.5-mHz transducer was used.

Figure 6–15

Sonogram of an adrenal cyst (arrow) in a dolphin. The adrenal gland had been removed and placed in a water bath for scanning. A 5-mHz transducer was used.

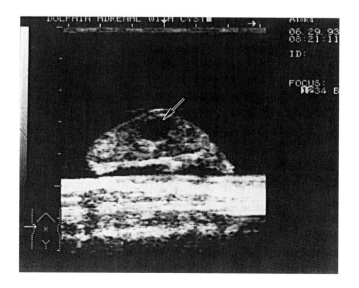

size of the adrenal gland is based tentatively on comparing the length-width ratios. A ratio of greater than 30% is suggestive of enlargement. Care should be taken in interpreting size estimations because the angle of the beam may affect the appearance. The maximum length and width should be obtained before the measurements are made.

In man, sonography has been used in the diagnosis of adrenal hyperplasia,[67] aldosteronism,[68] Cushing's syndrome,[69] cysts,[70] tumors,[71–74] calcifications,[75] hematomas,[76–78] and adrenal hemorrhage[79–81]. In two dolphin species,[82,83] cysts of the adrenal, which appeared as anechoic regions (Fig. 6–15), were diagnosed. In both man and animals, adrenal masses are usually rounded hypoechoic structures and may or may not contain echogenic areas with acoustic shadowing.

THE LYMPH NODES

Sonographic examination of lymph nodes in the cervical, abdominal, axillary, and pelvic areas is a routine procedure in man.[84–99] Although the sonographic examination of abdominal, aortic, and pelvic lymph nodes is routine in veterinary medicine, little has been written on the subject and little has been performed or written concerning the examination of the cervical and axillary lymph nodes of animals.

In man, lymph nodes are sonographically evaluated relative to their size, shape, echo pattern, and vascularity.[100] In veterinary medicine, size is usually the major criterion for diagnosis. In one report, enlarged cervical lymph nodes in man were described as round or ovoid with discrete hypoechoic nodules or multiple confluent heterogeneous or homogeneous hypoechoic masses.[84] Another report showed that a ratio of transverse diameter to longitudinal diameter of greater than 2 was predictive of metastatic disease in the cervical nodes.[85] In a slightly conflicting study, ultrasound was shown to be reliable in detecting enlargement but not as specific in diagnosing the character of the change in cervical lymph nodes and structures.[86] Changes in size of the cervical lymph node after therapy were easily monitored with ultrasound examinations.[87]

In one study of lymph nodes in general, a linear internal echo pattern was associated with benign lesions.[88] In a study of malignant lymphoma, linear or spotty areas of echogenicity were purported to be indicative of malignancy.[89] The pattern of internal echoes in lymph nodes from lung cancer victims appeared to be determined by the diffuse or local nature of the cancer.[90] In esophageal cancer, sonographic examination of the regional lymph nodes did not appear to be useful.[91,92] In the abdominal region, sonographic evaluation of lymph node enlargement, shape, and echo pattern was shown to be useful in detecting colorectal cancer,[93] gastric cancer,[94] chronic lymphocytic leukemia,[95] and hepatocellular damage.[96] Whereas the axillary lymph nodes were reported to be easily accessible with sonographic scanning, diagnosis of breast cancer using this technique was not reliable.[97–99] The use of ultrasound in the examination and biopsy of the pelvic lymph nodes was shown to be valuable in the diagnosis of gynecologic neoplasia.[100] Doppler pulsatility and resistivity indices (PI, RI) for benign and malignant lymph nodes indicated that abnormal PI and RI are predictive of malignancy.[101]

In one report, the canine regional cervical lymph nodes were characterized as round to oval hypoechoic structures.[102] Figure 6–16 shows the in vitro appearance of normal canine lymph nodes from two body regions. Figure 6–17 shows pathologically enlarged lymph nodes. Further studies are needed to examine echo patterns of specific disease processes in the lymph nodes of animals. Abdominal lymph nodes may be seen as hypoechoic structures within the relatively hyperechoic mesentery. The medial iliac nodes may be located by following the aorta to its bifurcation into the internal and external iliac arteries. The nodes appear as hypoechoic oval structures lateral to the vessels. Peripheral lymph nodes such as the axillary, superficial cervical, and popliteal may be located in the axillary space, cranial to the scapula and caudal to the femorotibial joint, and appear as mostly hypoechoic oval structures.

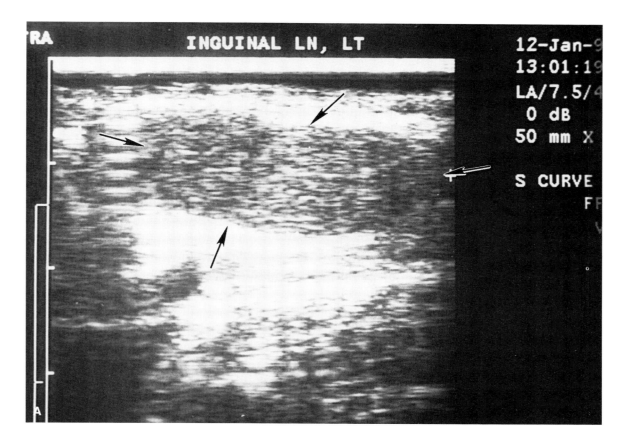

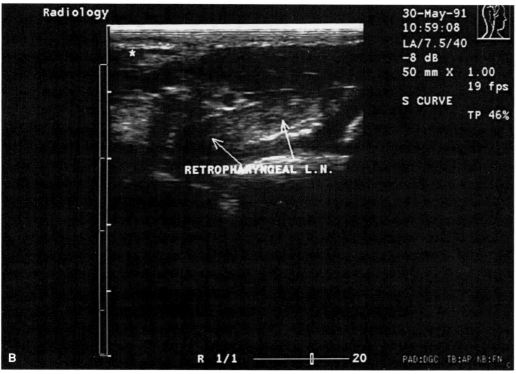

Figure 6–16

Sonograms of normal superficial inguinal **(A)** and retropharyngeal **(B)** lymph nodes of a dog. A 7.5-mHz transducer was used.

Figure 6–17

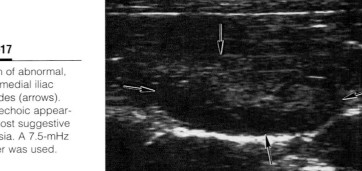

Sonogram of abnormal, enlarged medial iliac lymph nodes (arrows). The hypoechoic appearance is most suggestive of neoplasia. A 7.5-mHz transducer was used.

REFERENCES

1. Rinast E, et al: Digital subtraction sialography, conventional sialography high resolution ultrasonography and computed tomography in the diagnosis of salivary gland diseases. Eur J Radiol 9:224, 1989.
2. Takanami S, et al: A case of cavernous hemangioma with large hematoma. Jpn J Clin Radiol 33:613, 1988.
3. Gritzmann N: Sonography of the salivary glands. AJR Am J Roentgenol 153:161, 1989.
4. Zbaren P, Ducommon JC: Diagnosis of salivary gland disease using ultrasound and sialography: A comparison. Clin Otolaryngol 14:189, 1989.
5. D'alimonte P, et al: 1.5 TMR in the diagnosis of parotid masses: Comparison with ultrasonography. Radiol Med (Torino) 78:314, 1989.
6. Diederich S, et al: Diagnostic imaging of the salivary glands in children and adolescents. Radiologe 31:550, 1991.
7. Wisner ER, et al: Normal ultrasonographic anatomy of the canine neck. Vet Radiol 32:185, 1991.
8. Waldron DR, Smith NM: Salivary mucoceles. Probl Vet Med 3:270, 1991.
9. Brown ND: Salivary gland diseases: Diagnosis, treatment, and associated problems. Probl Vet Med 1:281, 1989.
10. Tsuchimochi M, et al: Magnetic resonance imaging of canine salivary glands after ductal ligation and stimulation by pilocarpine. Oral Surg Oral Med Oral Pathol 71:635, 1991.
11. Klima G, et al: Sonographically established thyroid volume in 7 to 11-year-old children. Acta Med Austriaca 13:1, 1986.
12. Yokoyama N, et al: Determination of the volume of the thyroid gland by a high resolutional ultrasonic scanner. J Nucl Med 27:1475, 1986.
13. Miki K: Determination of the thyroid volume using computerized ultrasonography and its clinical application. Nippon Naibunpi Gakkai Zasshi 62:97, 1986.
14. Brander A: Ultrasound appearances in de Quervain's subacute thyroiditis with long term follow-up. J Intern Med 232:321, 1992.
15. Miyakawa M, et al: Thyroid ultrasonography related to clinical and laboratory findings in patients with silent thyroiditis. J Endocrinol Invest 15:289, 1992.
16. Klingmuller V, Fiedler C, Otten A: Characteristics of thyroid sonography in infants and children. Radiologe 32:320, 1992.
17. Ueda D, et al: Sonographic imaging of the thyroid gland in congenital hypothyroidism. Pediatr Radiol 22:102, 1992.
18. Gooding GA, Clark OH: Use of color Doppler imaging in the distinction between thyroid and parathyroid lesions. Am J Surg 164:51, 1992.
19. Szebeni A, Beleznay E: New simple method for thyroid volume determination by ultrasonography. JCU 20:329, 1992.
20. Vitti P, et al: Thyroid hypoechoic pattern at ultrasonography as a tool for predicting recurrence of hyperthyroidism after medical treatment in patients with Graves disease. Acta Endocrinol (Copenh) 126:128, 1992.
21. Bromley B, et al: The fetal thyroid: Normal and abnormal sonographic measurements. J Ultrasound Med 11:25, 1992.
22. Hubsch P, et al: Color-coded Doppler sonography of the thyroid: An advance in carcinoma diagnosis? ROFO 156:125, 1992.

23. Aingmuller V, Otten A, Bodeker RH: Ultrasonographically determined thyroid gland volume in children. Monatsschr Kinderheilkd *139:*826, 1991.
24. Wisner ER, et al: Normal ultrasonographic anatomy of the canine neck. Vet Radiol *32:*185, 1991.
25. Wisner ER, et al: Ultrasonographic evaluation of the parathyroid glands in hypercalcemic dogs. Vet Radiol *34:*108, 1993.
26. Cartee RE, Finn-Bodner ST, Gray BW: Feline thyroid ultrasonography. J Diagn Med Sonogr *9:*323, 1993.
27. Lamb CR: Abdominal ultrasonography in small animals: Examination of the liver, spleen, and pancreas. J Small Anim Pract *31:*6, 1990.
28. Saunders HM, Pugh CR, Rhodes WH: Expanding applications of abdominal ultrasonography. J Am Anim Hosp Assoc *28:*369, 1992.
29. Evans HE, Christensen GC: *Miller's Anatomy of the Dog.* Philadelphia: WB Saunders, 1979, pp. 501–504.
30. Nyland TG, Mulvany MH, Strombeck DR: Ultrasonic features of experimentally induced acute pancreatitis in the dog. Vet Radiol *24:*260, 1983.
31. Murtaugh RJ, et al: Pancreatic ultrasonography in dogs with experimentally induced acute pancreatitis. Vet Radiol *26:*27, 1985.
32. Saunders HM: Ultrasonography of the pancreas. Probl Vet Med *3:*583, 1991.
33. Miles KG, et al: The use of intraperitoneal fluid as a simple technique for enhancing sonographic visualization of the canine pancreas. Vet Radiol *29:*258, 1988.
34. So CB, et al: Sonographic findings in pancreatic lipomatosis. AJR Am J Roentgenol *149:*67, 1987.
35. Mark WM, Filly RA, Callen PW: Ultrasound evaluation of normal pancreatic echogenicity and its relationship to fat deposition. Radiology *137:*475, 1980.
36. Worthen NJ, Beabeau D: Normal pancreatic echogenicity: Relation to age and body fat. AJR Am J Roentgenol *139:*1095, 1982.
37. Patel S, et al: Fat replacement of the exocrine pancreas. AJR Am J Roentgenol *135:*843, 1980.
38. Atri M, Finnegan PW: The pancreas. In *Diagnostic Ultrasound*, Vol. 1. Edited by CM Rumack, SR Wilson, JW Charboneau. St Louis: Mosby Year Book, 1991.
39. Saunders HM: Ultrasonographic detection and characterization of pancreatitis in dogs. Proceedings of the Annual Meeting of the American College of Veterinary Radiology, Chicago, IL, November, 1990, p. 66.
40. Edwards DF, et al: Pancreatic masses in seven dogs following acute pancreatitis. JAAHA *26:*189–198, 1990.
41. Lamb CR: Dilation of the pancreatic duct: An ultrasonographic finding in acute pancreatitis. J Small Anim Pract *30:*410, 1989.
42. Rutgers C, Herring DS, Orton C: Pancreatic pseudocyst associated with acute pancreatitis in a dog: Ultrasonographic diagnosis. JAAHA *21:*411, 1985.
43. Salisbury SK, et al: Pancreatic abscess in dogs: Six cases (1978–1986). J Am Vet Med Assoc *193:*1104, 1988.
44. Wolfsheimer KJ, Hedlund CS, Pechman Jr RD: Pancreatic pseudocyst in a dog with chronic pancreatitis. Canine Pract *16:*6, 1991.
45. Maier W: Echographic patterns of just evolving acute pancreatitis: An experimental study. Eur J Radiol *11:*145, 1990.
46. Salinas A, et al: The pathogenesis of pancreatic pseudocyst - a canine experimental model. Am J Gastroenterol *80:*126, 1985.
47. Kane MG, Krejs GJ: Pancreatic pseudocyst. Adv Intern Med *29:*271, 1984.
48. Jubb KVF, Kennedy PC, Palmer N: The pancreas. In *Pathology of Domestic Animals*, 3rd Ed.,Vol. 2. Orlando, Academic Press, 1985.
49. Saunders HM: The ultrasonographic appearance of canine pancreatic insulinomas: Three case reports. Proceedings of the Annual Meeting of the American College of Veterinary Radiology, Washington, DC, October, 1988, p. 2.
50. Yamakita N, Yasuda K, Miura K: Delineation of adrenals in controls and nontumorous adrenal disorders by real-time ultrasonic-scanner. Ultrasound Med Biol *12:*107, 1986.
51. Zappasodi F, Derchi LE, Rizzatto G: Ultrasonography of the normal adrenal glands: A study using linear-array real time equipment. Br J Radiol *59:*759, 1986.
52. Winkler P, Abel T, Helmke K: Sonographic imaging of normal adrenal glands in children and adolescents: An analysis of forms and reflex properties. Ultraschall Med *8:*271, 1987.
53. Senecail B, Bellet M: Ultrasonic study of the left adrenal gland by anterior transgastric approach. Ann Radiol (Paris) *29:*627, 1986.
54. Krebs CA, et al: Cava-suprarenal line: New position for sonographic imaging of left adrenal gland. JCU *14:*535, 1986.
55. Matter D, et al: Echographic study of the normal adrenal gland during development and in the adult. Morphol Med *3:*19, 1983.
56. Kangarloo H, et al: Sonography of adrenal glands in neonates and children: Changes in appearance with age. JCU *14:*43, 1986.
57. Ginther RW, Kelbel C, Lenner V: Real time ultrasound of normal adrenal glands and small tumors. JCU *12:*211, 1984.
58. Winkler P, Abel T, Helmke K: New signs for the echographic identification of the adrenal glands in children and adolescents. Fortschr Geb Rontgenstr Muselearmed *148:*150, 1988.
59. McGalron JP, Myracle MR: Adrenal hypertrophy: Possible pitfall in the sonographic diagnosis of renal agenesis. J Ultrasound Med *5:*265, 1986.

60. Hata K, Hata T, Kitao M: Ultrasonographic identification and measurement of the human fetal adrenal gland in utero: Clinical application. Gynecol Obstet Invest *25:*16, 1988.
61. Hata T, et al: Ultrasonographic assessment of fetal adrenal gland and placenta: Correlation with estrogen in maternal urine. Gynecol Obstet Invest *24:*80, 1987.
62. Huta K, et al: Ultrasonographic evaluation of adrenal involution during antenatal and neonatal periods. Gynecol Obstet Invest *26:*29, 1988.
63. Dubov I, Glukhorrets B, Kordivkov EV: Method of precise measurement of the volume of small biological objects. Arkhi Patol *47:*85, 1985.
64. Voorhout G: X-ray-computed tomography, nephrotomography and ultrasonography of the adrenal glands of healthy dogs. Am J Vet Res *51:*625, 1990.
65. Kontrowitz BM, Nyland TG, Feldman EC: Adrenal ultrasonography in the dog. Vet Radiol *27:*91, 1986.
66. Cartee RE, Finn-Bodner S, Gray BW: Ultrasonography of the normal feline adrenal gland. J Diagn Med Sonogr, Nov–Dec, 1993.
67. Guhiacy S, Dobbins PA, Boumer H: Ultrasound demonstration of congenital adrenal hyperplasia. JCU *13:*419, 1985.
68. Yammakita N, et al: Image diagnosis of adrenal disorders. I. CT images of control subjects and image diagnosis of primary aldosteronism. Nippon Naibunpi Gakkai Zasshi *61:*97, 1985.
69. Yammakita N, et al: Image diagnosis of adrenal disorders. II Cushings syndrome. Nippon Naibunpi Gakkai Zasshi *61:*112, 1985.
70. Marganti VJ, Anderson NG: Simple adrenal cysts in fetus, resolving spontaneously in neonate. J Ultrasound Med *10:*521, 1991.
71. Wan YL, Lee TY, Tsi CC: Ultrasonography of adrenal lesions. J Formosan Med Assoc *90:*392, 1991.
72. McVican M, Margouleff D, Cliendra M: Diagnosis and imaging of the fetal and neonatal abdominal mass: An integrated approach. Adv Pediatr *38:*135, 1991.
73. Billard L, et al: Adrenal masses discovered accidentally. Diagnostic and therapeutic approaches. Rev Praticien *41:*1006, 1991.
74. Gross MD, et al: Distinguishing benign from malignant adrenal masses. Ann Intern Med *109:*613, 1988.
75. Akhan O, Cekirge HS, Gulekon N: Bilateral triangular adrenal calcifications. AJR Am J Roentgenol *153:*1102, 1989.
76. Chevallier B, et al: An unusual echographic evaluation of an adrenal hematoma in a newborn infant. Ann Pediatr (Paris) *36:*262, 1989.
77. Zimmerman JM, et al: Unilateral hematoma of the adrenal gland. J Urol (Paris) *96:*399, 1990.
78. Liessi G, et al: Traumatic hematomas of the adrenal glands. CT and US findings in 3 cases. Radiol Med (Torino) *76:*610, 1988.
79. Challa S, et al: Haemorrhagic pseudocyst of the adrenal in an adult. Australas Radiol *33:*402, 1989.
80. Bergami G, et al: Echography in the follow-up of neonatal adrenal hemorrhage. Radiol Med (Torino) *79:*474, 1990.
81. Enriquez G, et al: Sonographic diagnosis of adrenal hemorrhage in patients with fulminant meningococcal septicemia. Acta Paediatr Scand *79:*1255, 1990.
82. Li Z: The adrenal gland of the Chinese River Dolphin (Lipotes Vexillifer). Acta Hydrobiol Sin *12:*59, 1988.
83. Cartee RE, et al: A case of cystic adrenal disease in a common dolpin (Delphinus dolphis). J Zoo Wildl Med, Submitted for publication, 1993.
84. Chang DB, et al: Ultrasonic evaluation of cervical lymphadenopathy. J Formosan Med Assoc *89:*286, 1990.
85. Steinkamp HI, et al: Cervical lymph node metastases. The sonographic demonstration of malignancy. ROFO *156:*135, 1992.
86. Borre A, et al: Ultrasonography in diseases of lymph nodes and soft tissues of the neck. Minerva Med *82:*349, 1991.
87. Hessling KH, et al: Use of sonography in the follow-up of preoperative irradiated efferent lymphatics of the neck in oropharyngeal tumors. J Craniomaxillofac Surg *19:*128, 1991.
88. Rubaltelli L, et al: Sonography of abnormal lymph nodes in vitro: Correlation of sonographic and histologic findings. AJR Am J Roentgenol *155:*1241, 1990.
89. Sakai F, et al: Computed tomography of neck lymph nodes involved with malignant lymphomas Comparison with ultrasound. Radiat Med *9:*203, 1991.
90. Lee N, et al: Patterns of internal echoes in lymph nodes in the diagnosis of lung cancer metastasis. World J Surg *16:*986, 1992.
91. Heintz A, et al: Endosonography of esophageal cancer. Results of a clinical study and in vitro analysis. Chirurg *63:*629, 1992.
92. Grimm H, et al: Enlarged lymph nodes: Malignant or not? Endoscopy *24*(Suppl 1):320, 1992.
93. Rafailson SR, Kronborg O, Fenger C: Echo pattern of lymph nodes in colorectal cancer: An in vitro study. Br J Radiol *65:*218, 1992.
94. Akahoshi K, et al: Regional lymph node metastasis in gastric cancer: Evaluation with endoscopic ultrasound. Radiology *182:*559, 1992.
95. Bessmel'tser SS, Abdulkadyrov KM: Ultrasonographic examination of the liver and abdominal lymph nodes in patients with chronic lymphocytic leukemia. Gematol Transfuziol *36:*9, 1991.
96. Lyttkens K, et al: Ultrasound, hepatic lymph nodes and primary biliary cirrhosis. J Hepatol *15:*136, 1992.
97. Hergan K, Amann T, Oser W: Sonographic anatomy of the axilla. Ultraschall Med *12:*236, 1991.

98. Pene CI, De Hooge P, Leguit P: Little extra information with ultrasonic studies of the axillary glands in patients with breast carcinoma. Ned Tijdschr Geneeskd *135:*1275, 1991.

99. Gordon PB, Gilko B: Sonographic appearance of normal intramammary lymph nodes. J Ultrasound Med *7:*545, 1988.

100. Nagano T, et al: Diagnosis of paraaortic and pelvic lymph node metastasis of gynecologic malignant tumors by ultrasound - guided percutaneous fine-needle aspiration biopsy. Cancer *68:*2571, 1991.

101. Tschammler A, et al: The diagnostic assessment of enlarged lymph nodes by the qualitative and semi-quantitative evaluation of lymph node perfusion with color-coded duplex sonography. ROFO *159:*414, 1991.

102. Wisner ER, et al: Normal ultrasonographic anatomy of the canine neck. Vet Radiol *32:*185, 1991.

CHAPTER 7

THE HEART, VESSELS, LUNGS, AND MEDIASTINUM

Robert E. Cartee

THE HEART

Because echocardiology is a subject that deserves a textbook of its own, this discussion is designed to acquaint the reader with the potential for its use in a routine nonspecialized practice. Detailed diagnosis based on M mode interpretations is not within the scope of this text. What is desired is a base that interested practitioners may use to expand their interest.

Echocardiography is the use of ultrasound in the imaging and assessment of the heart and cardiac function. Three modes of display are commonly used. Real-time gray scale B mode, M mode, and Doppler are combined on many instruments to allow a triplex display package. Both spectral analysis and color Doppler are used in these studies. Other systems may include only M mode or only a combination of B mode and M mode.

Although many of these instruments are designed to display complex measurement parameters, they are all basically used to determine the diameters of chambers, thickness and integrity of walls and valves, and contractile properties. Determination of flow patterns by Doppler is not a standard part of veterinary practice but it has application in university clinical settings. Direction and lamination of flow (depth-related velocities) can be determined using this technique. Measurements of velocity and resistance to flow are also possible. The variability of species and sizes of animals produces an additional variation in echocardiographic measurements with which human echocardiographers do not have to deal. For this reason, most reports of heart measurements of animals present ranges of values that are based on multiple observations.

History

As early as 1974, the dog was proposed as a long-term model for studying echocardiography.[1] Measurements of the canine ventricular dimensions using this technique were presented in 1976.[2] The use of ultrasound in the measurement of arterial blood pressure in Thoroughbred horses was also proposed in 1976.[3] Similar ultrasonic transducers were placed in the left ventricular walls of conscious dogs to measure thickness. In that 1976 study, a 31% increase in thickness was observed between end systole and end diastole.[4] That same year, a similar study showed the left ventricle to be a prolate ellipsoid and reported an ejection fraction of 42%.[5] In 1977, Pipers and Hamlin presented the first paper on M mode echocardiography in the horse. They reported the left ventricular wall thickness and diameter of the lumen were 3.2 cm and 9.3 cm (diastole) and 5.7 cm (systole), respectively. The aortic root was 7.7 cm and an ejection fraction of 38.6% was calculated.[6] In 1977, a study involving implantation of ultrasonic crystals in the left ventricular wall and papillary muscles of the dog heart showed that the papillary muscles shorten less during systole than do the circumferential fibers of the left ventricular free wall.[7] Also in 1977, Franklin and colleagues first proposed a closed chest method of B mode evaluation of the canine heart.[8] In an M mode study of the heart of the pig conducted in 1978, Pipers and co-workers compared the internal luminal dimensions of the left ventricle during diastole and systole. They noted a change of 44.8%, as well as a left ventricular wall thickness of 0.61 cm.[9] Also in 1978, the echocardiographic (M mode) appearance of endocarditis in a bull was reported. Superfluous echoes adjacent to the right atrioventricular (AV) valve and flattening of the slope of the valve motion indicated valvular stenosis consistent with vegetative endocarditis. Subsequent necropsy showed this to be the case.[10] Similar valve motions were seen in dogs with stenotic and thickened left AV valves. In this 1978 study, the authors used both transesophageal and transcutaneous placement of the ultrasound probe.[11]

The cat became the focus of a 1979 echocardiographic study. A normal shortening fraction of 41% was presented, as well as internal dimensions of the left ventricle and aorta.[12] That same year marked the echocardiographic detection of cardiovascular lesions in the horse.[13] In 1980, Baylen and co-workers presented evidence that left lateral supine positioning of the dog improved echocardiographic imaging.[14] Lacuata and others again described the echocardiographic appearance of endocarditis in the bovine species. They observed that endocarditis is more common in the right side of the heart in the bovine species and agreed with Pipers' finding of tricuspid valvular superfluous motion patterns and right ventricular enlargement.[15] Pipers and Hamlin described the echocardiographic appearance of clinical heart disease in the cat. They demonstrated the value of M mode echocardiography in the diagnosis of dilatory and hypertrophic cardiomyopathy and pericardial effusion. They also commented on the difficulty in making a diagnosis of a ventricular septal defect using the M mode technique.[16] Finally in 1980, Wingfield and colleagues assessed valve motion in horses with atrial fibrillation.[17]

In 1981, the use of echocardiography to detect abnormalities of the mitral valve of the dog was reported.[18] Bonagura and Pipers also reported the echocardiographic features of pericardial effusion in dogs. They described the echo-free separation of the visceral and parietal pericardium, dampening of the parietal pericardial motion, exaggerated paradoxic motion of intracardiac structures, and thickened epicardium.[19] In 1982, Allen published an account of the echocardiographic study of the anesthetized cat.[20] Also in 1982, Wingfield, Boon, and Miller described the echocardiographic features in dogs with atrial fibrillation: significant decreases in the size of the aorta, interventricular septum, and posterior left ventricular wall; decreased motion amplitude of the posterior left ventricular wall; and decreased fractional shortening.[21] The next year, these authors recorded the echocardiographic indices of the normal dog. In this study, they found a significant correlation between body surface area and some of the echocardiographic dimensions.[22] Also in 1982, Bonagura presented the basic principles of M mode echocardiography and described the diagnosis of cardiac lesions using contrast echocardiography.[23,24]

In 1983, several reports on echocardiography in cats were presented.[25–27] One of these reports dealt with the echocardiographic assessment of cats anesthetized with xylazine sodium pentobarbital.[25] Bond described the appearance of the heart in cats with hyperthyroidism.[26] Soderberg et al. described feline cardiomyopathy and reported abnormal mitral valve motion in cats with hypertrophic cardiomyopathy.[27] Yamaguchi and others reported that the echocardiographic appearance of bacterial vegetative endocarditis in cats was identical to that in other species.[28] Also in 1983, Lombard reported that bacterial vegetative endocarditis in dogs was similar in echocardiographic appearance to that in previous studies, but also discovered that the incidence was higher in (1) males, (2) dogs between 5 and 8 years of age, (3) German Shepherds, and (4) the aortic valve than in the mitral valve.[29] Bonagura described the appearance of aortic endocarditis in the dog, cow, and horse, and found no differences between the species.[30] Pipers described spurious echoes within the right ventricle of dogs infected with heartworms.[31]

In 1984, Lombard and Ackerman described sonographically determined right heart enlargement in heartworm-infected dogs.[32] Lombard also described the normal M mode values for the dog.[33] In that same year, Thomas described the two-dimensional real-time determined values and standardized scanning techniques in the dog.[34] He also reported on the detection of cardiac masses using two-dimensional echocardiography.[35] In studies of horses, the echocardiographically determined dimensions of the heart of foals were found to be directly related to age and body weight.[36,37] Rantanan later described the use of spontaneous contrast echocardiography to diagnose mass lesions in the hearts of race horses.[38]

In 1985, two-dimensional echocardiography of the normal cat was compared to M mode techniques and found to be similar and equally as quantifiable.[39] Also in this year, the diagnostic value of contrast echocardiography in the horse was reported.[40] Echocardiographic measurements of the equine heart were compared to the autopsy measurements and found to be reasonably accurate.[41] In 1986, O'Grady and others reported that, using two-dimensional echocardiography in the dog, left- and right-sided positioning of the probe are equally effective.[42] In a study in 1987, Carlsten found that the use of a sedative before scanning the heart of the horse did not affect image quality.[43] In 1989, Hay et al. reported the echocardiographic findings of a peritoneopericardial diaphragmatic hernia in dogs and cats.[44] Also in 1989, a report of the echocardiographic measurement of the swine heart showed positive correlations between body weight and age and cardiac dimensions.[45] In several vascular studies, investigators presented information on the sonographic determination of portal vein flow in dogs and in cranial mesenteric artery evaluation in horses.[46–49]

In two studies in 1990, Voros and others reconfirmed that two-dimensional echocardiographic measurements of the equine heart correlated well with actual physical measurements taken at autopsy, and that the left ventricular volume could be accurately calculated using sonographic measurements and the formula for determining the volume of a truncated cone.[50,51] In 1990, a study of two-dimensional sonographic measurements of the carotid artery in the goat showed an increase in diameter after the use of xylazine sedation.[52] In 1991, two studies of two-dimensional and M mode echocardiography in calves confirmed its applicability in analyzing dimensions and that age and body weight affected these dimensions significantly.[53,54]

In studies of horses conducted in 1991, Long and others presented standardized techniques for use in adult horses and showed no correlation of measurements with body weight, no difference in measurements taken in left or right positioning, and no significant daily variation in measurements.[55] In another study in 1991, Voros reported a correlation between body weight and some echocardiographically determined dimensions.[56] In a review of equine echocardiography, Reef confirmed the use of this technology in the diagnosis of heart disease in the horse, and reported on the use of contrast echocardiography in the diagnosis of some diseases.[57] In 1992, Mahoney and colleagues reported that spontaneous echocardiographic contrast was common in the Thoroughbred but that the incidence was high in bleeders.[58] A 1992 study by Stadler reaffirmed the use of echocardiography in the diagnosis of heart disease in horses, and a 1993 study showed an echocardiographically determined increase in heart muscle mass in horses relative to the level of their physical training regimen.[59,60]

Positioning and Preparation of the Animals

In both human and veterinary echocardiography, the planes of section of the heart are similar. In animals, long axis (LAX = sagittal or frontal plane) and short axis (SAX = transverse plane) are the two most reliable examinations (Figs. 7–1 and 7–2). The apical

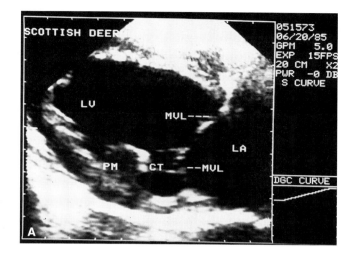

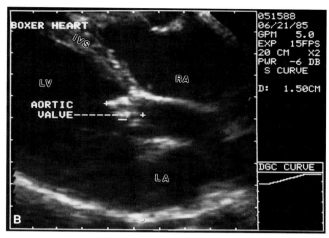

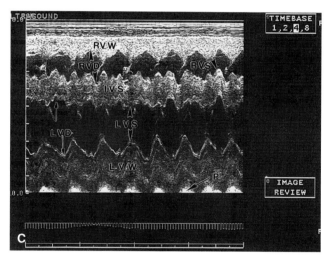

Figure 7–1

A, Long axis, parasternal B mode image of the left side of the canine heart. MVL, mitral valve; CT, chordae tendinae; PM, papillary muscle; LA, left atrium; LV, left ventricle. **B,** At the level of the aortic valve (thickened). RA, right atrium; LA, left atrium; LV, left ventricle; IVS, interventricular septum. **C,** M mode tracing. RVW, right ventricular wall; LVW, left ventricular wall; IVS, interventricular septum; LVS, lumen of the left ventricle during systole; LVD, lumen of the left ventricle during diastole; RVD, lumen of the right ventricle during diastole; RVS, lumen of the right ventricle during systole; P, pericardium.

view is sometimes possible but it is not consistently useful. Parasternal and subcostal positions are commonly used in veterinary medicine. In the attempt to make this chapter useful and practical, the actual value ranges for both normal and abnormal conditions are presented in Table 7–1.

Cardiac sonography can be performed while the animal is standing, with the ipsilateral forelimb advanced and the head turned contralaterally from the side being scanned. Turning the head stretches the trachea and esophagus and pulls the heart closer to the opposite thoracic wall. The cardiac notch between the lungs on the right side makes this side more useful, but the left side is also used. In dogs and cats, the animal is usually positioned in lateral recumbency over an opening in the table. The probe is then placed on the thoracic wall on the down side (usually the right side). Sometimes, anesthesia or sedation is needed. Good restraint is always necessary. Clipping of the hair in the area over the heart (ribs 3 to 7) is helpful before saturating the area with a contact gel. The use of alcohol saturation before the gel as a substitute for clipping the hair has been suggested. Simultaneous electrocardiographic (ECG) recording is recommended.

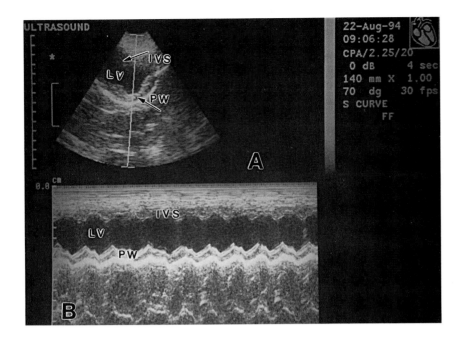

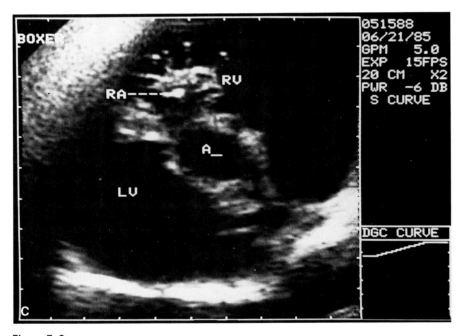

Figure 7-2

A, Short axis, parasternal B mode image of canine ventricles through the heart at the papillary muscle area. Note the position of the M mode cursor line. **B,** M mode trace of **A.** IVS, interventricular septum; PW, posterior wall; LV, left ventricle; **C,** Short axis B mode scan at the level of the aorta. RA, right atrium; RV, right ventricle; A, aorta; LV, left ventricle.

Probe Types and Placement

Sector (mechanical or electronic) annular or curvilinear transducer probe configurations are commonly used in cardiac studies. Straight linear probes are difficult to use because their size prevents good positioning between intercostal spaces. The 4th or 5th intercostal space is located and the heart is visualized from both sides. Usually a 5-mHz transducer is satisfactory for most dogs, a 7-mHz probe for cats, and a 3- to 2.25-mHz probe for horses, ruminants, and very large dogs.

Parasternal positioning of the probe on the right side of the thorax with a long axis view (apex to the left and atria and great vessels to the right) best shows the left ventricular inflow and mitral valve, but not all of the aortic valve cusps are visible and it is not possible to see the left atrium and the aorta in the same image. The left parasternal long axis view best shows the left ventricular outflow tract, three aortic valve cusps, the right ventricular inflow and outflow tracts, and the pulmonary valve and artery. Right and left parasternal short axis views are comparable to the respective long axis views of the same structures. Apical views are not really productive in most animals and are best obtained

TABLE 7–1
Normal Heart Measurements Based on Sonographic Evaluations

	mm Dog	mm Cat	mm Horse	mm Pig	mm Calf	Increase	Decrease
LVDd*	23–46 (42)†	11–21 (14)	105–134 (55)	38.5 (45)	51.3 (53)	Dilatation	Hypertrophy
LVDs	17–37 (42)	6–16 (12)	61–87 (55)	24.5 (45)	29.1 (53)	Dilatation	Hypertrophy
LVPWd	4–11 (42)	30 (61)	32 (6)	8–11 (45)	11.9 (53)	Hypertrophy	Dilatation
LVPWs	6–14 (42)	60 (61)	33–56 (55)	NA	20.5 (53)	Hypertrophy	Dilatation
LVPWTF%	15–73 (42)	15–72 (61)	NA	NA	76.1 (53)	Wall stress	
LVEF%	50–71 (42)	58 (61)	41–35 (55)	38 (45)	43 (53)	Mitral regurgitation	Dilatation
FS%	21–34 (42)	23–56 (12)	29–47 (55)	36.5 (45)	43.1 (53)		
LVET (SFC)	.12–.15 (14)	.11–.19 (12)	3.4 (36)	NA	NA		Systemic hypertension Aortic stenosis
LVWE	5–17 (42)	NA	NA	NA	NA		
LVSV	7–52 (42)	NA	NA	NA	NA		
IVSd	5–10 (42)	31 (61)	27–37 (55)	9–12 (45)	12.4		
IVSs	6–14 (12)	58 (61)	33–56 (55)	NA	19.9 (53)		
IVSTF%	22–92 (42)	15–72 (61)	49	NA	60.4 (53)		
AO (sinus)	10–24 (42)	7–11 (61)	77–95 (55)	21.5 (45)	31.5 (53)	Aneurysm, insufficiency	
LAd (ml)	18–50 (42)	7–13 (61)	11–81 (56)	17.5 (45)	25.9 (53)	Mitral regurgitation/VSD	
RA	NA	NA	NA	NA	NA		
RVd	5–17 (33)	12–75 (61)	22–54 (55)	NA	NA		
RVs	12–75 (61)	10–49 (55)	NA	NA	NA		

* See text for abbreviations; NA, not available.
† Numbers in parenthesis are references cited in the text.

from a subcostal position in smaller animals (e.g., cats and small dogs). When apical views can be obtained, they clearly show all four chambers and make Doppler evaluation more credible.

Included in this chapter are positions and axes and the cardiac structures that are best seen given these positions. Only data relating to the cat, dog, and horse are given because data for other species is not yet available (Tables 7–2 and 7–3). Table 7–3 summarizes the normal ranges of measurement of the cardiac structures in the major animal species and also indicates the implications of an increase or decrease in the normal measurement.

The ability to display both B mode and M mode simultaneously increases the accuracy of measurements by optimizing the positioning of the cursor for measurements. Most measurements of ventricular dimensions and thickness are determined using M mode tracings with simultaneous ECG coordination. Although analysis of valvular motions from M mode tracings is possible and preferred, they are not used routinely in clinical veterinary medicine. Rather, subjective evaluation based on B mode images is often used in clinical practice. For research purposes, most ultrasound equipment now has the capability to perform multiple calculations based on the measurements possible from both M mode and B mode images (Fig. 7–3). The addition of Doppler analysis to the other two functions has increased the ability to assess both cardiac function and peripheral vasculature flow features (e.g., resistance to flow, pulsatility). Spectral analysis of flow and color analysis of flow have become separate fields of study and evaluation of the heart, although neither has become sufficiently standardized for veterinary medicine to allow routine use.

TABLE 7–2
Canine/Feline[61]—Normal Structures Visible Using Various Modes and Positions for Sonography of the Heart

Position	Mode	Structure Visible
RLAX*	M/B	LV; MV; LVOT; AV; Ao; LA; IVS
RSAX	M/B	LV; Chordae tendinae
LAX	M/B	LV; MV; LA; RV; RA
LLAX	M/B	LVOT; AV; Ao; RVIT; TV; RVOT; PV; PA
LASX	M/B	RVIT; Ao; Av

* See text for abbreviations.

TABLE 7–3
Equine[43]—Normal Structures Visible Using Various Modes and Positions for Sonography of the Heart

Position	Mode	Structure Visible
SAX (4–5 ICS)*	B	RV; TV; IVS; LV; MV; LA; A; AV
RCdLAX (4–5 ICS)	B	RV; RA; TV; IVS; LV; MV; LA
RCrSAX (2–3 ICS)	B	RV; TV; PV; IVS; LA; A; AV; LV; MV
RCrLAX (2–3 ICS)	B	RV; RA; TV; IVS; LV; MV; LA; A; AV
LCdSAX (4–5 ICS)	B	RV; IVS; LV; MV
LCdLAX (4–5 ICS)	B	LV; MV; LA; A; AV
LCdSAX (2–3 ICS)	B	RV; TV; IVS
LCrLAX (2–3 ICS)	B	LV; MV; LA; A; AV

* See text for abbreviations.

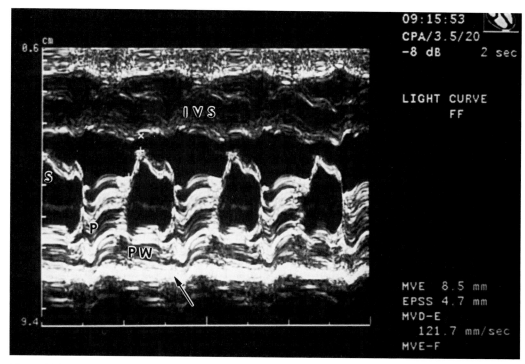

Figure 7–3

A, M mode pattern through the canine heart below the level of the mitral valve on a short axis. IVS, interventricular septum; S, septal leaflet; P, posterior leaflet; PW, posterior wall.

DEFINITION OF TERMS

Cardiac Parameters

Left ventricle diameter diastolic (LVDd): Diameter of the lumen of the left ventricle during diastole. Usually made from M mode image (MM).

Left ventricle diameter systolic (LVDS): Diameter of the lumen of the left ventricle during systole. M mode usually (MM).

Left ventricle ejection time (LVET): Time from opening of the aortic valve until its closing. M mode.

Shortening fraction (%) (SF): The percentage of change in the diameter of the left ventricle from diastole to systole. Calculated.

Aortic root dimension (Ao): Diameter of the aortic root. M mode or B mode. End of diastole.

Interventricular septal wall thickness diastole (IVSd): Thickness of IVS end diastole. M mode or B mode.

Interventricular septal wall thickness systole (IVSs): Thickness of IVS end systole. M mode or B mode.

Left ventricular posterior wall thickness diastole (PWd): Self explanatory. M mode or B mode.

Left ventricular posterior wall thickness systole (PWs): Self explanatory. M mode or B mode.

Left atrial diameter (diastole LAd, systole LAs): Self explanatory. M mode or B mode.

Heart rate (HR): Self explanatory.

Cardiac output (CO): Amount of blood ejected from left ventricle at end of systole or for 1 minute.

Left atrium diameter aortic ratio (LAD/AO): Divide LA diameter by aortic diameter. M mode or B mode.

Ejection fraction (EF): The fractional volume of blood pumped out of the left ventricle during systole.

Left ventricle stroke volume (LVSV): Volume of blood pumped from the left ventricle during systole.

Left ventricle posterior wall thickening fraction (LVPWTF) (%): Percent change of wall thickness from diastole to systole. Calculated from M mode.

$$\frac{LVPWs - LVPWd}{LVPWS} \times 100$$

Left ventricle wall excursion (LVWE): Initial excursion to peak excursion. M mode.

Interventricular septal thickness fraction (IVSTF) (%): Percent change of thickness from diastole to systole.

Right ventricle diameter diastole (RVDd): see above.

Right ventricle diameter systole (RVDs): see above.

Right ventricle free wall diastole (RVFWd): see above.

Right ventricle free wall systole (RVFWs): see above.

Right ventricle free wall thickening fraction (RVFWTF): see above.

Pericardial effusion (PE): Distance between pericardium and heart.

Heart Disease[62,63]

Atrial Septal Defect (Ostium Secundum)
1. Dilatation of hyperdynamic right ventricle, right atrium, and pulmonary artery
2. Paradoxic motion of IVS
3. Visual defect
4. One third of cases have mitral valve prolapse

Atrial Septal Defect (Ostium Primum)
1. Dilatation of left ventricle
2. Defects of left and right AV valves
3. Defects of both IVS, IAS
4. Pulmonary artery hypertension

Patent Ductus Arteriosus
1. Dilatation of left atrium and ventricle
2. Hyperdynamic left ventricle or IVS
3. Possible visualization of ductus
4. Reduced fractional shortening

Coarctation of Aorta
1. Left ventricular hypertrophy

Pulmonary Valve Stenosis
1. "a" dip on M mode
2. Thickened more prominent valve on B mode
3. Dilatation of right ventricle and atrium
4. Right ventricular hypertrophy, IVS, hypertrophy

Tetralogy of Fallot
1. Visualize VSD (B mode)
2. Overriding aorta visualization (B mode)
3. Right ventricular enlargement
4. Right ventricular outflow obstruction
5. Septal hypertrophy with paradoxic motion

Pulmonary Hypertension
1. Right ventricular hypertrophy (M mode, B mode)

Aortic Stenosis
1. Thickened/calcified aortic valve leaflets (B mode)
2. Left ventricular hypertrophy (B mode, M mode)
3. LA/AV ratio increased

Aortic Regurgitation
1. Aortic value vegetation or dysfunction
2. Diastolic fluttering of mitral valve
3. Premature mitral closure
4. Left ventricular dilatation

Mitral Stenosis
1. Valve thickened (EF slope decreased on M mode)
2. Posterior leaflet drawn ventrally during diastole (B mode, M mode)
3. Mitral calcification possible (B mode)
4. Left atrial enlargement (B mode, M mode)
5. Pulmonary trunk enlargement (B mode, M mode)

Mitral Regurgitation (Fig. 7–4)
1. Hyperactive IVS
2. Left atrial dilatation
3. Prolapsed valve (B mode)

Tricuspid Stenosis
1. Dilated right atrium
2. Hypertrophy of right ventricle

Tricuspid Regurgitation
1. Dilated right atrium and ventricle
2. Abnormal Doppler flow or valve motion

Pulmonary Regurgitation
1. Dilatation of right ventricle

Endocarditis
1. Vegetation B mode (90% sensitive)

Myocarditis
1. May be normal
2. May see atrial and ventricular dilatation (B mode, M mode)
3. Ventricular hypokinesis (B mode, M mode)
4. Mitral and/or tricuspid regurgitation (B mode, M mode)
5. Pericardial effusion (B mode, M mode)

Dilatory Cardiomyopathy
1. Dilatation of ventricles and atria (B mode, M mode)
2. Ventricular systolic and diastolic dysfunction (B mode, M mode)
3. Hypokinesis especially in left ventricle (B mode, M mode)

Hypertrophic Cardiomyopathy
1. Disproportionate thickening of IVS and/or left ventricular free wall
2. End systolic diameter of lumen of left ventricle is decreased
3. Left atrium enlarged

Restrictive Cardiomyopathy
1. Hyperechoic endocardium
2. Some pericardial effusion
3. Ventricular wall thrombus (echogenic focus)
4. Myocardial "sparkle" with amyloidosis

Pericardial Effusion
1. Echo-free space around left and/or right ventricle

Cardiac Tamponade
1. Diastolic collapse of right atrium and right ventricle
2. Swinging of heart in pericardial sac

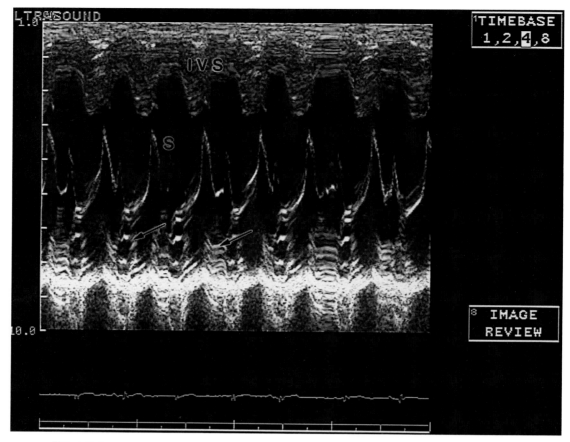

Figure 7–4

M mode tracing of the canine heart with severe mitral regurgitation. Note the large deviation of motion of the interventricular septum (IVS). Fluttering of the posterior leaflet is also seen (arrow). The septal leaflet (S) shows a normal pattern.

Constrictive Pericarditis
1. Thickened pericardium
2. Abnormal motion of IVS
3. Short steep E to F slope of anterior leaflet of mitral valve

ARTERIES AND VEINS

Free flowing blood is anechoic in all vessels. Arterial pulse may be used to distinguish arteries and veins. In some cases, the proximity of the artery to the vein may cause the appearance of a pulse in the vein. Color and pulsed Doppler examination may quickly distinguish the two vessels. In the event that these capabilities are not available, it is possible to rotate the probe so that a cross-sectional image is presented. Physical compression of the area may also be informative in that the vein is more compressible.

Thrombi within vessels usually appear echogenic in part because of enhancement from the anechoic adjacent free-flowing blood. A thrombus may also be seen to oscillate in the stream of flow. In horses that have a higher incidence of rouleaux formation, slow blood flow in large veins or obstructed flow may cause the clumping and "chaining" of red blood cells, which appear in the stream of flow as echogenic foci. Thrombi in major arteries are also echogenic and may appear pulsatile as the proximal arterial pulse of blood strikes the thrombus (Fig. 7–5). Collateral dilatation of blood vessels may also be evident.

Aneurysms are rare in most animals, with the exception of the horse. Aneurysms appear as hypoechoic dilatations of the cranial mesenteric artery in the horse. Normal standards of diameter, flow, and pulsatility and resistivity to flow have not been established in animals.

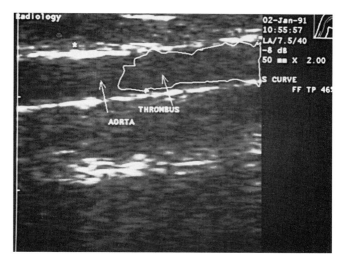

Figure 7–5

B mode image of a thrombus in the aorta of a dog.

THE AORTA

The ascending aorta and the aortic arch are routinely examined using echocardiography. Standard sizes and ratios to left atrial size have been established in some species (see Table 7–1). The thoracic aorta is not usually visualized sonographically. The abdominal aorta is examined by positioning the probe parallel to the sublumbar muscles and slightly ventral to them on the left side (Fig. 7–6). Rotating the probe dorsally and ventrally as it is moved caudally allows examination of the celiac, cranial mesenteric, renal, phrenicoabdominal, and iliac arteries (Fig. 7–7). The caudal vena cava lies parallel to and to the right of the aorta (Fig. 7–8). The renal vein extends into the kidney from the caudal vena cava. The caudal vena cava may be followed cranially on the right side, extending into the liver. The portal vein is visualized by rotating the probe medially from the caudal vena cava (Figs. 7–8 and 7–9). The portal vein characteristically has walls that are more hyperechoic than those of the caudal vena cava.

The carotid arteries in all species except the pig are accessible parallel to the trachea. The external jugular vein can be scanned parallel and superficial to the carotid artery. In horses, the median artery and veins and their distal branches may be followed down the forelimb. The femoral artery and vein are visible in the dog and horse and may be followed to the popliteal vessels. In the horse, the plantar branches of the cranial tibial may also be seen on the medial and lateral sides of the metacarpal region. Work is continuing in the evaluation of blood vessels of animals using sonography.

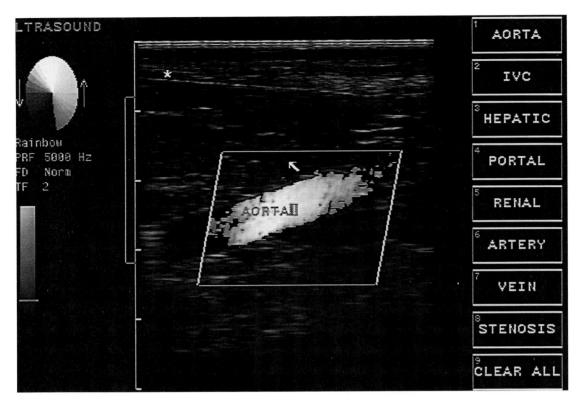

Figure 7–6

Duplex Doppler/B mode image of the canine aorta scanned parallel to the sublumbar muscles (arrow) on the left side.

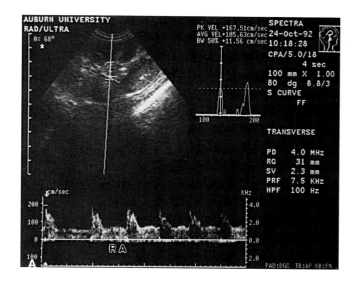

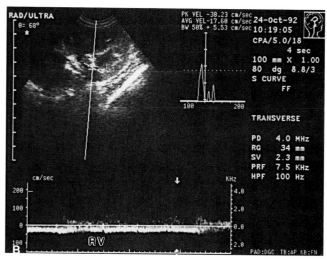

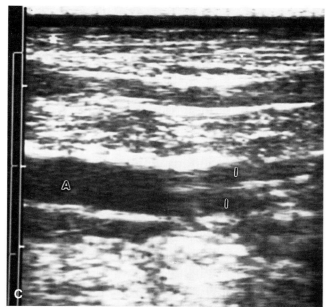

Figure 7–7

B mode images of canine abdominal vessels. Renal artery **(A)** and vein **(B).** RA, right atrium; RV, right ventricle. Pulsed Doppler flow shown above label. **C**, Iliac bifurcation of the aorta. A, aorta; I, iliac.

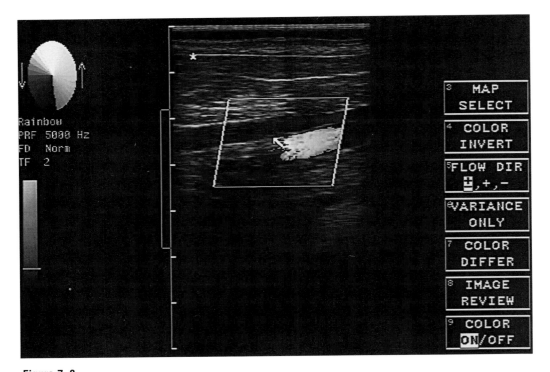

Figure 7–8

Duplex Doppler/B mode image (right longitudinal plane) of the caudal vena cava (blue, arrow); red, aorta.

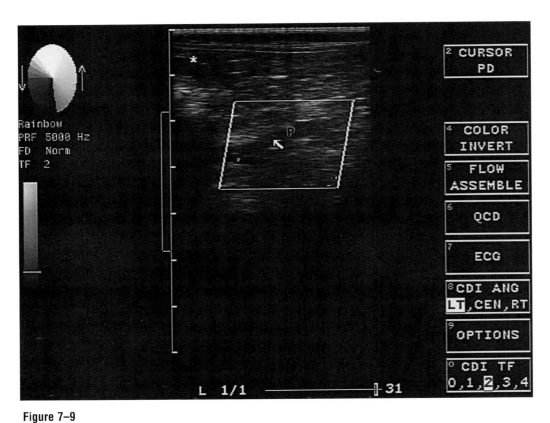

Figure 7–9

B mode image of the extrahepatic portal vein (P, arrow).

THE LUNGS AND MEDIASTINUM

Sonographic examination of the lungs is not performed routinely. The lung area may be scanned over the chest wall through the intercostal spaces. Although the reverberation pattern created by the normal lung surface prevents examination of deeper structures, this pattern may indicate that the lung surface is normal (Fig. 7–10).[64] Consolidated lung tissue appears hypoechoic with variable amounts of internal echogenic structures such as bronchi or air pockets (Fig. 7–11). Consolidated lung has also been reported to be vascular compared to lung tumors.[65] Tumors of the lungs have been described as having variable echogenicity, irregular borders, vascularity, and dystrophic calcification (Fig. 7–12).[65]

Pleural effusion creates an anechoic area between the thoracic wall and both lung and mediastinal structures (Fig. 7–13). An ultrasound examination may show the best site for thoracentesis of fluid as well as thickening of the pleura.[65–67] Gas echoes within pleural fluid are highly suggestive of anaerobic bacterial infection from pleuropneumonia and pulmonary abscessation.[68,69] The presence of a gas-filled structure within the pleural cavity has been reported to signify the possibility of a diaphragmatic hernia.[70] The hyperechoic diaphragmatic interface should be carefully examined for interruptions.[71] One report concerning mediastinal masses of dogs and cats indicated that neoplasms of the mediastinal structures varied in echogenicity. Lymphosarcomas were mostly hypochoic but some were hyperechoic. Thymomas were routinely echogenic.[72] Biopsy of mediastinal masses is possible using ultrasound guidance.[65] The presence of pleural effusion is helpful in locating the mass for biopsy. In man, transesophageal probe placement has enhanced the visualization of the lungs and mediastinal structures as well as of the heart.

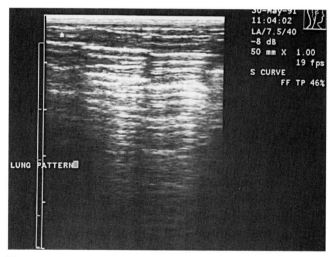

Figure 7–10

Sonographic image of normal lung surface reverberation pattern (5-mHz CL probe).

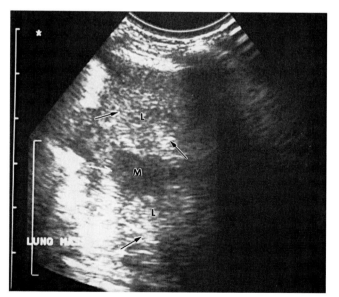

Figure 7–11

Sonographic image of consolidated lung lobe (L) and mass (M, white arrows) with echogenic air pockets (black arrows).

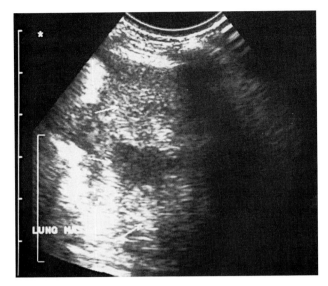

Figure 7–12

Lung tumor (arrows) with an inhomogeneous echogenic pattern and irregular border.

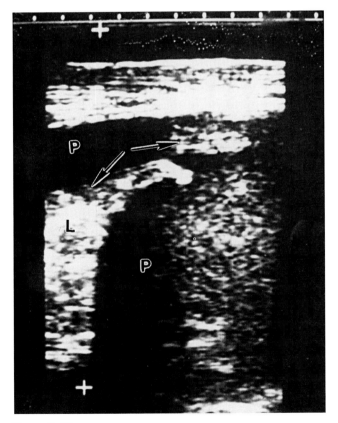

Figure 7–13

Pleural effusion (P). Note the surface of the lung (L) and mediastinal structures (arrow).

REFERENCES

1. Meyerowitz DP, et al: Long term canine model for echocardiography. Am J Cardiol 34:72, 1974.
2. Mashiro I, et al: Ventricular dimensions measured non-invisibly by echocardiography in the awake dog. J Appl Physiol 41:953, 1976.
3. Johnson JH, Garner HE, Hutcheson DP: Ultrasonic measurement of arterial blood pressure in conditioned Thoroughbreds. Equine Vet J 8:55, 1976.
4. Shigetake S, et al: Dynamic changes in left ventricular wall thickness and their use in analyzing cardiac function in the conscious dog. Am J Cardiol 38:870, 1976.
5. Rankin JS, et al: The three-dimensional dynamic geometry of the left ventricle in the conscious dog. Circ Res 39:304, 1977.
6. Pipers FS, Hamlin RL: Echocardiography in the horse. J Am Vet Med Assoc 170:815, 1977.
7. Hirakawa S, et al: In situ measurement of papillary muscle dynamics in the dog left ventricle. Am J Physiol 233:389, 1977.
8. Franklin TD, Weyman AE, Egenes KM: A closed chest canine model for cross sectional echocardiographic study. Am J Physiol 23:417, 1977.
9. Pipers FS, Muir WW, Hamlin RL: Echocardiography in swine. J Am Vet Med Assoc 39:707, 1978.
10. Pipers FS, et al: Echocardiographic diagnosis of endocarditis in a bull. J Am Vet Med Assoc 172:1313, 1978.
11. Dennis MO, et al: Echocardiographic assessment of normal and abnormal valvular function in beagle dogs. Am J Vet Res 39:1591, 1978.
12. Pipers FS, Reef V, Hamlin RL: Echocardiography in the domestic cat. J Am Vet Med Assoc 40:882, 1979.
13. Pipers FS, Hamlin RL, Reef V: Echocardiographic detection of cardiovascular lesions in the horse. J Eq Med Surg 3:68, 1979.
14. Baylen BG, et al: Improved echocardiographic evaluation of the closed chest canine. Methods and anatomic observations. JCU 8:335, 1980.
15. Lacuata AQ, et al: Electrocardiographic and echocardiographic findings in four cases of bovine endocarditis. J Am Vet Med Assoc 176:1355, 1980.
16. Pipers FS, Hamlin RL: Clinical use of echocardiography in the domestic cat. J Am Vet Med Assoc 176:57, 1980.
17. Wingfield WE, et al: Echocardiography in assessing mitral valve motion in 3 horses with atrial fibrillation. Equine Vet J 12:181, 1980.
18. Pipers FS, et al: Echocardiographic abnormalities of the mitral valve associated with left sided heart disease in the dog. J Am Vet Med Assoc 179:580, 1981.
19. Bonagura JD, Pipers FS: Echocardiographic features of pericardial effusion in dogs. J Am Vet Med Assoc 179:49, 1981.
20. Allen DG: Echocardiographic study of the anesthetized cat. Can J Comp Med 46:115, 1982.
21. Wingfield WE, Boon J, Miller CW: Echocardiographic assessment of mitral valve function, cardiac structures and ventricular function in dogs with atrial fibrillation. J Am Vet Med Assoc 181:7, 1982.
22. Boon J, Wingfield WE, Miller CW: Echocardiographic indices in the normal dog. Vet Radiol 24:214, 1983.
23. Bonagura JD: M-mode echocardiography: Basic principles. Vet Clin North Am Small Anim Pract 13:299, 1983.
24. Bonagura JD, Pipers FJ: Diagnosis of cardiac lesions by contrast echocardiography. J Am Vet Med Assoc 182:396, 1983.
25. Allen DG, Downey RS: Echocardiographic assessment of cats anesthetized with xylozine-sodium pentobarbital. Can J Comp Med 47:281, 1983.
26. Bond BR, Fox PR, Peterson ME: Echocardiographic evaluation of 45 cats with hyperthyroidism. J Am Institute Ultrasound Med Proc 2:184, 1983.
27. Soderberg SF, et al: M-mode echocardiography as a diagnostic aid for feline cardiomyopathy. Vet Radiol 24:66, 1983.
28. Yamagrechi RA, Pipers FS, Gamble DA: Echocardiographic evaluation of a cat with bacterial vegetative endocarditis. J Am Vet Med Assoc 183:118, 1983.
29. Lombard CW, Bvergelt CD: Vegetative bacterial endocarditis in dogs; echocardiographic diagnosis and clinical signs. J Small Anim Pract 24:325, 1983.
30. Bonagura JD, Pipers FS: Echocardiographic features of aortic valve endocarditis in a dog, a cow and a horse. J Am Vet Med Assoc 182:595, 1983.
31. Pipers FS: Detection of Dirofilaria immitis in the canine right ventricle by echocardiography. Heartworm Symposium, 1983, personal communication.
32. Lombard CW, Ackerman N: Right heart enlargement in heartworm-infected dogs. Vet Radiol 25:210, 1984.
33. Lombard CW: Normal valves of the canine M-mode echocardiogram. Am J Vet Res 45:2015, 1984.
34. Thomas WP: Two dimensional real-time echocardiography in the dog. Vet Radiol 25:50, 1984.
35. Thomas WP, et al: Detection of cardiac masses in dogs by two-dimensional echocardiography. Vet Radiol 25:65, 1984.

36. Stewart JH, Rose RJ, Barks AM: Echocardiography in foals from birth to three months old. Equine Vet J *16:*332, 1984.
37. Lombard CW, et al: Blood pressure, electrocardiogram and echocardiogram measurements in the growing pony foal. Equine Vet J *16:*342, 1984.
38. Rantanen NW, et al: Spontaneous contrast and mass lesions in the hearts of race horses: Ultrasound diagnosis—preliminary data. Equine Vet Sci *4:*220, 1984.
39. Demadron E, Bonagura JD, Hening DS: Two dimensional echocardiography in the normal cat. Vet Radiol *26:*149, 1985.
40. Kvart C, et al: Diagnostic value of contrast echocardiography in the horse. Equine Vet J *17:*357, 1985.
41. O'Callaghan MW: Comparison of echocardiographic and autopsy measurements of cardiac dimensions in the horse. Equine Vet J *17:*361, 1985.
42. O'Grady MR, et al: Quantitative cross-sectional echocardiography in the normal dog. Vet Radiol *27(2):*76, 1987.
43. Carlsten JC: Two dimensional real-time echocardiography in the horse. Vet Radiol *28:*76, 1987.
44. Hay WH, Woodfield JA, Moon MA: Clinical, echocardiographic, and radiographic findings of peritoneopericardial diaphragmatic hernia in two dogs and a cat. J Am Vet Med Assoc *195:*1245, 1989.
45. Gwathmey JK, et al: Echocardiographic assessment of cardiac chamber size and functional performance in swine. Am J Vet Res *50:*192, 1989.
46. Kantrowitz BM, Nyland TG, Fisher P: Estimation of portal blood flow using duplex real-time and pulsed doppler ultrasound imaging in the dog. Vet Radiol *30:*222, 1989.
47. Wallace KD, et al: Transrectal ultrasonography of the cranial mesenteric artery of the horse. Am J Vet Res *50:*1699, 1989.
48. Wallace KD, et al: In vitro ultrasonographic appearance of the normal and verminous equine aorta, cranial mesenteric artery and its branches. Am J Vet Res *50:*1774, 1989.
49. Wallace KD, Selcer BA, Becket JL: Technique for transrectal ultrasonography of the cranial mesenteric artery of the horse. Am J Vet Res *50:*1695, 1989.
50. Voros K, Holmes JR, Gibbs C: Anatomical validation of two-dimensional echocardiography in the horse. Equine Vet J *22:*392, 1990.
51. Voros K, Holmes JR, Gibbs C: Left ventricular volume determination in the horse by two-dimensional echocardiography. Equine Vet J *22:*398, 1990.
52. Lee SW, et al: Comparative study of ultrasonography and arteriography of the carotid artery of xylazine-sedated and halothane-anesthetized goats. Am J Vet Res *51:*109, 1990.
53. Amary H, Jakovljevic S, Lekeux P: Quantitative M-mode and two dimensional echocardiography in calves. Vet Rec *128:*25, 1991.
54. Amary H, Lekeux P: Effects of growth on functional and morphological echocardiographic variables in friesian calves. Vet Rec *128:*349, 1991.
55. Long KJ, Bonagura JD, Darke PGG: Standardized imaging technique for guided M-mode and doppler echocardiography in the horse. Equine Vet J *24:*226, 1992.
56. Voros K, Holmes JR, Gibbs C: Measurement of cardiac dimensions with two dimensional echocardiography in the living horse. Equine Vet J *23:*461, 1991.
57. Reef VB: Advances in echocardiography. Vet Clinics North Am *7:*435, 1991.
58. Mahoney C, et al: Spontaneous echocardiographic contrast in the Thoroughbred. Equine Vet J *24:*129, 1992.
59. Stadler P, et al: B mode, M mode and Doppler sonographic findings in mitral valve insufficiency of horses. Zentralbl Veterinarmed [A] *39:*704, 1992.
60. Stadler P, Newel A, Deagen E: M mode echocardiography in dressage horses, class S jumping horses and intrained horses. Zentralbl Veterinarmed *40:*292, 1993.
61. Lusk RH, Ettinger SJ: Echocardiographic techniques in the dog and cat. In *Handbook of the Heart.* Edited by RC Schlant, JW Hurst. New York: McGraw-Hill Book, 1988.
62. Schlant RC, Hurst JW: *Handbook of the Heart.* New York: McGraw-Hill Book, 1988.
63. Moise NS: *Echocardiography in Canine and Feline Cardiology.* Edited by PR Fox, New York: Churchill Livingstone, 1988.
64. Rantanen NW: Ultrasound appearance of normal long borders and adjacent viscera in the horse. Vet Radiol *22:*217, 1981.
65. Stowater JL, Lamb CR: Ultrasonography of non-cardiac thoracic diseases in small animals. J Am Vet Med Assoc *195:*514, 1989.
66. Stadtbarmer G: Sonography in pleural effusion of horses. Tierarztl Prax *17:*395, 1989.
67. Rantanen NW, Gage L, Paradis MR: Ultrasonography as a diagnostic aid in pleural effusion of horses. Vet Radiol *22:*211, 1981.
68. Reimer JM, Reef VB, Spencer PA: Ultrasonography as a diagnostic aid in horses with anaerobic bacterial pleuropneumonia and/or pulmonary abscessation: 27 cases. J Am Vet Med Assoc *194:*278, 1989.
69. Osler GE, du Preez PM: Application of ultrasound in the diagnosis and treatment of empyema and mediastinal abscess in a dog. S Afr Med J *76:*174, 1989.

70. Hartzband LE, Karr DV, Morris EA: Ultrasonographic diagnosis of diaphragmatic rupture in a horse. Vet Radiol *3:*42, 1990.

71. Lamb CR, Mason GD, Wallace MK: Ultrasonographic diagnosis of peritoneopericardial diaphragmatic hernia in a Persian cat. Vet Rec *125:*186, 1989.

72. Konde LJ, Spaulding K: Sonographic evaluation of the cranial mediastinum in small animals. Vet Radiol *32:*178, 1991.

THE LIVER AND GALLBLADDER

Barbara A. Selcer

Hepatic sonography has gained widespread acceptance since its introduction as a diagnostic tool for veterinary medicine in the late 1970s. As sonographic equipment has improved, so has image quality, making ultrasound an important part of the diagnostic process. Sonography provides a noninvasive means of examining the liver and should be used as an ancillary procedure to complement radiography and other diagnostic procedures. Unlike some diagnostic tests, such as cholecystography and certain forms of hepatic scintigraphy, that rely on a degree of normal hepatic function, sonography can be performed on almost any patient. This technique is sensitive as a detector of hepatic abnormality and is extremely helpful in determining certain morphologic information, especially solid from cystic disease and focal (multifocal) from diffuse disease. Many sonographic patterns of hepatic disease are nonspecific, however, and sonography should therefore not be used to render histologic diagnoses.

Sonography is indicated when liver disease is suspected on the basis of patient history or findings from the physical examination. It may also be of benefit in characterizing and identifying abdominal masses, monitoring response to hepatic therapy, or examining the diaphragm for a possible diaphragmatic hernia. If neoplasia with potential hepatic metastasis is suspected, sonographic evaluation may provide noninvasive diagnostic information. Furthermore, ultrasound can be used when abdominal radiographic detail is poor because of insufficient intra-abdominal fat or ascites. Finally, percutaneous liver biopsies are facilitated by using ultrasound guidance.

ANATOMY

The solid parenchymal nature of the liver makes it highly amenable to sonographic evaluation. The normal liver has smooth sharp borders and a homogeneous, slightly coarse, medium level echo texture. Because assessment of echogenicity is somewhat subjective, liver echogenicity (Fig. 8–1) should be compared to that of the spleen and renal cortices at the same level and with the same machine gain and intensity settings. The normal liver is hypoechoic when compared to normal spleen and is isoechoic to slightly hyperechoic when compared to normal renal cortex. The echo texture of the liver is created by differences in the acoustic impedance of the components of hepatic parenchyma (hepatocytes, fat, collagen, and blood). The fibrous components and the fat content provide the greatest reflective surfaces.[1–3]

In addition to the hepatic parenchyma, the biliary system provides internal reflectivity. The normal gallbladder (Fig. 8–2) is usually an anechoic, smooth-margined, thin-walled structure within the liver just to the right of midline. Acoustic enhancement is visible distal to the gallbladder. Bile within the gallbladder has a lower protein content than blood. Therefore, bile attenuates sound less than blood and exhibits acoustic enhancement.[4-7] The size of the gallbladder varies with patient preparation and condition; generally, it is smaller in patients fed recently than in those that have fasted or are anorexic. The neck of the gallbladder is visualized only occasionally. Recognition of the common bile duct or cystic ducts in the normal dog is difficult. Intrahepatic bile ducts are not normally seen.

The hepatic vasculature (Figs. 8–2 and 8–3) may be recognized as anechoic tubular structures within the parenchyma. Variable segmental lengths are seen on individual scans; both longitudinal and cross-sectional segments may be identified. Hepatic veins can be differentiated from portal veins: in general, vessels with hyperechoic walls are por-

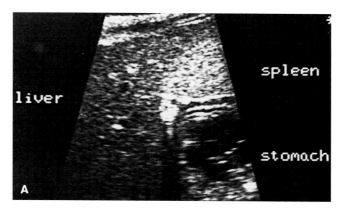

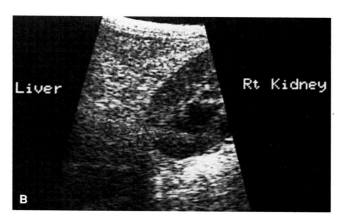

Figure 8–1

A, Left sagittal scan. The normal liver is hypoechoic compared to the normal spleen. **B,** Right sagittal scan of the liver. The echogenicity of the liver is usually either isoechoic or hyperechoic when compared to renal cortical echogenicity.

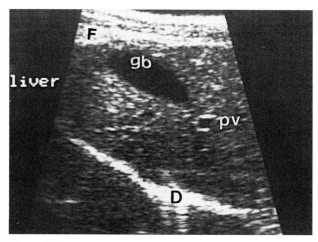

Figure 8–2

Right sagittal scan of the normal liver. The gallbladder (gb) is normally seen as an anechoic structure, the walls of which are thin or nonvisualized. The diaphragm (D) is represented by the echogenic curvilinear line marking the hepatic lung interface. Portal veins (pv) are characterized by highly echogenic walls with anechoic lumens. Falciform fat (F) is hyperechoic and seen in the extreme near field.

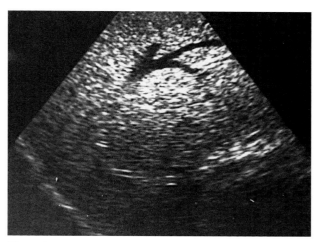

Figure 8–3

Midsagittal scan of the liver demonstrates dilated hepatic veins. Note the lack of echogenic walls (compare to the portal veins in Fig. 7–2).

tal veins and those without detectable walls are hepatic veins. Normal hepatic arteries are not seen. Large hepatic veins, especially near the porta hepatis, may appear to have hyperechoic walls. The caudal vena cava, which can be traced to the diaphragm and into the thoracic cavity, is identified as an anechoic tubular structure dorsal and to the right of midline. A spatial relationship exists among the caudal vena cava, portal vein, and common bile duct (identified if enlarged). The common bile duct lies ventral to the portal vein with the caudal vena cava dorsal and slightly to the right of the portal vein at the porta hepatis.

Determination of liver size is subjective and is often best determined radiographically. Sonographically, visualization of the liver well beyond its expected boundary in the cranial abdomen is indicative of hepatomegaly. Conversely, a small liver may be difficult to image because it is situated well beneath the rib cage. More direct liver measurement techniques have been proposed.[8–10] Godshalk et al. measured liver depth on sonograms and found no reliable correlation to liver weight.[8] On the other hand, Barr found a significant correlation between a single linear measurement made from scans of the tip of the ventral liver lobes to the diaphragm and liver mass.[9,10]

Additional anatomic structures identified in sonographic assessment of the liver include the diaphragm and ventral falciform fat (see Fig. 8–2). The diaphragm appears sonographically as a continuous, curvilinear hyperechoic structure along the cranial and dorsal boundary of the liver. Diaphragmatic integrity can be examined. Falciform fat is present in most dogs and cats in the extreme near field and is intensely hyperechoic.

TECHNIQUE

The early reports of veterinary hepatic sonography referred to the use of static B mode images.[11–13] Sonographic technology has improved, however, and most equipment in use today displays real-time images. Overall, diagnostic scan quality depends on proper transducer selection (frequency and scan head size), proper adjustment of machine settings (gain and intensity), individual patient conformation and cooperation, patient preparation, location of an adequate scan "window," and a systematic scanning technique to thoroughly evaluate the liver.

Examination of the canine or feline liver is best performed using a sector or curvilinear transducer. These scanners have small scan heads and allow the use of smaller areas of skin surface contact than do linear array transducers. Also, because of the small scan head, they may be more appropriate for scanning between ribs or "tucked-up" behind the xiphoid process or costal arch.

For most canine or feline patients, 5- to 7.5-mHz transducers are appropriate. In large dogs, a 5-mHz transducer may be needed to see dorsal structures within the liver. More superficial regions are best visualized with a 7.5-mHz transducer, providing greater resolution. A complete evaluation often requires more than one frequency transducer. In all examinations, properly adjusted gain and intensity settings should be used.

Preparation for the scan requires clipping of the hair in the area. Acoustic coupling gel is used for good transducer-skin contact. For hepatic sonography, most patients require little or no sedation unless a biopsy is to accompany the procedure. In general, fasting the patient facilitates visualization of the liver adjacent to the stomach. It is also wise to delay scanning by several hours if enemas were given recently to decrease the possibility of gas interference during the examination.

In all patients, the liver should be evaluated systematically. With the patient in dorsal recumbency, scans are made in sagittal and transverse planes with the transducer placed just caudal to the xiphoid process and the beam directed dorsocranially. If the liver is small or located well beneath the rib cage, an intercostal approach may be useful. Visualization of dilated bile ducts may require an intercostal approach.[4] General anesthesia with positive pressure ventilation may improve liver visualization by caudal displacement of the liver.[14] If gallstones are suspected, repositioning the patient to allow gravitational movement of the suspected stones can be helpful.

With most equipment, sonographic images are displayed as black on white or white on black. The more commonly accepted mode is white on black, i.e., white representing returning echoes and black representing sonolucent areas.

ARTIFACTS

Several sonographic artifacts are commonly encountered in hepatic sonography. A mirror-image artifact (Fig. 8–4) is identified when "liver" is falsely recognized cranial to the diaphragm. These phantom liver images are created when structures that are on one side of a strong reflector (such as lung/diaphragm) are artificially reproduced on the other side.[15] Slice thickness artifacts (Fig. 8–5) can occur when examining the gallbladder. Echoes from adjacent liver parenchyma may be added to the anechoic gallbladder lumen creating a false area of increased luminal echogenicity. This situation occurs as returning echoes from the parenchyma at a given depth in the ultrasound beam are aver-

Figure 8–4

Right sagittal scan of the liver. The sonolucent region (A) represents a mirror image artifact. In this instance, the gallbladder (gb) is artificially seen cranial to the diaphragm as well as in its normal position behind the diaphragm.

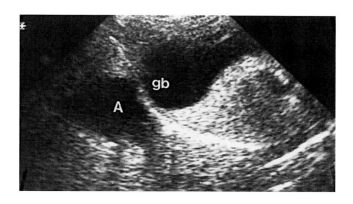

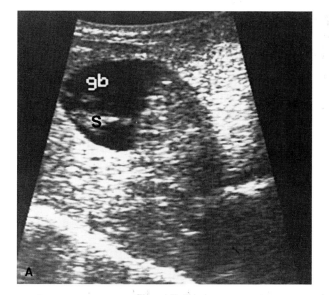

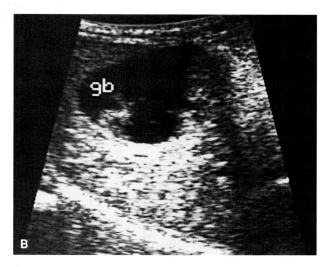

Figure 8–5

A, Right sagittal scan of the liver demonstrates a slice thickness artifact. Medium level echoes are present in the caudal one third of the gallbladder (gb) lumen. These echoes are artifactual and are the result of adjacent liver parenchymal echoes added to the gallbladder lumen (compare to **B**). Gallbladder sludge (S) is seen in the cranial portion of the gallbladder. **B,** Same gallbladder (gb) as in **A.** The transducer has been moved slightly to partially eliminate the slice thickness artifact.

Figure 8–6

Right sagittal scan of the liver demonstrates acoustic enhancement deep to the gallbladder (gb). The liver echogenicity immediately deep to the gallbladder is increased because fewer echoes are reflected in the fluid-filled gallbladder and therefore sound transmission through it is greater compared to the adjacent liver parenchyma.

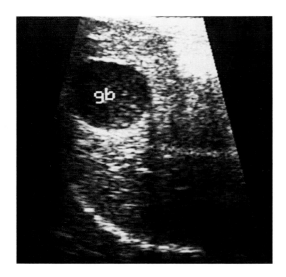

Figure 8–7

Right sagittal scan of the liver demonstrates acoustic shadowing (between arrows). Hyperechoic foci in the dependent portion of the gallbladder (gb) represent mineralized gallbladder calculi (c). The hypoechoic to anechoic region immediately beneath the calculi illustrates the sonographic phenomenon of acoustic shadowing. There is less through transmission of sound deep to the mineralized calculi.

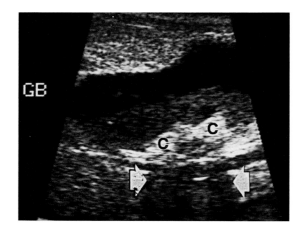

aged with luminal echoes to create a false image.[16] Side-lobe artifacts can be seen in the gallbladder when echoes that appear to originate within the true ultrasound beam (i.e., gallbladder lumen) are in fact created by adjacent strong reflectors such a bowel gas.[6] The latter two artifacts can be minimized by repositioning the patient or changing the angle of the transducer and ultrasound beam.

In addition to these artifacts, diagnostic hepatic sonography uses the physical sonographic properties of acoustic enhancement and acoustic shadowing to help characterize normal hepatic anatomy and some liver abnormalities. Acoustic enhancement (Fig. 8–6) results in increased echogenicity distal to cystic or sonolucent structures such as the gallbladder or hepatic cysts. Dilated bile ducts may also show acoustic enhancement.[4–6] Acoustic shadowing (Fig. 8–7) results in decreased transmission of sound deep to strong reflectors or attenuators of sound. In hepatic sonography, this situation may be encountered in cases of gallbladder calculi or hepatic mineralization.

HEPATOBILIARY DISORDERS

Sonography can be used to assist in the diagnosis of many different kinds of liver disease. It is generally accepted, however, that the sonographic changes of most hepatobiliary diseases in man and in animals are nonspecific.[2,6,11,12,17-25] Recognition of liver lesions depends on a knowledge of normal sonographic anatomy, adequate equipment, proper equipment use, and user experience. Lesion distinction depends on acoustic impedance differences between normal and abnormal tissue. As a result, small lesions with greater disparity in acoustic impedance may be recognized more readily than larger isoechoic lesions.[5] Most sonographic abnormalities are described in terms of (1) tissue echogenicity (hypoechoic, isoechoic, hyperechoic); (2) distribution (diffuse, focal, multifocal); (3) the presence of acoustic enhancement or acoustic shadowing; and (4) alteration of surface shape or contour. In addition, the size and shape of the liver, the gallbladder, the hepatic vasculature, and the hepatic ducts (if visible) may be evaluated. Again, although nonspecific, ultrasound is regarded as sensitive when establishing the presence of an abnormality.[2,26,27]

Hepatobiliary abnormalities can be sonographically separated into liver parenchymal lesions, hepatic vascular lesions, and lesions involving the gallbladder and biliary tree.

Hepatic Parenchymal Diseases

Hepatic parenchymal diseases are classified as benign or malignant.

Benign Lesions

The predominant forms of benign liver disease with reported sonographic findings include hepatic lipidosis (fatty liver), nodular hyperplasia, steroid hepatopathy, cirrhosis, passive congestion, hepatitis (chronic and acute), liver abscessation, hepatic cysts, and benign neoplasia.

The most common benign diffuse liver disease in dogs and cats is hepatic lipidosis[28] (Fig. 8-8). Fatty infiltration of the liver usually results in excess accumulation of fat in the form of triglycerides. Important causes of hepatic lipidosis include starvation, diabetes mellitus, obesity, and toxic or drug-related reactions.[28] Hepatomegaly is usually seen both radiographically and sonographically. The sonographic findings are characterized by diffuse increased liver parenchymal echogenicity when compared to renal cortical or splenic echogenicity.[1,5,17,21,26,29-33] Sound reflected and attenuated at strong echogenic interfaces between fat and water or fat and non-fat tissue is responsible for this appearance.[34] In fact, lipid content in soft tissue is a prime attenuator of sound, rendering it more echogenic than connective tissue.[3,31,35] A consequence of the overall increased echogenicity is decreased visualization of the echogenic portal vein walls.

Studies in man suggest ultrasound is 88% accurate in distinguishing between fatty (bright) livers and diffuse disease resulting in decreased echogenicity.[26] Not surprisingly, accuracy increases in patients with moderate to severe hepatic lipidosis relative to those with mild disease. The false-positive rate for identification of fatty infiltration is

Figure 8-8

Left sagittal scan of the liver in a dog with hepatic lipidosis. The echogenicity of the liver (black arrows) is greater than that of the spleen (white arrow).

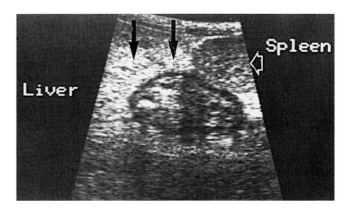

low.[21] Sonography is reported to be a sensitive and specific test (91% sensitive and 100% specific) in cats with hepatic lipidosis.[30] The liver in these cats is hyperechoic compared to the echogenicity of falciform fat.[30] Similarly, dogs and cats with steroid hepatopathy demonstrate diffuse increased liver echogenicity attributable to glycogen accumulation.[1,28,31]

Nodular hyperplasia (Fig. 8–9) is a common finding in aged dogs and is not associated with clinical signs.[28] Unfortunately, the sonographic appearance of nodular hyperplasia is not specific and can mimic both primary neoplasia and metastatic neoplasia. Its sonographic patterns range from normal to focal/multifocal hypoechoic or mixed hypoechoic and hyperechoic lesions, often with associated severe liver architectural rearrangement.[5,20,27,29] In man, a "halo sign" (see subsequent section) has been reported to be a highly sensitive finding (88% sensitivity and 86% specificity)[27] in patients with hepatic metastasis. Ironically, the same authors reported this sign in three of three patients with nodular hyperplasia. Whether the halo sign is also true in dogs has not been determined.

Another disease with a diffuse increased echogenic pattern is hepatic cirrhosis.[1,2,21,26,29,31–33] Unlike hepatic lipidosis in which smooth-margined hepatomegaly is common, cirrhotic livers are often smaller than normal and have irregular margins[1,2,29] (Fig. 8–10). This difference may help to distinguish the two abnormalities. The increased echogenicity seen in liver cirrhosis may in fact be attributable to associated fatty infiltration.[31,33]

Benign causes of diffuse decreased liver echogenicity include chronic passive congestion (Fig. 8–11) resulting from dilatation of hepatic sinusoids and hepatitis (Fig. 8–12) owing to swelling of hepatocytes.[1,2,5,6,29,33] Decreased echogenicity is most readily apparent when the echogenicity of the liver is compared to that of the renal cortex (especially those lobes adjacent to the right kidney). With decreased echogenicity in the liver, the walls of the portal vein become increasingly prominent (increased periportal echogenicity).[5,26,29,33,36] In man, amyloidosis is another disease with a sonographic appearance of diffuse decreased echogenicity.[5] Similar reports are not found in the veterinary literature.

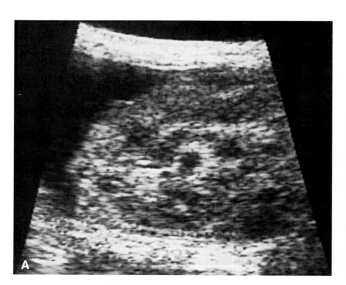 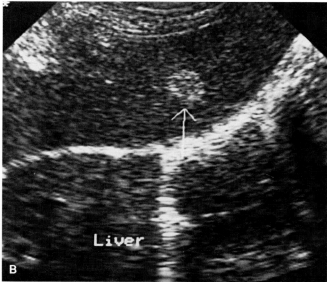

Figure 8–9

A, Left sagittal scan of the liver in a dog with hepatic nodular hyperplasia. Numerous hypoechoic to anechoic foci are diffusely present within the liver. **B,** Transverse scan of the left lobes of the liver in a dog with a solitary hyperechoic hepatic nodule (arrow). The histologic diagnosis was nodular hyperplasia.

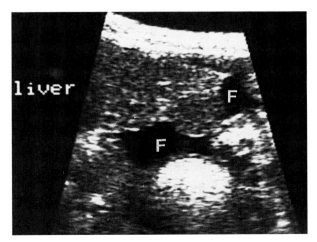

Figure 8–10

Right sagittal scan of the liver in a dog with hepatic cirrhosis and abdominal effusion (F). Note the irregular liver margination (arrows).

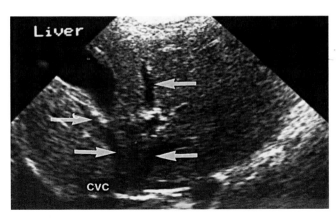

Figure 8–11

Transverse scan of the liver in a dog with congestive heart failure. The liver is enlarged with diffuse, slightly decreased echogenicity. The hepatic veins (arrows) are dilated as they join the caudal vena cava (cvc).

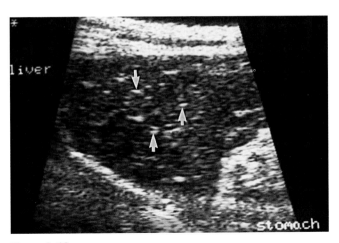

Figure 8–12

Left sagittal scan of the liver in a dog with chronic hepatitis. Liver echogenicity is decreased and periportal echogenicity is increased as the hyperechoic portal vein walls are more readily visible (arrows).

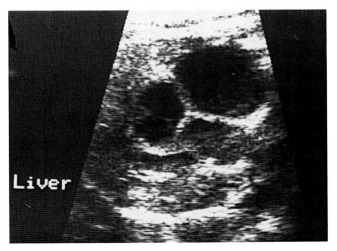

Figure 8–13

Right sagittal scan of the liver in a dog with hepatic cysts. Acoustic enhancement is seen deep to the large, sonolucent, septated cystic structure.

Hepatic abscessation has a varied sonographic appearance depending on abscess composition. If primarily liquid, abscesses can appear hypoechoic to anechoic. Abscesses detected early may appear solid and echogenic.[5,24,37] The walls of abscesses range in appearance from ill-defined to irregular and thick.[24] If gas-forming organisms are present within the abscess, small echogenic foci may be seen gas reverberation artifact.[24] Disease processes with a similar sonographic appearance include parasitic infestations (in man, amebic and echinococcal), cysts, cavitary or necrotic neoplasms, and hemorrhage or hematoma.[2,5,12,29]

Hepatic cysts (Fig. 8–13) are occasionally identified in dogs and cats. In most instances, they are congenital.[28] Fluid-filled hepatic cysts can be focal or multifocal. The fluid-filled cavity is sonolucent and acoustic enhancement is usually present.[5,12,29] Thin walls occasionally are recognized. Larger cysts may contain internal septations.

Some infrequently reported benign diseases that are evaluated sonographically include fungal disease, extramedullary hematopoiesis, and hepatocellular adenoma. The sonographic appearance of hepatic fungal disease is not well established. In one veterinary series of cases, a dog with "generalized mycosis" was described as having a multifocal nodular lesion.[17] The liver can also be a site of extramedullary hematopoiesis. Sonographic findings identified in human subjects with this diagnosis include hepatomegaly with either multiple hyperechoic foci or a mixed echogenic solitary mass-like lesion.[38] Hepatocellular adenomas have been reported in two cases.[11] In both animals, a large mixed echogenic mass was identified sonographically.[11]

Malignant Lesions

The liver is a site of both primary and secondary neoplasia. The most common primary hepatic tumors in dogs and cats are hepatocellular carcinoma and cholangiocellular carcinoma.[28] The liver is also a frequent site of metastasis; the portal circulation provides an additional pathway for metastasis from gastrointestinal neoplasia. In addition to metastases from gastrointestinal tumors such as pancreatic carcinoma, the liver is a common site of metastatic hematopoietic neoplasia, lymphosarcoma, and mesenchymal neoplasia (hemangiosarcoma).[28]

It is important to remember that sonography alone should not be used to differentiate benign from malignant liver disease.[1,2,11,12,17,23,25] The following sonographic descriptions of neoplastic disease should be used as examples. Like the benign diseases, malignant diseases are described according to echogenicity, distribution, overall liver size and contour, and the presence of acoustic enhancement or shadowing. The advantages and limitations of ultrasound as a diagnostic tool should be noted. Studies in man have generated conflicting results regarding the accuracy, sensitivity, and specificity of ultrasound in the detection or characterization of neoplastic hepatic lesions.[24,25,27,37,39] As a result, most authors state that ultrasound findings alone in man and animals cannot predict histologic cell type.[2,11,12,17,23–25] A negative sonographic examination (i.e., normal) does not preclude the presence of disease. The inability of ultrasound to detect isoechoic or small nodules has probably contributed to a reported false-negative detection rate of up to 50% for liver metastases in people.[25] Small focal lesions may be detected, but their identification is more difficult if they are less than 2 cm in diameter or isoechoic with normal tissue.[2,24]

Whalen compared sonography with magnetic resonance imaging (MRI) and CT in man and found no significant difference in the sensitivity of three diagnostic techniques (MRI, 80%; CT, 77%; sonography, 73%),[37] although MRI was significantly better at lesion characterization.[37] Whalen cited another study in which the MRI, CT, and sonography were compared in terms of their ability to differentiate malignant from benign lesions. No significant difference was found.[37] Authors of other reports suggest no apparent relationship exists between the echogenicity of liver lesions and their histologic appearance, and therefore differentiation of benign (e.g., focal nodular hyperplasia) from malignant nodules is unreliable.[24,25] On the other hand, findings from one human study suggest it is possible to distinguish benign and malignant multifocal lesions with approximately 86% accuracy.[27] A hypoechoic "halo" is seen along the border of malignant hyperechoic or isoechoic lesions.[27] This halo effect is created by an intratumoral rim of proliferating tumor cells and adjacent extratumoral compressed liver parenchyma.[40] Whether a similar finding can be used in animals has not been established. Research is underway to evaluate the benefits of pulsed Doppler, color Doppler, and sonographic contrast agents to enhance lesion detection and characterization[39,41- 45] (see the last section in this chapter).

In the dog, hepatocellular carcinoma (Fig. 8–14) is the most common primary hepatic neoplasm.[28] This tumor has a varied sonographic appearance; in veterinary reports, it is described as a solitary hyperechoic mass,[23] hyperechoic multifocal masses,[2] and hypoechoic or mixed multifocal masses.[17] By far the largest retrospective study of the sonographic appearance of canine hepatic tumors suggests that most hepatocellular carcinomas appear as solitary hyperechoic masses.[23] In man, this tumor also has a varied sonographic appearance, ranging from solitary to multifocal and diffuse with both hyperechoic and hypoechoic masses.[29] The hypoechoic "halo sign" often seen in malignant diseases is not a common finding in human hepatocellular carcinoma.[27]

Cholangiocellular carcinoma (Fig. 8–15) is a primary hepatic neoplasm most commonly arising from intrahepatic bile duct epithelium.[28] This tumor is relatively rare in humans but has been included in a number of retrospective veterinary sonographic liver evaluations.[2,11,13,23] Sonographic findings are not specific. It is most often described as multifocal in distribution and either hyperechoic or hypoechoic.[2,11,13,23] Mixed echo texture patterns have also been seen.[23]

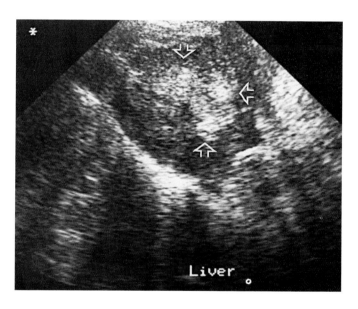

Figure 8–14

Sagittal midline scan of the liver in a dog with hepatocellular carcinoma. The liver is of mixed echogenicity with a large, moderately well-defined hyperechoic mass (arrows).

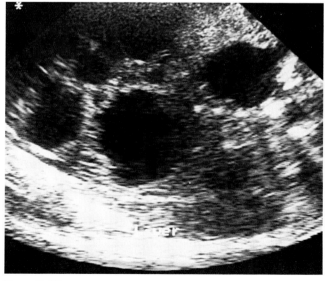

Figure 8–15

Right sagittal scan of the liver in a dog with cholangiocellular carcinoma. Multifocal hypoechoic to anechoic, variably sized masses are present within the liver.

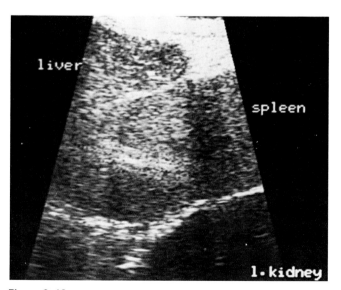

Figure 8–16

Left sagittal scan of the liver in a dog with diffuse hepatic lymphosarcoma. The liver is diffusely hyperechoic with its echogenicity equal to or greater than that of the spleen.

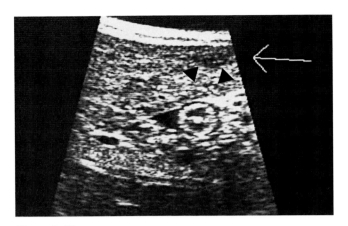

Figure 8–17

Right sagittal scan of the liver in a dog with lymphosarcoma. Variably sized, 1- to 3-cm hypoechoic masses are see throughout the liver (arrowheads).

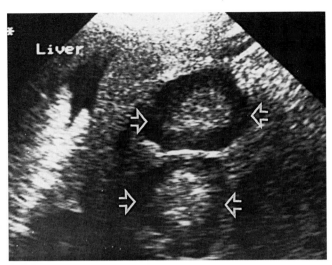

Figure 8–18

Dorsal plane scan of the liver in a dog with multifocal hepatic lymphosarcoma. Two large "target" lesions (arrows) have an isoechoic to hyperechoic center and are bordered by a hypoechoic rim.

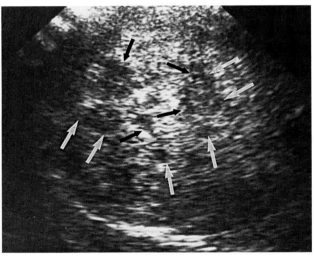

Figure 8–19

Right sagittal scan of the liver in a dog with metastatic pancreatic carcinoma. Multifocal, irregularly shaped hypoechoic foci are present throughout the liver parenchyma (arrows).

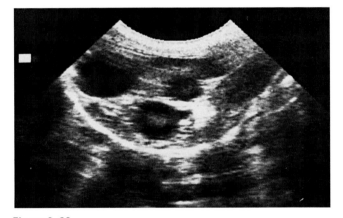

Figure 8–20

Right sagittal scan of the liver in a dog with multifocal "target" lesions related to cholangiocellular carcinoma. Note the target or bulls-eye appearance of the lesions.

Lymphosarcoma is the most common metastatic liver tumor.[28] The sonographic appearance of hepatic lymphosarcoma is highly variable (Figs. 8–16 to 8–18). The reported sonographic findings vary from normal to diffuse echo texture or multifocal lesions.[2,11,18,19,22,23,46] Lamb et al. state that sonography is not a good screening test for hepatic lymphosarcoma,[18] basing their observation on a retrospective study in which only 3 of 14 proven hepatic lymphosarcoma patients had identifiable lesions on sonograms.[18] Sonographic patterns of hepatic lymphosarcoma identified in the human and veterinary literature can be summarized as follows: normal,[11,19,29] diffuse hyperechoic,[11,17,23] diffuse hypoechoic,[5,18] multifocal hypoechoic,[2,11,18,19,23,46] and multifocal hyperechoic.[2,46]

Retrospective studies in man involving large total patient populations have found that the multifocal hypoechoic lesion is the most common pattern.[22,29,46]

Overall, metastatic liver disease is more common than primary neoplasia.[23,28,29] Sonography can be an important screening tool for most veterinary practitioners because it is better than radiography in the detection of diffuse or focal parenchymal disease. Most metastatic liver lesions are described sonographically as focal or multifocal masses[2,11,12,17–19,23,29] (Fig. 8–19). Diffuse lymphosarcoma is an exception.[2,11,17,18,23] Multifocal/focal hyperechoic and multifocal mixed echogenic patterns most likely represent carcinomas.[23,29] Metastatic carcinomas, sarcomas, hemangiosarcomas, lymphosarcomas, and primary hepatic neoplasms can all show multifocal hypoechoic patterns.[2,11,18,19,22–24,27,29,46] A target or bull's eye appearance (see Figs. 8–18 and 8–20) has been associated with some multifocal lesions.[11, 19, 22, 46] This pattern is not specific; it can be seen with primary or secondary neoplasia and with non-neoplastic conditions.[19,29]

Hepatic Vascular Disease

Portasystemic shunts (Fig. 8–21) can be congenital or acquired. Congenital shunts are more common.[47] They may be intrahepatic or extrahepatic and usually involve a single, large communicating vessel, frequently a patent ductus venosus. Acquired shunts on the other hand are usually the result of multiple collateral shunting vessels.[28] Large breed dogs typically have intrahepatic shunts, whereas small breed dogs and cats more frequently have extrahepatic shunts.[47]

Ultrasound may be useful in establishing or confirming a diagnosis of a portasystemic shunt. Sonograms usually reveal a small hypovascular (few hepatic and portal veins) liver.[14,48,49] The actual vascular communication between the portal vein and the caudal vena cava may be identified as a large anechoic dilated venous structure[2,12,14,49,50] (see Fig. 8–21). Acquired shunts may show tortuous dilated portal vasculature.[49] The veterinary literature suggests that intrahepatic shunts may be easier to identify than extrahepatic shunts.[14,49]

Not all shunts are visualized. In patients with a small liver, scanning can be difficult because of interference by the ribs and overlying gas-filled bowel. Positive pressure ventilation can improve sonographic accuracy in the identification of portasystemic shunts by caudally displacing the liver and dilating the intrahepatic veins and caudal vena cava.[14,48] Pulsed Doppler and intraoperative sonography may also be beneficial in the sonographic diagnosis of shunts.[14,48]

Ultrasound has also been used in the diagnosis of congenital hepatic arteriovenous fistula in dogs.[51] This condition is characterized sonographically by recognition of enlarged tortuous, anechoic tubular vascular structures or anechoic irregular "lakes" within the liver parenchyma.[51] The use of pulsed Doppler confirms unidirectional flow within the arteriovenous fistula.[51]

Figure 8–21

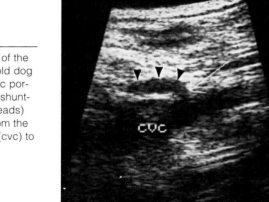

Right sagittal scan of the liver in a 4-month-old dog with an extrahepatic portacaval shunt. The shunting vessel (arrowheads) could be traced from the caudal vena cava (cvc) to the portal vein (not illustrated).

Hepatic venous distention frequently accompanies right ventricular failure or caudal caval obstruction. In these patients, the hepatic veins and the caudal vena cava are dilated[2,12] (see Figs. 8–3 and 8–22). The sonographic features of a Budd-Chiari-like syndrome, hepatic vein obstruction, have been reported in the dog and include mild hypoechoic liver enlargement.[52] The intrahepatic caudal vena cava was slightly narrowed and the hepatic veins were small and thickened compared to the dilated intrahepatic portal veins.[52]

Portal vein blood flow and velocity have been determined in normal dogs using pulsed Doppler ultrasound combined with real-time B mode imaging.[53] Scans are best performed at the right lateral 11th or 12th intercostal space.[53] The normal mean portal vein blood flow as measured with pulsed duplex Doppler is 31.06 ± 9.1 ml/min/kg using a portal vein diameter method.[54] Normal portal blood flow velocity is 18.1 ± 7.6 cm/sec.[54] These values have been compared with values obtained in dogs with induced cirrhosis, and the results showed decreased portal velocity and flow in cirrhotic patients.[54]

Disease of the Biliary Tract

Sonography can be useful in the diagnosis of cholelithiasis, biliary obstruction, and cholecystitis. In man, sonography has virtually replaced oral cholecystography, demonstrating a 95% success rate in the identification of gallbladder disease.[55]

Unlike survey radiography, sonography can be used to identify both radiopaque and nonradiopaque gallbladder calculi.[12,49,56–58] Choleliths are recognized as hyperechoic foci within the dependent lumen of the gallbladder (Fig. 8–23). Some degree of posterior shadowing is usually seen. Both radiopaque and radiolucent stones can exhibit posterior shadowing.[12,49,56–58] In fact, current reports suggest that neither stone size nor chemical composition play significant roles in sonographic detectability.[56–58] The physical relationship of the stone to the sonographic beam and the resolution of the transducer are the primary factors determining whether acoustic shadowing is displayed.[56,58,59] Irregular hypoechoic to hyperechoic matter in the form of sludge can also be identified within the gallbladder (Fig. 8–24). This material may be tenacious or freely movable. Posterior acoustic shadowing is usually absent. Sonography may also be used to distinguish hepatic parenchymal mineralization from calculi within the biliary tract.

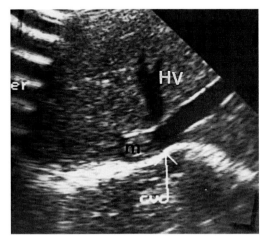

Figure 8–22

Right sagittal scan of the liver in a dog with a large, medium level echogenic mass (m) within the caudal vena cava at the level of the diaphragm. The hepatic vein (HV) is large and dilated.

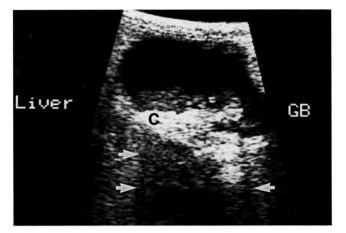

Figure 8–23

Right sagittal scan of the liver in a dog with cholelithiasis. The calculi (C) are hyperechoic and lie within the dependent portion of the gallbladder (GB). Posterior shadowing (arrows) is evident deep to the calculi.

In jaundiced patients, sonography may help to differentiate hepatocellular disease from biliary obstruction. Biliary obstruction can be the result of extrahepatic disease such as neoplasia; inflammation of the pancreas, duodenum, or extrahepatic biliary tract; or intraluminal obstruction owing to cholelithiasis or parasitic disease such as Platynosomum concinnum.[60,61]

Sonographic features of biliary obstruction vary depending on the level of the obstruction, i.e., hepatic duct, cystic duct, or common bile duct (Fig. 8–25). Experimental ligation of the common bile duct produced rapid dilatation of the gallbladder followed by dilatation of the common bile duct (24 to 48 hours) and peripheral ducts (5 to 7 days).[4] Normally, the common bile duct is not easily identified; however, when distended, it can be seen ventral to the portal vein. The best window for visualization of a dilated common bile duct is found along the right side cranial to the xiphoid and dorsal to the sternum.[4] Dilated intrahepatic bile ducts can be differentiated from portal veins,[62] and may have the following characteristics: irregular tortuous walls, an irregular tortuous branching pattern, posterior acoustic enhancement, and, in man, a "stellate" appearance where several large ducts converge.[6,49,62] In addition, seeing too many tubular structures in the area of the intrahepatic portal vessels (double-barrel gunshot sign) is suggestive of, although not definitive for, biliary tract enlargement.[49,63,64] Partial obstruction may modify the sonographic appearance. Ductal dilatation alone can be an unreliable sign of current biliary obstruction because dilatation can persist following prior obstruction.[65,66]

More complete diagnostic information can be obtained by combining the sonographic evaluation with synthetic cholecystokinin-induced gallbladder emptying.[65] Normal dogs empty at least 40% of the gallbladder volume within 1 hour after synthetic cholecystokinin intravenous injection. In dogs with obstructed gallbladders, less than 20% of gallbladder volume is emptied within 1 hour.[65]

A veterinary case report describes the sonographic findings in a cat with extrahepatic biliary obstruction related to the parasite Platynosomum concinnum.[60] In this cat, the gallbladder and common bile duct were dilated but the intrahepatic bile ducts and liver parenchyma were normal.[60]

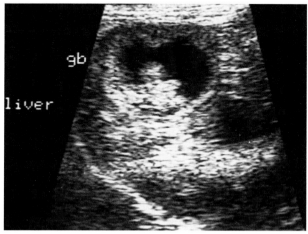

Figure 8–24

Right sagittal scan of the liver of a dog with irregular sludge accumulation. The gallbladder (gb) wall is thickened. Note the lack of posterior shadowing.

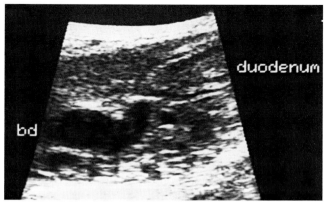

Figure 8–25

Right sagittal scan of the liver in a cat with obstruction of the common bile duct (bd). The dilated common bile duct is seen as it curves toward the duodenum.

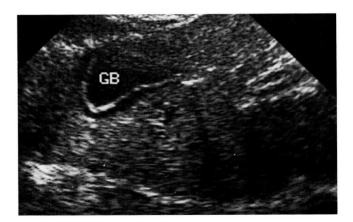

Figure 8–26

Right sagittal scan of the liver in a dog with a double-layered, thick-walled gallbladder (GB). Note the internal hyperechoic layer and the hypoechoic outer layer. The cause for this appearance was not determined.

Acute or chronic cholecystitis is a difficult disease to diagnose in small animals and therefore is rarely reported.[61] Its sonographic appearance is not well defined. In man, gallbladder wall thickening may be sign of cholecystitis, although gallbladder wall thickening (Fig. 8–26) itself can also be seen in association with other conditions such as ascites, hypoproteinemia, acute pyelonephritis, portal hypertension, chronic renal disease, and hepatitis.[49,67–69] In dogs, it has been identified in conjunction with cholangiohepatitis.[12]

The sonographic appearance of emphysematous cholecystitis reportedly resembles "champagne bubbles" with small echogenic foci rising from the dependent portion of the gallbladder lumen.[70] An interesting human study showed a high degree of sensitivity (80.6%) and specificity (93.9%) when gallbladder wall thickness is used to classify malignant versus benign ascites.[71] A single-layered nonthickened wall was usually associated with malignant disease, whereas a single-layered thick wall or double-layered thick wall corresponded to benign causes of ascites.[71] Whether the same is true in small animals has not been determined.

ULTRASOUND-GUIDED LIVER BIOPSY

Percutaneous liver biopsy is performed routinely in small animals. Ultrasound guidance facilitates the procedure by allowing accurate biopsy site determination and needle monitoring to improve the accuracy of the biopsy sample and permit focal lesion biopsy. Another advantage of this technique is visualization of the site after the procedure for detection of possible complications. Complications are infrequent, however, if clotting profiles are routinely performed before the biopsy to identify patients with bleeding disorders.[72,73]

Ultrasound-guided liver biopsies can be performed with or without (free-hand style) a transducer attachment. Use of this attachment during biopsy provides a visualized "tract" on the ultrasound monitor as well as a fixed angle and approach for the needle during the puncture (Fig. 8–27). The free-hand style may be useful if odd angles of approach to the biopsy site preclude the use of the fixed path provided by the guide.

Ultrasound-guided liver biopsy can be performed using conventional manual biopsy needles or automatic biopsy devices.[72–76] Manual ultrasound-guided biopsies are usually performed using True-Cut needles (Travenol Laboratories, Inc., Deerfield, IL). Automated devices have been used successfully for ultrasound-guided liver biopsy,[73–76] and in general are equal or superior to manual devices.[73,76,77] The automated devices reliably obtain a tissue core, increasing both the quality of the biopsy sample and the quantity of sample volume.[75,77] When four available automatic biopsy devices were eval-

Figure 8–27

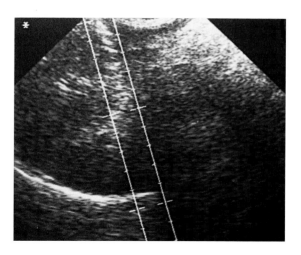

Center sagittal scan of the liver in a dog during an ultrasound-guided biopsy. Use of a transducer guide enables the operator to visualize the path of the needle during the procedure. The hyperechoic line within the parallel tracts represents the biopsy needle.

TABLE 8–1
Automatic Biopsy Devices

Biopsy Device	Manufacturer	Needle Specification
Biopty with Inrad Needle (Grand Rapids, MI)	Bard Urological, Covington, GA	18-gauge, 20-cm length needle (23-mm penetration, 16.7-mm sample notch)
Monopty	Bard Urological, Covington, GA	18-gauge, 20-cm length needle (22-mm penetration, 16.6-mm sample notch)
ASAP18	Microvasix I/Boxton Scientific, Watertown, MA	18-gauge, 21-cm length needle (22-mm penetration, 16.6-mm sample notch)
Ultra-Cut	Medical Device Technologies, Gainesville, FL	18-gauge, 14-cm length needle (22-mm penetration, 16.6-mm sample notch)

uated, no significant difference was found in overall quality of the biopsy specimen.[73] The four instruments tested are listed in Table 8–1.

Regardless of individual preference for a particular ultrasound-guided technique, certain steps should be followed in the biopsy procedure. Before the biopsy, the liver is scanned to determine whether an appropriate window for biopsy is present. Fasting the patient decreases the possibility of an enlarged stomach encroaching on the liver and obscuring large portions of the anatomy. A small liver or the presence of overlying gas can severely limit potential liver biopsy sites. Sterile technique is used for percutaneous ultrasound-guided biopsy. The ultrasound transducer can be placed within a sterile rubber sleeve. A small stab incision in the skin permits easy penetration and advancement of the needle, which can be monitored sonographically. An accurate biopsy site and biopsy depth can then be determined.

ADVANCED HEPATIC SONOGRAPHIC TECHNIQUES

The use of duplex Doppler sonography was mentioned previously in regard to the evaluation of portasystemic shunts. Color Doppler has also yielded good results when used in human patients to identify portosystemic shunts.[78] Few case reports in the veterinary literature cite the use of duplex Doppler to evaluate diseases other than shunts.[50,51,54] Duplex Doppler capabilities were used in dogs with induced hepatic cirrhosis.[54] In these dogs, Doppler ultrasound demonstrated decreased portal vein velocity and flow.[54]

In man, duplex Doppler has been used to differentiate hepatocellular carcinoma from other tumors.[42,43] High velocity duplex Doppler signals (greater than 5 kHz) are reportedly found in the periphery of hepatocellular carcinoma because of arterioportal shunting.[42,43] Hypoechoic metastases frequently have no detectable Doppler shift signal and rarely exceed 4 kHz when present.[42]

Like two-dimensional sonographic liver imaging, duplex Doppler imaging of the portal circulation can be complicated by artifacts. Mirror image artifacts can occur when the Doppler signal is present on both sides of the zero base line and erroneously suggest bidirectional flow.[79] Another pitfall, the flip artifact, has been described when a unidirectional Doppler signal suddenly flips from one side of the zero base line to the other.[79] An absent or poorly detectable Doppler signal can be the result of overlying gas or small vessel size.[79] The latter difficulty is exaggerated by patient motion and respiration.[79]

In an effort to sonographically distinguish isoechoic lesions within the hepatic parenchyma, the use of several contrast agents has been proposed.[41,44,45,80] Iodipimide ethyl ester (IDE) was used experimentally in rabbits to visualize otherwise isoechoic tumors.[41] The small IDE particles are collected by Kupffer cells in the liver where they cause scattering sites during sonography and result in overall increased liver echogenicity. Regions within the liver that lack Kupffer cells (i.e., tumors) appear relatively hypoechoic.[41] Perflubron emulsion has also been used clinically to increase tumor echogenicity after intravenous injection.[44] This contrast agent is taken up selectively by the liver and the spleen.[44] In human subjects, side effects have included flu-like symptoms, mild fever, and back pain.[44] In another human clinical trial, hepatic arterial injection of carbon dioxide microbubbles was used to enhance and distinguish liver tumors on sonograms.[45] This particular technique would appear to have limited veterinary application because of its invasive nature. Finally, an experimental study involving rat liver tumors suggests that intravenous lipid-coated microbubbles may be used as a contrast agent to increase the echogenicity of liver tumors.[80] This technique is associated with leakage and accumulation of the lipid-coated microbubbles by the tumor.[80] The rationale and efficacy for the use of similar agents in dogs and cats has yet to be established.

REFERENCES

1. Biller DS, Kantrowitz B, Miyabayashi T: Ultrasonography of diffuse liver disease. J Vet Intern Med 6:71, 1992.
2. Lamb CR: Abdominal ultrasonography in small animals: Examination of the liver, spleen, and pancreas. J Small Anim Pract 31:6, 1990.
3. Layer G, et al: Computerized ultrasound B-scan texture analysis of experimental diffuse parenchymal liver disease: Correlation with histopathology and tissue composition. JCU 19:193, 1991.
4. Nyland TG, Gillett NA: Sonographic evaluation of experimental bile duct legation in the dog. Vet Radiol 23:252, 1982.
5. Leopold GR: Abdominal Ultrasonography. New York: John Wiley and Sons, 1984, pp. 81–120.
6. Laing FC: Diagnostic Ultrasound. St Louis: Mosby Year Book, 1991, pp. 106–144.
7. Filly RA, Sommer FG, Minton MJ: Characterization of biological fluids by ultrasound and computed tomography. Radiology 134:167, 1980.
8. Godshalk CP, et al: Quantitative ultrasonic assessment of liver size in the dog. Vet Radiol 29:162, 1988.
9. Barr F: Normal hepatic measurements in mature dogs. J Small Anim Pract 33:367, 1992.
10. Barr F: Ultrasonographic assessment of liver size in the dog. J Small Anim Pract 33:359, 1992.
11. Feeney DA, Johnston GR, Hardy RM: Two-dimensional, gray-scale ultrasonography for assessment of hepatic and splenic neoplasia in the dog and cat. J Am Vet Med Assoc 184:68, 1984.
12. Nyland TG, Park RD: Hepatic ultrasonography in the dog. Vet Radiol 24:74, 1983.
13. Nyland TG, et al: Gray-scale ultrasonography of the canine abdomen. Vet Radiol 22:220, 1981.
14. Wrigley RH, et al: Ultrasonographic diagnosis of portocaval shunts in young dogs. J Am Vet Med Assoc 191:421, 1987.
15. Nguyen KT, Sauerbrei EE, Nolan RL: Diagnostic Ultrasound. St. Louis: Mosby Year Book, 1991, pp. 365–382.
16. Jakovljenic S: Veterinary Diagnostic Ultrasound. West Lafayette, IN: Purdue University, 1991, pp. 16–20.
17. Voros K, et al: Correction of ultrasonographic and pathomorphological findings in canine hepatic diseases. J Small Anim Pract 32:627, 1991.
18. Lamb CR, et al: Ultrasonographic findings in hepatic and splenic lymphosarcoma in dogs and cats. Vet Radiol 32:117, 1991.

105

19. Nyland TG: Ultrasonic patterns of canine hepatic lymphosarcoma. Vet Radiol 25:167, 1984.
20. Stowater JL, Lamb CR, Schelling SH: Ultrasonographic features of canine hepatic nodular hyperplasia. Vet Radiol 31:268, 1990.
21. Foster KJ, et al: The accuracy of ultrasound in the detection of fatty infiltration of the liver. Br J Radiol 53:440, 1980.
22. Wernecke K, Peters PE, Kruger KG: Ultrasonographic patterns of focal hepatic and splenic lesions in Hodgkin's and non-Hodgkin's lymphoma. Br J Radiol 60:655, 1987.
23. Whitely MB, et al: Ultrasonographic appearance of primary and metastatic canine hepatic tumors: A review of 48 cases. J Ultrasound Med 8:621, 1989.
24. Zeman RK, et al: Hepatic imaging: Current status. Radiol Clin North Am 23:473, 1985.
25. Ferrucci JT: Liver tumor imaging: Current concepts. AJR Am J Roentgenol 155:473, 1990.
26. Needleman L, et al: Sonography of diffuse benign liver disease: Accuracy of pattern recognition and grading. AJR Am J Roentgenol 146:1011, 1986.
27. Wernecke K, et al: The distinction between benign and malignant liver tumors on sonography: Value of a hypoechoic halo. AJR Am J Roentgenol 159:1005, 1992.
28. Hardy RM: *Textbook of Veterinary Internal Medicine*. Philadelphia: WB Saunders, 1989, pp. 1479–1527.
29. Withers CE, Wilson SR: *Diagnostic Ultrasound*. St Louis: Mosby Year Book, 1991, pp. 45–86.
30. Yeager AE, Mohammed H: Accuracy of ultrasonography in the detection of severe hepatic lipidosis in cats. Am J Vet Res 53:597, 1992.
31. Garra BS, et al: Quantitative estimation of liver attenuation and echogenicity: Normal state versus diffuse liver disease. Radiology 162:61, 1987.
32. Joseph AE, Dewbury KC, McGuire PG: Ultrasound in the detection of chronic liver disease (the "bright liver"). Br J Radiol 52:184, 1979.
33. Scott WW, Donovan PJ, Sanders RC: The sonography of diffuse liver disease. Semin Ultrasound 2:219, 1981.
34. Behan M, Kazam E: The echographic characteristics of fatty tissues and tumors. Radiology 129:143, 1978.
35. Taylor KJ, et al: Quantitative US attenuation in normal liver and in patients with diffuse liver disease: Importance of fat. Radiology 160:65, 1986.
36. Kurtz AB, et al: Ultrasound findings in hepatitis. Radiology 136:717, 1980.
37. Whalen E: Liver imaging-current trends in MRI, CT, and US: International symposium and course. AJR Am J Roentgenol 155:1125, 1990.
38. Bradley MJ, Metreweli C: Ultrasound appearances of extramedullary hematopoiesis in the liver and spleen. Br J Radiol 63:816, 1990.
39. Numata K, et al: Flow characteristics of hepatic tumors at color Doppler sonography: Correlation with arteriographic findings. AJR Am J Roentgenol 160:515, 1993.
40. Wernecke K, et al: Pathologic explanation for hypoechoic halo seen in sonograms of malignant liver tumors: An in vitro correlative study. AJR Am J Roentgenol 159:1011, 1992.
41. Parker KJ, et al: Ultrasound contrast for hepatic tumors using IDE particles. Invest Radiol 25:1135, 1990.
42. Taylor JW, et al: Focal liver masses: Differential diagnosis with pulsed Doppler US. Radiology 164:643, 1987.
43. Lin Z-Y, et al: Duplex pulsed Doppler sonography in the differential diagnosis of hepatocellular carcinoma and other common hepatic tumors. Br J Radiol 65:202, 1992.
44. Behan M, et al: Perfluorooctylbromide as a contrast agent for CT and sonography: Preliminary clinical results. AJR Am J Roentgenol 160:399, 1993.
45. Matsuda Y, Yabuuchi I: Hepatic tumors: US contrast enhancement with CO_2 microbubbles. Radiology 161:701, 1986.
46. Ginaldi S, et al: Ultrasonographic patterns of hepatic lymphoma. Radiology 136:427, 1980.
47. Breznock EM, Whiting PG: *Textbook of Small Animal Surgery*. Philadelphia: WB Saunders, 1985, p. 1156.
48. Moon ML: Diagnostic imaging of portosystemic shunts. Semin Vet Med Surg (Small Anim) 5:120, 1990.
49. Nyland TG, Hager DA: Sonography of the liver, gallbladder, and spleen. Vet Clin North Am 15:1123, 1985.
50. Partington BP, et al: Transvenous coil embolization for treatment of patent ductus venosus in a dog. J Am Vet Med Assoc 202:281, 1993.
51. Bailey MQ, et al: Ultrasonographic findings associated with congenital hepatic arteriovenous fistula in three dogs. J Am Vet Med Assoc 192:1099, 1988.
52. Cohn LA, et al: Intrahepatic postsinusoidal venous obstruction in a dog. J Vet Intern Med 5:317, 1991.
53. Kantrowitz BM, Nyland TG, Fisher P: Estimation of portal blood flow using duplex real-time and pulsed Doppler ultrasound imaging in the dog. Vet Radiol 30:222, 1989.
54. Nyland TG, Fisher PE: Evaluation of experimentally induced canine hepatic cirrhosis using duplex Doppler ultrasound. Vet Radiol 31:189, 1990.
55. Turner MA: Diagnostic methods and pitfalls in the gallbladder. Semin Roentgenol 26:197, 1991.
56. Baron RL: Gallstone characterization: The role of imaging. Semin Roentgenol 26:216, 1991.
57. Carroll BA: Gallstones: In vitro comparison of physical, radiographic, and ultrasonic characteristics. AJR Am J Roentgenol 131:223, 1978.
58. Filly RA, Moss AA, Way LW: In vitro investigation of gallstone shadowing with ultrasound tomography. JCU 7:255, 1979.
59. Colhoun EN, Fitzgerald EJ, McKnight L: The importance of appropriate frequency selection in sonographic gallstone detection. Br J Radiol 60:645, 1987.

60. Jenkins CC, et al: Extrahepatic biliary obstruction association with Platynosomum concinnum in a cat. Compend Contin Educ Pract Vet *10:*628, 1988.

61. Hager DA: *Textbook of Veterinary Internal Medicine.* Philadelphia: WB Saunders, 1989, pp. 1555–1558.

62. Laing FC, London LA, Filly RA: Ultrasonographic identification of dilated intrahepatic bile ducts and their differentiation from portal venous structures. JCU *6:*90, 1978.

63. Wing VW, et al: Sonographic differentiation of enlarged hepatic arteries from dilated intrahepatic bile ducts. AJR Am J Roentgenol *145:*57, 1985.

64. Bressler EL, Rubin JM, McCracken S: Sonographic parallel channel sign: A reappraisal. Radiology *164:*343, 1987.

65. Finn ST, et al: Ultrasonographic assessment of sincalide-induced canine gallbladder emptying: An aid to the diagnosis of biliary obstruction. Vet Radiol *32:*269, 1991.

66. Huntington DK, Hill MC, Steinberg W: Biliary tract dilation in chronic pancreatitis: CT and sonographic findings. Radiology *172:*47, 1989.

67. Saverymuttu SH, et al: Gallbladder wall thickening (congestive cholecystopathy) in chronic liver disease: A sign of portal hypertension. Br J Radiol *63:*922, 1990.

68. Talarico HP, Rubens D: Gallbladder wall thickening in acute pyelonephritis. JCU *18:*653, 1990.

69. Teefey SA, Baron RL, Bigler SA: Sonography of the gallbladder: Significance of striated (layered) thickening of the gallbladder wall. AJR Am J Roentgenol *156:*945, 1991.

70. Nemcek AA, et al: The effervescent gallbladder: A sonographic sign of emphysematous cholecystitis. AJR Am J Roentgenol *150:*575, 1988.

71. Huang Y-S, et al: Utility of sonographic gallbladder wall patterns in differentiating malignant from cirrhotic ascites. JCU *17:*187, 1989.

72. Hager DA, Nyland TG, Fisher P: Ultrasound-guided biopsy of the canine liver, kidney, and prostate. Vet Radiol *26:*82, 1985.

73. Mladinich CR, et al: Evaluation and comparison of automated biopsy devices. Radiology *184:*845, 1992.

74. Selcer B, Cornelius LM: Percutaneous liver biopsy using the ultrasound guided Biopty instrument. Vet Med Report *1:*412, 1989.

75. Hoppe FE, et al: A comparison of manual and automatic ultrasound-guided biopsy techniques. Vet Radiol *27:*99, 1986.

76. Hopper KD, et al: Efficacy of automated biopsy guns versus conventional biopsy needles in the pygmy pig. Radiology *176:*671, 1990.

77. Bernardino ME: Automated biopsy devices: Significance and safety. Radiology *176:*615, 1990.

78. Grant EG, et al: Color Doppler imaging of portosystemic shunts. AJR Am J Roentgenol *154:*393, 1990.

79. Parvey HR, et al: Duplex sonography of the portal venous system: Pitfalls and limitation. AJR Am J Roentgenol *152:*765, 1989.

80. D'Arrigo JS, Ho S-Y, Simm RH: Detection of experimental rat liver tumors by contrast assisted ultrasonography. Invest Radiol *28:*218, 1993.

THE GASTROINTESTINAL TRACT

Judith A. Hudson and Mary B. Mahaffey

INDICATIONS

Sonography is a useful adjunct to abdominal radiography for evaluation of the gastrointestinal (GI) tract. It has been used to detect and evaluate foreign bodies,[1-3] tumors,[2,4-6] pyloric obstruction,[2] intussusceptions,[2,5,7,8] and enteric duplication.[9] Ultrasound-guided aspiration or biopsy can be performed if the lesion or wall thickening is sufficiently large.[10] Although ultrasonic examination cannot totally replace positive contrast examination of the GI tract, it may eliminate the need for an upper GI series in many patients, and sonography is less expensive and quicker to perform. Intraluminal contents, however, may limit the ability to evaluate the entire gastrointestinal wall. Gas may completely obscure the far wall of the stomach or intestine, and ingesta and fecal material can create artifacts that obscure the wall or mimic mural masses. Repeat sonographic evaluation or a GI series might be beneficial in these cases.

TECHNIQUE

A 5.0- or 7.5-mHz transducer can be used, but the higher resolution 7.5-mHz transducer is preferred when possible. Scanning should be done in both longitudinal and transverse planes. Luminal contents, wall thickness, and GI motility should be noted. In general, it is best to scan the GI tract after fasting and before enema administration to decrease the amount of intraluminal gas. In one study, however, no obvious differences in the quality of intestinal scans was found between dogs fasted for 12 hours and nonfasted dogs.[11] For evaluation of the stomach, much of the gas can be removed using an orogastric tube. The stomach is then distended with fluid to aid in visualization of the layers of the far wall.[4,11] Gas in intestinal loops located near the surface can be displaced by applying pressure with the probe. Another way to avoid gas is to place the probe on the dependent surface of the intestine.

Sonography can be performed on animals without delay after a barium GI series. Sonograms made after administration of barium have been shown to be similar or superior in quality to pre-barium sonograms.[12] Previous reports suggesting a deleterious effect of barium on the sonographic image[13] were based on the use of equipment that is now outdated. Also, the greater particulate nature of older barium suspensions may have played a role, perhaps by trapping more air than occurs with modern barium contrast

It is best to sample all regions of the gastrointestinal tract. A scanning protocol should be established to avoid omitting interrogation of any abdominal organ. In one protocol,

107

scanning begins in the region of the left kidney, left adrenal gland, and spleen with the patient in right lateral recumbency. The small intestine can be sampled in this region. The probe is moved caudally along the aorta to the aortic bifurcation and the urinary bladder where the descending colon and pelvic organs are investigated. The patient is moved to dorsal recumbency to allow further investigation of the pelvic organs and midabdomen, including additional small and large intestines. The probe can be moved cranially from the pelvic inlet along the descending colon, from left to right along the transverse colon, and caudally along the ascending colon to the ileum. The patient is moved to left lateral recumbency and the probe is moved cranially along the right side where the right kidney and adrenal gland are imaged. The probe is rotated medially from a plane that shows the right kidney. The duodenum is located in this region and can be followed caudally to the caudal duodenal flexure and cranially to the pylorus. The pancreas lies deep to the duodenum and pylorus. The examination concludes with investigation of the stomach, liver, and gallbladder, remembering to obtain both transverse and longitudinal images. The patient is repositioned as necessary. Regional lymph nodes, including the mesenteric lymph nodes, are investigated as each area of the abdomen is explored. The vascular supply is also evaluated when Doppler sonography is available.

Ultrasonic examination of adult horses can be made transabdominally using a 3.0-mHz probe for deeper structures and a 5.0-mHz probe for intestinal wall close to the body surface. The 5.0-mHz probe is also used for examination of foals. The sonographic appearance of gastrointestinal neoplasia and ileus in horses has been described.[14] Transrectal sonography can provide clear visualization of structures, including intestines, in the pelvic and caudal abdominal cavities.[15]

NORMAL APPEARANCE

The Oropharynx

The oropharynx is best examined by other methods because the presence of a large amount of air impedes sonographic examination. The retropharyngeal space can be examined, although the anatomy of this region has not been well described.

The Esophagus

The anatomy of the neck of dogs was described on the basis of sonographic findings from eight normal adult dogs. The esophagus was seen inconsistently as a poorly defined structure with a hyperechoic, stellate center representing intraluminal mucus and air. Identification of the esophagus is facilitated by movement of an esophageal stethoscope in an anesthetized dog and by observation of swallowing in a conscious dog (Fig. 9–1).[16]

Although not performed routinely in veterinary practice, endoscopic sonography with a high-resolution transducer[17,18] is being used in man for close inspection of the wall of the esophagus in addition to the gastrointestinal tract and the pancreas.[19] In man, the esophagus has a five-layered appearance similar to that seen with the stomach and intestines.[19] Use of this technique in animals might be valuable to further define the esophagus.

The Stomach and Small Intestine

The appearance of the stomach (Fig. 9–2) and small intestine (Fig. 9–3) of dogs is similar to that described for man.[17,20] Five layers of alternating hyperechoic and hypoechoic

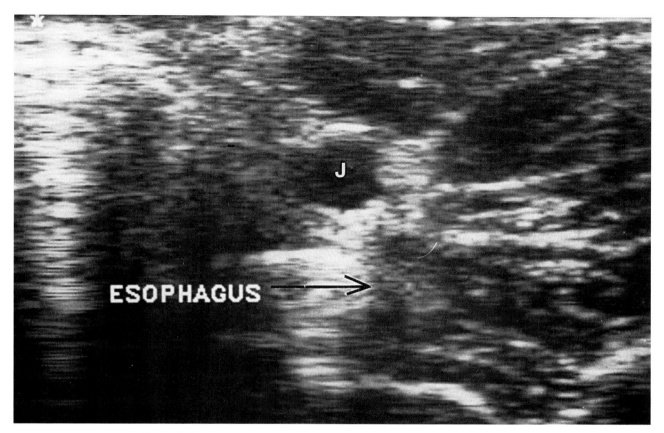

Figure 9–1

Transverse sonogram of the neck of a normal dog. The esophagus (arrow) appears as a small hyperechoic focus with a hypoechoic center. Identification was possible only by moving an esophageal stethoscope back and forth within the esophagus. J, jugular vein.

echoes include an inner hyperechoic layer, representing the mucosal surface, a central hyperechoic layer (the submucosa), and an outer hyperechoic layer (the subserosa and serosa). The inner hypoechoic layer is the mucosa and the outer hypoechoic layer is the muscularis propria.[11] In transverse images, the appearance may vary from a bull's eye with an echogenic center within a hypoechoic rim to identification of all five layers.[21] The difference in echogenicity is related to a larger amount of collagen or fat in the more echogenic layers. The thickness of each layer does not exactly equal the thickness of the corresponding histologic layer. The ultrasound image results from echoes created at an interface because of differences in acoustic impedance between layers and from echoes created by the internal structure of tissue layers.[17] The mucosal layer is the thickest layer, however, in both histologic sections[22] and sonograms. This characteristic is most noticeable in the small intestine.

Normal wall thickness depends on the degree of distention. The thickness of the stomach from the inner hyperechoic surface to the outer hyperechoic surface varies from 3.0 to 5.0 mm and may be greater in large breed dogs. The thickness of the small intestine varies from 2.0 to 3.0 mm (Fig. 9–4). Measurements of gastric wall thickness greater than 6.0 to 7.0 mm and of intestinal wall thickness greater than 5.0 mm are considered abnormal.[11]

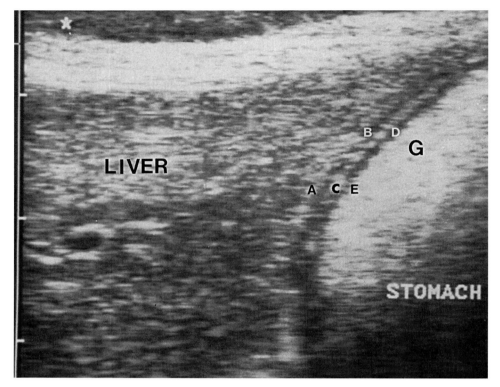

Figure 9–2

Sonogram of the gastric wall of a normal dog. The wall appears as five layers of alternating hyperechoic and hypoechoic echoes. From the outer hyperechoic layer to the inner hyperechoic layers, the layers are: serosa (hyperechoic), muscularis propria (hypoechoic), submucosa (hyperechoic), mucosa (hypoechoic), and mucosal surface (hyperechoic). The hyperechoic mucosal surface blends with hyperechoic gas in the gastric lumen. Compare the appearance of the normal gastric wall to that of the small intestine in Figure 9–3. A, serosa; B, muscularis propria; C, submucosa; D, mucosa; E, mucosal surface; G, gas in the gastric lumen.

Figure 9–3

Sagittal sonogram of the small intestinal wall of a normal dog. Compare the appearance of the normal intestinal wall to that of the stomach (see Fig. 9–2). The mucosal layer of the intestinal wall is thicker than the other layers of the wall.

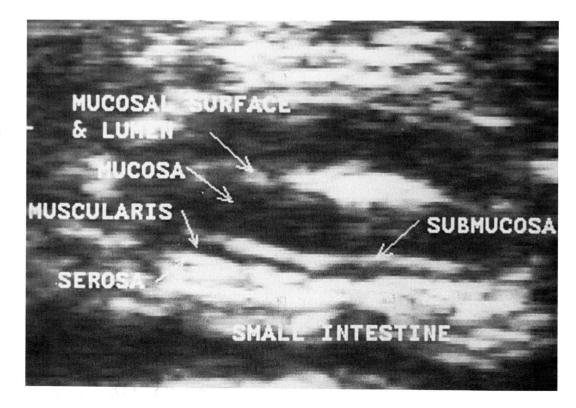

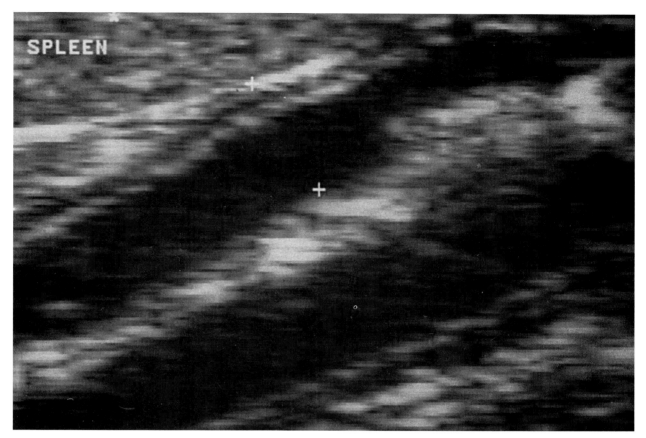

Figure 9–4

Sagittal sonogram of the small intestinal wall of a normal dog. The intestine is deep to the spleen. Calipers measure the near wall of the small intestine from the serosa to the mucosal surface.

Normal luminal contents include mucus, gas, and fluid. Mucus is echogenic without acoustic shadowing (Fig. 9–5). Gas is hyperechoic with distal acoustic shadowing or ring down artifact (Figs. 9–6 and 9–7).[2] The acoustic shadow deep to gas has been described as "dirty" because reverberations between the transducer and gas appear as artifactual lines within the shadow.[1,23] Intraluminal fluid is anechoic (Fig. 9–8).[11] In one study, mucus or fluid allowed visualization of the mucosa and muscularis propria as hypoechoic layers but gas impeded scanning, causing the wall to appear hyperechoic.[11] Water can be administered through an orogastric tube to improve imaging of the gastric wall.[11] An empty stomach has a star-shaped appearance with gastric fluid between rugal folds appearing hyperechoic (Fig. 9–9).

Gastrointestinal motility can be evaluated using ultrasound. The normal peristaltic contraction rate in the stomach and proximal duodenum of normal dogs is four to five contractions per minute. In small intestine in the central abdomen, the rate is one to three per minute. When water is given by orogastric tube into the stomach, the peristaltic rate in the stomach and proximal duodenum increases by approximately one contraction per minute. Any change in the rate in the central small intestine is minimal.[11]

The Large Intestine

The colon is usually hyperechoic with no through transmission[24] because of the presence of a large amount of gas (Fig. 9–10). The wall of the colon has a layered appearance similar to that of the stomach and small intestine, but large amounts of intraluminal gas may prevent accurate measurement. When measurable, the thickness of the colon is between 2.0 and 3.0 mm. The mucosal layer of the colon is not as thick as that of the stomach and small intestine.[22] Contractions may not be seen in the descending colon.[11]

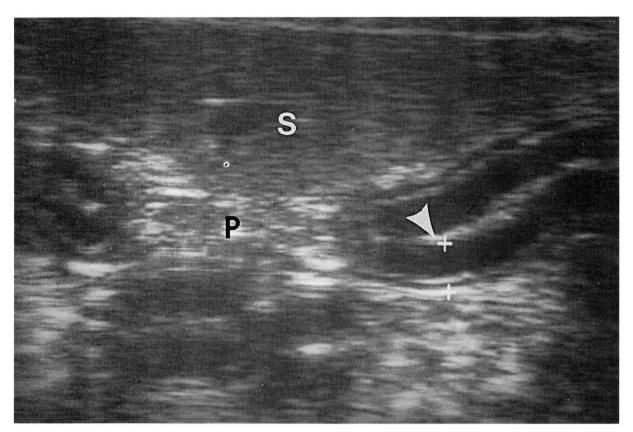

Figure 9–5

Sagittal sonogram of the small intestine of a normal dog scanned on the left side of the abdomen deep to the spleen (S). Calipers measure the far wall of the intestine from the mucosal surface to the serosa. Note the peristaltic wave (P) proximal to the measured area of small intestine. Mucus within the lumen (arrowhead) is hyperechoic without acoustic shadowing, allowing visualization of the layers of the far bowel wall.

Figure 9–6

Sagittal sonogram of the duodenum of a normal dog, scanned lateral to the right limb of the pancreas. Intraluminal gas is hyperechoic with a "dirty" acoustic shadow, causing a loss of visualization of the far wall of the intestine. P, pancreas; V, pancreaticoduodenal vein; G, intraluminal gas; S, acoustic shadow caused by intraluminal gas.

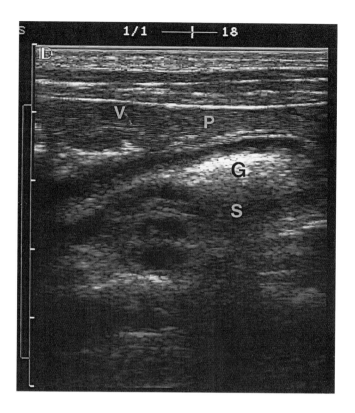

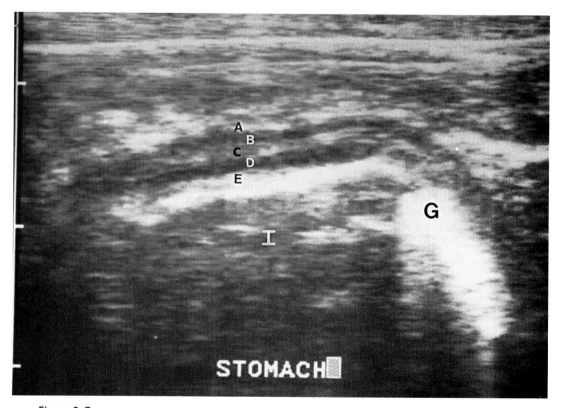

Figure 9–7

Sonogram of a normal full stomach of a dog. A, serosa; B, muscularis propria; C, submucosa; D, mucosa; E, mucosal surface; I, ingesta; G, gas.

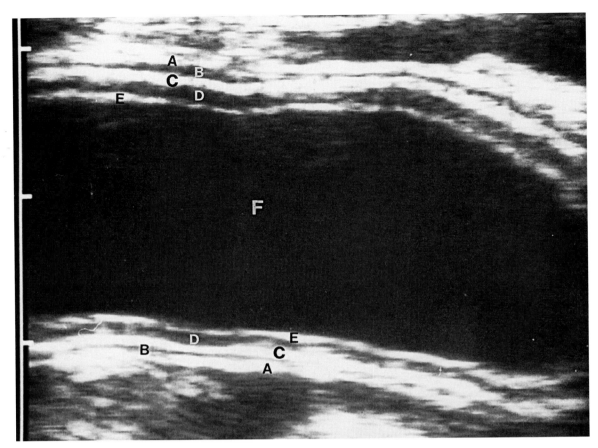

Figure 9–8

Sagittal sonogram of a dilated loop of small intestine in a dog with peritoneal effusion. Intraluminal fluid (F) is anechoic. Note the alternating hyperechoic and hypoechoic layers of the intestinal wall. A, serosa; B, muscularis propria; C, submucosa; D, mucosa; E, mucosal surface.

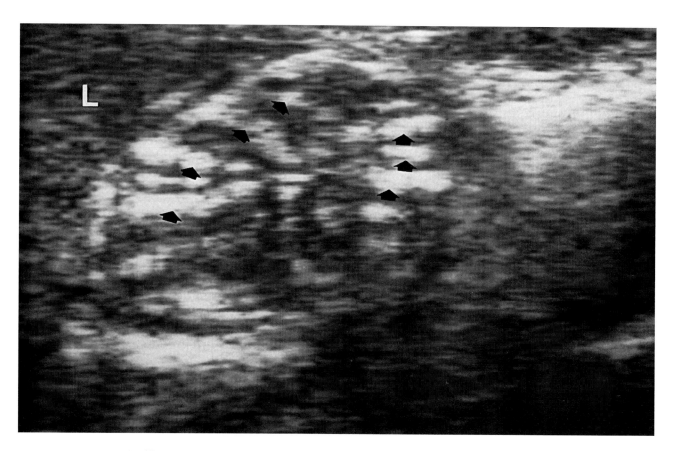

Figure 9-9

Sonogram of the empty stomach of a normal dog. Normal hyperechoic gastric fluids (arrows) between rugal folds gives the stomach a stellate appearance. Compare with the appearance of a full stomach in Figure 9-7. L, liver.

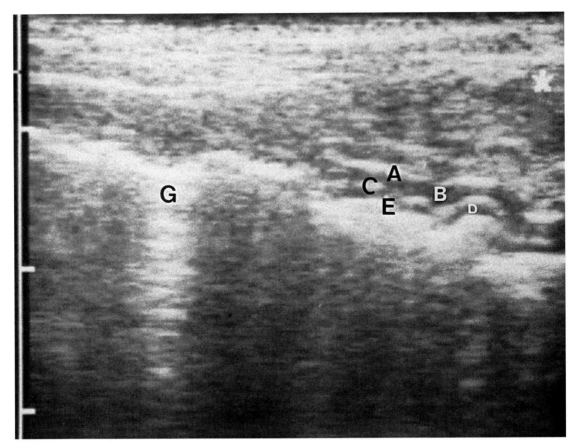

Figure 9–10

Sagittal sonogram of a normal canine colon. Note that the colonic wall has a layered appearance similar to that of the stomach and small intestine, but the mucosal layer is not disproportionately thick. A, serosa; B, muscularis propria; C, submucosa; D, mucosa; E, mucosal surface; G, gas causing a "dirty" acoustic shadow and loss of visualization of structures deep to the colon.

DISEASE PROCESSES

Foreign Body

Sonography can be used to identify or remove foreign bodies in the retropharyngeal region. A piece of wire in the retropharyngeal region of a Quarter horse mare was identified radiographically but intraoperative ultrasound was useful to guide surgical dissection and removal of the wire.[25]

The appearance of gastrointestinal foreign bodies varies with the composition of the object and its ability to transmit or attenuate sound (Fig. 9–11). A reflective near interface might cause a hyperechoic near border with deep acoustic shadowing, as has been seen with rocks, a sewing needle, an acorn, and some rubber balls.[1,2] The shape of the near interface (semicircular with a rubber ball, straight with a sewing needle) might aid in identification of the object. Other objects, such as a rubber toy, might attenuate sound with minimal reflection, causing acoustic shadowing but no hyperechoic near border. Others foreign bodies transmit sufficient sound to allow visualization of their shape. A rubber ball might appear as a homogeneous, circular echodensity or as a hyperechoic circular object with an anechoic center. The curved margins of fragment of a tennis ball caused refraction and reflection of the ultrasound beam, resulting in edge shadowing.[1] The presence of intraluminal fluid can help determine the shape of a foreign body.[2] Fluid can be administered if sufficient intraluminal fluid is not present.[1]

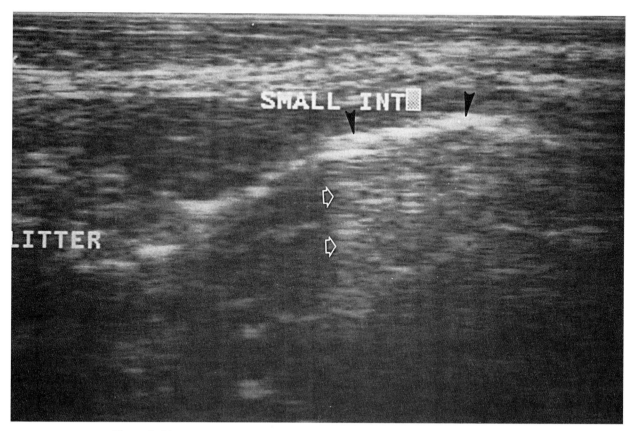

Figure 9–11

Sagittal sonogram of foreign material (cat litter) within the small bowel of the cat. The cat litter shows as an echogenic mass (LITTER) distending a segment of small intestine. Intraluminal gas (arrowheads) with a "dirty" acoustic shadow (arrows) is seen within normal bowel located more distally.

The character of acoustic shadowing can help identify a foreign body. A "clean" or crisp complete shadow is more likely to occur with a soft tissue-bone interface or a soft tissue-foreign body interface. A "dirty" shadow may be caused by reverberations between the transducer and intraluminal gas.[1]

Foreign objects can lead to obstruction of the gastrointestinal tract and mechanical ileus. Distention of the stomach or intestine with decreased or absent motility might be seen proximal to the obstruction.[1,2] Hyperperistalsis and intestinal plication have been reported with linear foreign bodies.[1] In some cases, obstruction is accompanied by findings related to other organs, including pancreatitis with enlargement of the pancreas, free peritoneal fluid, and enlarged mesenteric lymph nodes.[1]

Neoplasia

Abnormalities found using operative sonography to investigate gastric neoplasia in man include thickening of the gastric wall, altered echogenicity, and destruction of the normal layers of the gastric wall. Most neoplasms were hypoechoic but some were hyperechoic. The muscularis propria and subserosa-serosal layer were preserved in early neoplasia, whereas all layers were involved in advanced neoplasia.[20]

Similar findings have been reported in a series of dogs with gastric neoplasia. Wall thickening was described as symmetric or asymmetric and localized or generalized. Although parameters for wall thickening did not allow distinction between neoplasia and inflammation, disruption of wall layers is more likely with neoplasia.[2] A gastric leiomyoma in one dog and a gastric leiomyosarcoma in another resulted in disruption of wall layers at the site of each mass, although wall layers were identifiable in adjacent areas. Only the mucosal layers appeared intact when the masses were scanned in a water bath after surgical removal.[2] Gastric adenocarcinoma in a Tibetan terrier caused thickening of the gastric wall with a loss of visualization of normal wall layers (Fig. 9–12). A hyperechoic or complex mass may be found in some cases (Fig. 9–13).

Intestinal masses also show thickening and disruption of wall layers. In one study, feline intestinal lymphosarcoma caused segmental thickening of the intestinal wall with loss of visualization of discrete wall layers. Only one equivocal intestinal adenocarcinoma showed preservation of wall layers with thickening of just the muscularis propria. Diagnosis of neoplasia in this cat was based on lymph node histopathology, but histopathologic analysis of the intestinal wall revealed idiopathic muscular hyperplasia.[2] Figure 9–14 illustrates a sonogram of a midventral abdominal mass in a 7-year-old Labrador Retriever. The mass appeared to be within or associated with the intestine and on the basis of the histopathologic findings was identified as a papillary adenocarcinoma in the jejunal mucosa with extension through the muscular tunic to the serosa and mesentery. Mineralization can occur within intestinal neoplasms (Figs. 9–15 and 9–16). Destruction of wall layers may be incomplete (Fig. 9–15) or complete (Fig. 9–17). Mesenteric lymphadenopathy can be an indication of metastasis (Fig. 9–18).

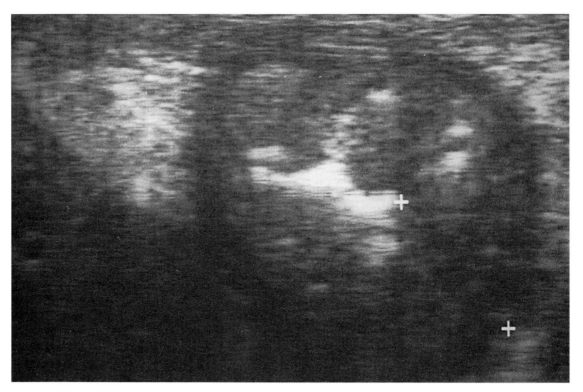

Figure 9–12

Sonogram of the empty stomach of a Tibetan terrier with gastric adenocarcinoma. The gastric wall is thickened, measuring 10.6 mm in this scan. Layers of the gastric wall cannot be distinguished.

Ulceration can occur with neoplasia but may be present also in conjunction with inflammatory conditions. Ulcers are typically hyperechoic because of gas trapped at the site of the ulcer crater. Ileus associated with neoplasia may be recognized by the presence of decreased motility and increased fluid and mucus retention.[2]

Carcinomatosis has been described in horses resulting from gastric squamous cell carcinoma and colonic adenocarcinoma. Ultrasonic examination can locate the primary neoplasm and demonstrate tumor implants on the serosal surfaces of other organs.[14] Figure 9–19 shows a sonogram of a large, mixed echogenic mass in the mid- and caudal abdomen of a cat. Multiple, small hypoechoic areas within the mass represent intestinal loops incorporated within the mass. Histopathologic analysis confirmed carcinomatosis.

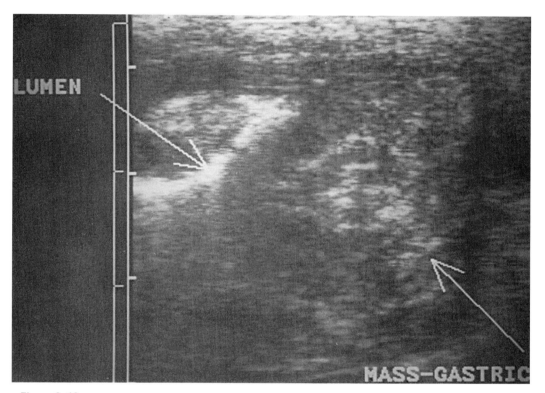

Figure 9–13

Sonogram of the stomach of a 6-year-old spayed female Basset hound with a complex mass in the gastric wall of the pyloric area of the stomach. Note the hyperechoic change in the gastric wall and loss of visualization of normal layers. Biopsy of the mass during exploratory laparotomy confirmed the presence of gastric adenocarcinoma.

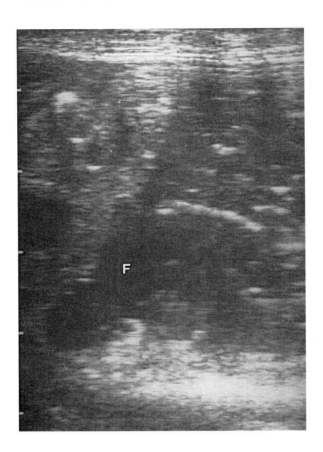

Figure 9–14

Sagittal sonogram of a jejunal papillary adenocarcinoma in a 7-year-old Labrador Retriever. No normal intestinal architecture can be recognized. The mass is complex with areas of mixed echogenicity. Anechoic areas may have represented fluid within the lumen or fluid pockets within the wall. The mass appeared to arise from the mucosa with extension through the muscular tunic to the serosa and mesentery. Mesenteric lymphadenopathy also was present. F, fluid.

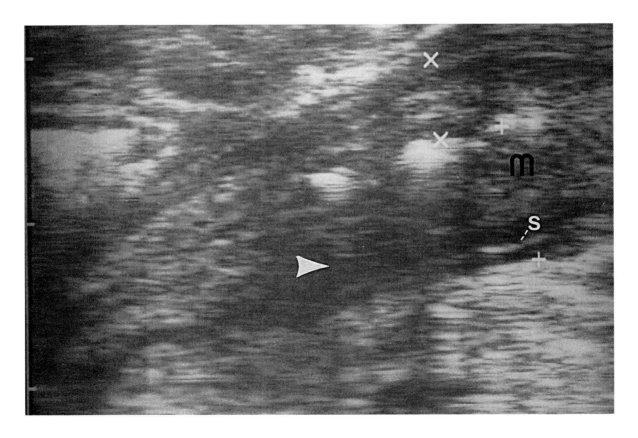

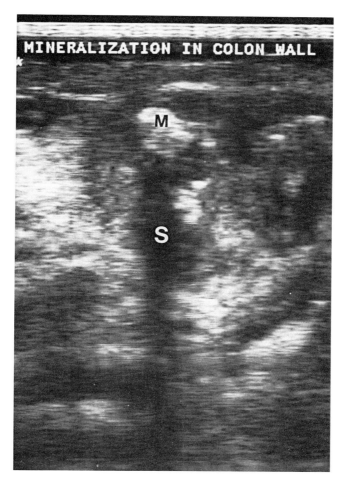

Figure 9–16

Sonogram of the colon of the same Yorkshire terrier as in Figure 9–15. Note the disruption of wall layers. A clean acoustic shadow deep to a hyperechoic area in the mucosa represents mineralization. M, mineralization in colonic wall; S, acoustic shadow.

Figure 9–15

Sonogram of the colon of a 10-year-old intact male Yorkshire terrier that had diarrhea and weight loss for 3 to 4 months. Calipers measure the near and far walls from the serosa to the mucosal surface. The colonic wall is thickened, measuring 8.4 mm in some areas. Nodular hyperechoic change is evident in the mucosa. Clean acoustic shadowing is noted in some areas, suggesting mineralization. Normal wall layering is apparent in some areas. Complete destruction of the internal architecture of the wall was present in only a few areas. S, submucosa; M, mucosa with hyperechoic change; arrowhead, small acoustic shadow.

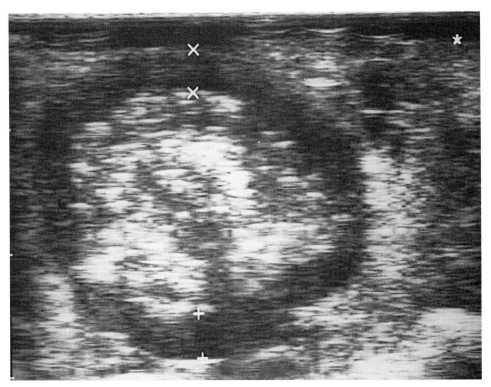

Figure 9–17

Transverse sonogram of the colon of a castrated male cat with alimentary lymphosarcoma. The colonic wall is thickened with loss of visualization of normal wall layering. Calipers measure the thickness of the near and far walls. Fecal material is present within the lumen.

Figure 9–18

Sagittal sonogram of mesenteric lymphadenopathy in a dog with an intestinal mass. Calipers measure the length of two mesenteric lymph nodes. Loss of wall layering was incomplete in this scan but complete in others. A, serosa; B, muscularis propria; C, submucosa; D, mucosa; E, mucosal surface; arrows, enlarged mesenteric lymph nodes.

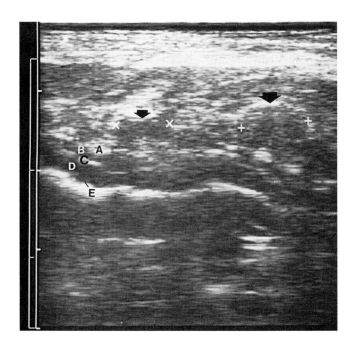

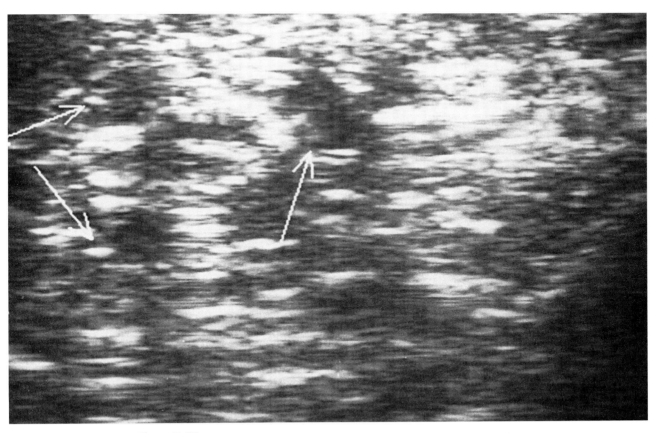

Figure 9–19

Sonogram of a large, mixed echogenic mass in the mid- and caudal abdomen of a 7-year-old spayed female cat with carcinomatosis. Multiple, small hypoechoic areas (arrows) are seen within the mass. The hypoechoic areas may represent small masses or loops of bowel incorporated within the mass. The appearance suggests carcinomatosis, peritonitis, or a large abdominal mass incorporating loops of bowel.

Ileus

Ileus, which is a lack of movement of intestinal contents, is categorized as focal or generalized, depending on the proportion of small intestine involved.[26] The degree of intestinal dilatation is variable. Radiographically, ileus is classified as mild when the intestinal diameter is approximately three to four times the width of a rib and extensive when the diameter is five to six rib widths.[26] Mechanical (dynamic, obstructive) ileus occurs when the lumen is obstructed by such things as a mass, foreign body, or intussusception.[27] Functional (adynamic, paralytic) ileus occurs when the neuromuscular functioning of the intestine is disturbed (Figs. 9–8 and 9–20). Functional ileus can be related to mechanical ileus or it can occur in diverse circumstances such as in neoplasia and after trauma.[27]

Sonography can be used easily to evaluate gastrointestinal motility. Decreased motility is often attended by increased fluid and mucus within the lumen.[2] Ileus has been recognized using sonography in man with diseases such as gastrointestinal foreign body, neoplasia, pancreatitis, and parvovirus enteritis.[2]

Figure 9–20

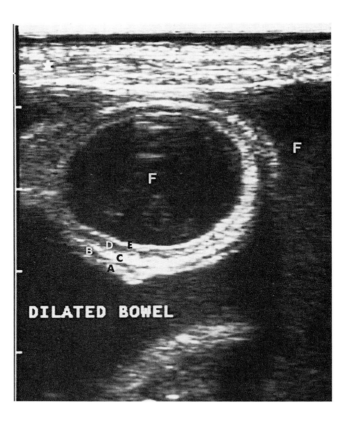

Transverse sonogram of a dilated loop of small intestine in a dog with peritoneal effusion. A sagittal image is shown in Figure 9–8. Intraluminal and extraluminal fluid (F) is anechoic. Note the alternating hyperechoic and hypoechoic layers of the intestinal wall. A, serosa; B, muscularis propria; C, submucosa; D, mucosa; E, mucosal surface.

Intussusception

Intussusception occurs when a portion of intestine invaginates into an adjacent segment. The invaginated segment is the intussusceptum and the receiving segment is the intussuscipiens.[27] Intussusception characteristically shows as multiple concentric rings surrounding an echogenic core in transverse images (Fig. 9–21) and as multiple layers in longitudinal images (Fig. 9–22).[2,5,7,8] Duodenojejunal intussusception in two dogs was seen in transverse scans as two concentric hypoechoic rings surrounding a hyperechoic center.[5,7] In longitudinal sonograms, alternating parallel hyperechoic and hypoechoic lines were noted.[5,7] Three patterns were seen in transverse sonograms of three foals with intussusception.[28] Scans made through the apex of the intussusception showed a target-like pattern with a sonolucent center. A thick hypoechoic rim was attributed to severe edema of the inner and outer walls of the intussusceptum. In a second pattern seen more proximally, edema was less severe, allowing recognition of two concentric rings (representing the inner and outer walls of the intussusceptum) in addition to the inner hypoechoic circular area. The third pattern was similar, with double hypoechoic concentric rings but with a hyperechoic center. The variation in pattern was attributed to the degree of edema, luminal fluid content, and scanning location. A sonolucent center reflected the presence of fluid in the lumen of the intussuscipiens. The intussusceptum was hyperechoic. In longitudinal sonograms, two hyperechoic areas alternating with three hypoechoic areas were described.[28]

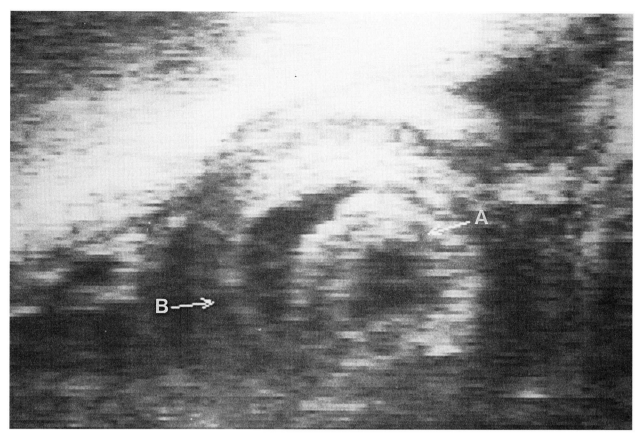

Figure 9–21

Transverse sonogram of bowel of a dog with gas-filled dilated loops of small intestine seen on radiographs. A segment of small intestine contains an intussuscepted loop of bowel. The intussusceptum (intussuscepted loop) appears as two hyperechoic concentric rings with a hypoechoic center. The concentric rings represent the inner and outer walls of the intussusceptum. Jejunal intussusception was confirmed during exploratory surgery. The dog was discharged after resection of the involved area of intestine and anastomosis of healthy intestine. A, intussusceptum; B, intussuscipiens.

A "target" or "bull's eye" appearance is seen also in transverse sonograms of intussusception in man. Hypoechoic, edematous intestinal wall alternates with hyperechoic mucosa in which trapped air bubbles may contribute to increased echogenicity. Longitudinal sonograms of intussuscepted bowel can resemble sonograms of a kidney, so the appearance in longitudinal section has been called a "pseudokidney".[29] Variations in the appearance of transverse sonograms occur because of the plane of scanning, degree of edema, and nature of the invaginated contents. Invaginated mesentery at the proximal aspect of the intussusception appears as a larger central hyperechoic area. An enlarged lymph node in this area can appear as a hypoechoic nodule within the hyperechoic center.[30]

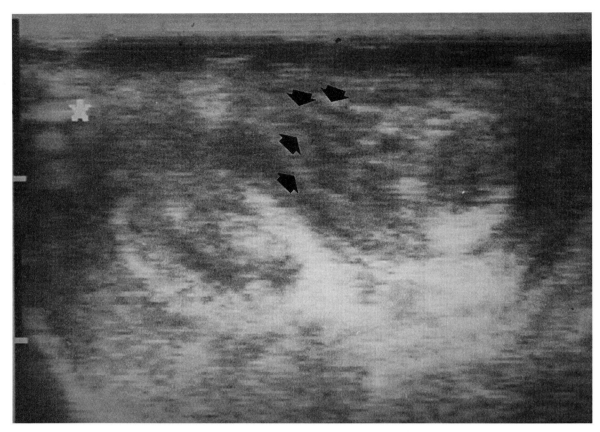

Figure 9-22

Sagittal sonogram of the jejunal intussusception in Figure 9–21. Arrows, multiple layers of an intussuscepted loop.

Inflammation

Inflammation can be accompanied by normal or increased wall thickness. The intestine in a dog with parvovirus enteritis exhibited normal wall thickness, fluid distention, and a lack of motility. Gastritis in another dog was accompanied by diffuse thickening of the gastric wall with localized ulceration. Normal wall layers are generally preserved with nonfungal inflammation, unlike with neoplasia (Fig. 9–23).[2] Exocrine pancreatic insufficiency can be accompanied by thickening of intestinal wall with preservation of normal wall layers. Corrugation (spasticity) and increased echogenicity can occur but they are nonspecific findings (Fig. 9–24). Acute hemorrhagic pancreatitis can result in hemorrhage in adjacent intestine with loss of the normal layered appearance.[2] Fungal enteritis in dogs may involve only the mucosa or all wall layers. Involved organisms include Candida albicans, Histoplasma capsulatum, Aspergilla, and Phycomycetes. Dramatic thickening of bowel wall may occur diffusely or involving specific segments. The normal wall architecture may be replaced by a thick homogeneous wall with increased echogenicity. Mesenteric, gastric, and colic lymph nodes may be enlarged. Phycomycetes

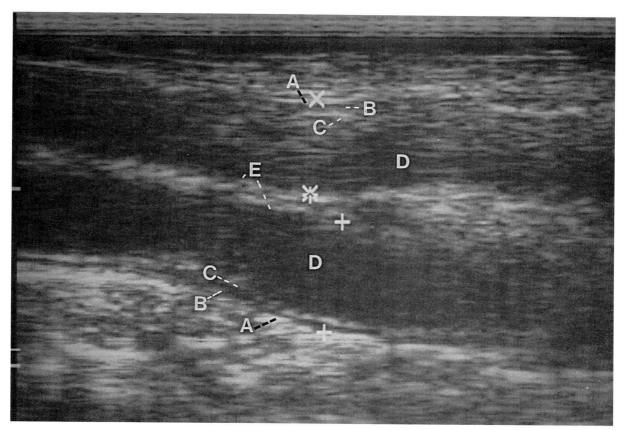

Figure 9–23

Sagittal sonogram of a dog with a 2-year history of diarrhea. Echogenicity of the mucosal layer of the small intestinal wall is increased. Numerous loops are thickened (5.5 to 6.8 mm). Wall layers remain visible. Peristalsis occurred with a back-and-forth motion instead of the usual aboral progression. Histopathologic analysis showed edema and mild diffuse infiltration of the lamina propria with lymphocytes and plasma cells. Lymphangiectasia was present. A, serosa; B, muscularis propria; C, submucosa; D, mucosa; E, mucosal surface.

(Figs. 9–25 and 9–26) may cause a palpable abdominal mass requiring differentiation from intussusception or foreign body obstruction.[31] Feline infectious peritonitis is a pyogranulomatous disease that produces similar changes in intestines of cats (Fig. 9–27). Concurrent increased echogenicity of the kidney and renal capsule (Fig. 9–28) increases suspicion of this disorder (Finn-Bodner ST, personal communication). Adhesions of the bowel have been diagnosed in horses suffering from intermittent bouts of colic. Examination for a significant length of time showed no independent movement of involved segments of the intestine. Ileus was not always present.[15]

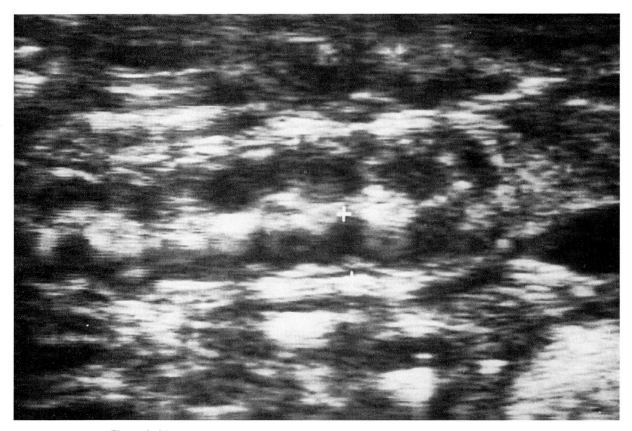

Figure 9–24

Sagittal sonogram of a loop of small intestine of a 6-month-old female Schnauzer with retarded growth and anorexia caused by exocrine pancreatic insufficiency. Multiple areas of small bowel appeared thickened with hyperechoic change in the mucosal layer. The wall of the intestinal loop has a corrugated appearance, which was noted throughout the examination. Calipers measure wall thickness, which is normal.

Figure 9–25

Transverse sonogram of the small intestine of a dog with granulomatous enteritis caused by Pythium. A large hetero-echoic mass involves the small intestine in the mid-abdomen. The intestinal wall was thickened, up to 2.1 cm, and showed disruption of wall layers. Calipers measure wall thickness, which was 11.4 mm in this sonogram. Histopathologic analysis showed that the mucosa, submucosa, and muscularis propria contained confluent granulomas. Gridley's fungal stain revealed many hyphae within the granulomas.

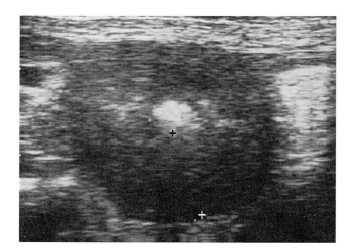

Figure 9–26

Sagittal sonogram of the small intestine of the dog in Figure 9–25. Reverberation (arrows) from gas in the bowel lumen can be seen in the central portion of the granulomatous mass involving the small intestine. G, gas in intestinal lumen.

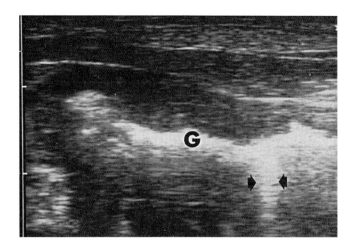

Figure 9–27

Transverse sonogram of the small intestine of a cat with feline infectious peritonitis (FIP). Calipers measure the thickness of the intestinal wall. The complete loss of the normal layering pattern indicates infiltrative disease (such as neoplasia, mycosis, FIP). Both kidneys appeared enlarged with thickened, hyperechoic cortices and increased capsular echogenicity (see Figure 9–28).

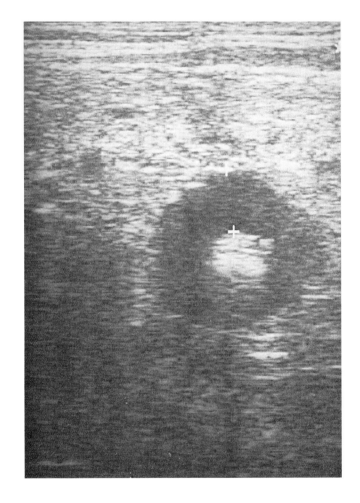

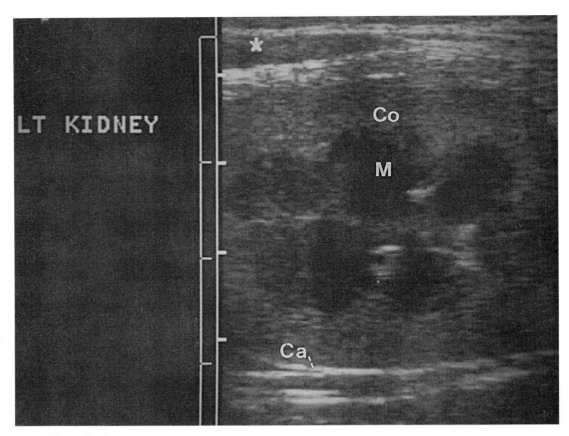

Figure 9–28

Lateral sagittal image of the left kidney of the cat pictured in Figure 9–27. Note the enlargement of the kidney with increased echogenicity of the cortex and capsule. Co, cortex; M, medulla; Ca, capsule.

Mesenteric Vascular Disease

The technique and results of transrectal sonography have been described for evaluation of the cranial mesenteric artery in normal horses and horses with verminous arteritis.[32,33] The sensitivity for the detection of normal arteries was 90% and the specificity of detection of abnormal arteries was 86%. In man, endoscopic sonography using prototype Doppler 5- and 10-mHz transducers was performed to record flow velocities in vessels within and surrounding the gastrointestinal tract.[34] Use of color flow Doppler imaging and Doppler spectral analysis, when available, during routine abdominal sonography will allow the eventual use of these techniques to gain information regarding gastrointestinal vascularity.

Displacement of Bowel

Sonography can help to identify placement of abdominal organs. For example, cranial or caudal displacement of the gastrointestinal tract could indicate microhepatic or hepatic enlargement, respectively. Diaphragmatic herniations are recognized by following the cranial edge of the liver and diaphragm from side to side, although some minimal herniations are difficult to appreciate. Inguinal hernias have a "tornado" appearance. Loops of bowel can be followed to the hernial contents if intestinal herniation has occurred (Fig. 9–29). The appearance of congenital peritoneopericardial herniation has been described.[35,36] Observation of the beating heart adjacent to the cranial aspect of the liver and diaphragmatic discontinuity is diagnostic (Figs. 9–30 to 9–32).[35,36]

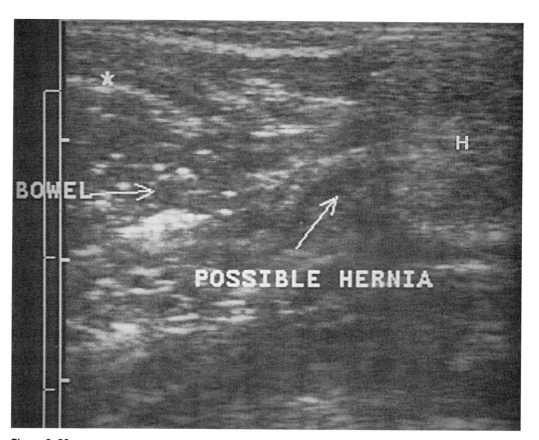

Figure 9–29

Sagittal sonogram of a male dog with suspected inguinal herniation. Bowel could be followed to an area of disruption of the abdominal wall (POSSIBLE HERNIA). Inguinal herniation of the distal jejunum was confirmed at surgery. Note the "tornado" appearance where the intestine passes through the abdominal wall. H, herniated loop of small intestine.

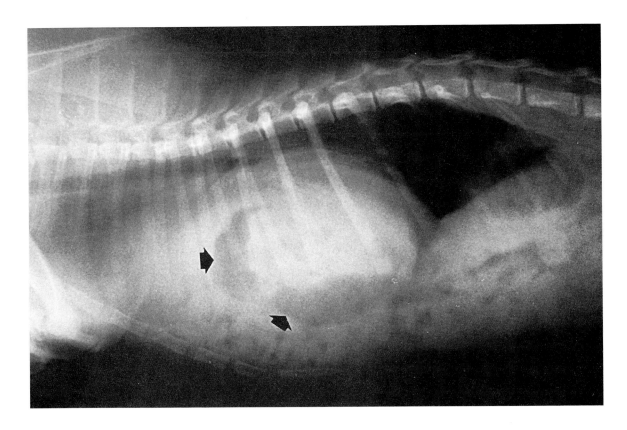

Figure 9–31

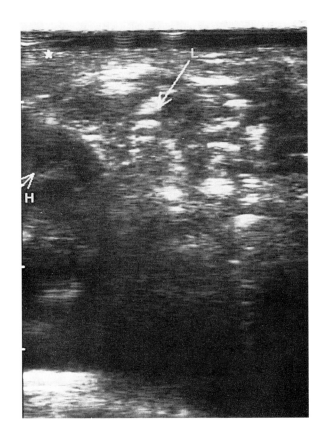

Sagittal sonogram of the left thorax of the cat in Figures 9–30 and 9–32. L indicates a loop of small intestine. Wall layering is normal. H indicates the heart. Real-time images are interpreted more easily than static images because peristaltic waves and cardiac motion allow better identification of the intestine and heart, respectively.

Figure 9–30

Lateral radiograph of a cat with a peritoneopericardial herniation. A dilated loop of small intestine (arrows) is located within the pericardial sac. Multiple other loops are seen ventrally. Congenital peritoneopericardial herniation with torsion of a herniated loop of small intestine was confirmed at surgery.

Figure 9–32

Sagittal sonogram of the right thorax of the cat in Figures 9–30 and 9–31. Liver (L) is visualized in the pericardial sac. As noted in Figure 9–31, cardiac motion during real-time sonography allows easier identification of the heart (H) than is possible when viewing still images. R, acoustic shadow deep to a rib.

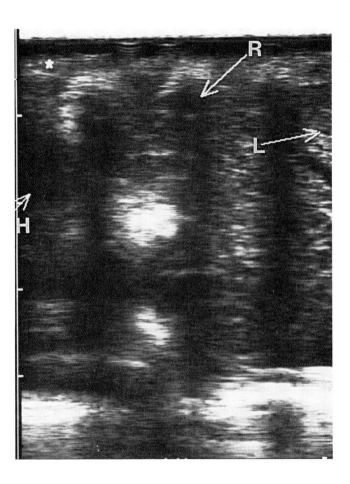

Congenital Anomalies

The sonographic appearance of enteric duplication in two dogs was reported.[9] Enteric duplication is a rare anomaly involving a cyst-like formation adjacent to a bowel segment. These structures share a common wall, and the muscular layer of the free wall of the cyst and the bowel are continuous. The cyst may contain hypoechoic fluid. Three of the five layers of intestinal wall may be identified sonographically in the free wall of the cyst.

REFERENCES

1. Tidwell AS, Penninck DG: Ultrasonography of gastrointestinal foreign bodies. Vet Radiol Ultrasound *33*:160, 1992.
2. Penninck DG, et al: Ultrasonographic evaluation of gastrointestinal diseases in small animals. Vet Radiol *31*:134, 1990.
3. Spaulding KA, et al: Veterinary case of the day. J Ultrasound Med *9*:S103, 1990.
4. Lamb CR: Abdominal ultrasonography in small animals: Intestinal tract and mesentery, kidneys, adrenal glands, uterus, and prostate. J Small Anim Pract *31*:295, 1990.

5. Watson DE, Mahaffey MB, Neuwirth LA: Ultrasonographic detection of duodenojejunal intussusception in a dog. J Am Anim Hosp Assoc 27:367, 1991.

6. Nyland TG, et al: Gray-scale ultrasonography of the canine abdomen. Vet Radiol 22:220, 1981.

7. Kantrowicz B, et al: Ultrasonographic detection of jejunal intussusception and acute renal failure due to ethylene glycol toxicity in a dog. J Am Anim Hosp Assoc 24:697, 1987.

8. Kleine LJ, Lamb CR: Comparative organ imaging: The gastrointestinal tract. Vet Radiol 30:133, 1989.

9. Spaulding KA, et al: Enteric duplication in two dogs. Vet Radiol 31:83, 1990.

10. Saunders HM, Pugh CR, Rhodes WH: Expanding applications of abdominal ultrasonography. J Am Anim Hosp Assoc 28:369, 1992.

11. Penninck DG, et al: Ultrasonography of the normal canine gastrointestinal tract. Vet Radiol 30:272, 1989.

12. Elam EA, et al: The lack of sonographic image degradation after barium upper gastrointestinal examination. AJR Am J Roentgenol 153:993, 1989.

13. Leopold GR, Asher WM: Deleterious effects of gastrointestinal contrast material on abdominal echography. Radiology 98:637, 1971.

14. Rantanen NW: Diseases of the abdomen: Diagnostic ultrasound. Vet Clin North Am Equine Pract 2:67, 1986.

15. Schmidt AR: Transrectal ultrasonography of the caudal portion of abdominal and pelvic cavities in horses. J Am Vet Med Assoc 194:365, 1989.

16. Wisner ER, et al: Normal ultrasonographic anatomy of the canine neck. Vet Radiol 32:185, 1991.

17. Kimmey MB, et al: Histologic correlates of gastrointestinal ultrasound images. Gastroenterology 96:433, 1989.

18. Kimmey MB, Martin RW, Silverstein FE: Endoscopic ultrasound probes. (Review). Gastrointest Endosc 36:S40, 1990.

19. Botet JF, Lightdale C: Endoscopic ultrasonography of the upper gastrointestinal tract. Radiol Clin North Am 30:1067, 1992.

20. Machi J, et al: Normal stomach wall and gastric cancer: Evaluation with high-resolution operative ultrasound. Radiology 159:85, 1986.

21. Wilson SR: *The gastrointestinal tract.* In *Diagnostic Ultrasound,* Vol 1. Edited by CM Rumack, SR Wilson, JW Charboneau. St Louis: Mosby Year Book, 1991.

22. Trautman A, Fiebiger J: *Fundamentals of the Histology of Domestic Animals.* Ithaca: Comstock Publishing Associates, 1952, p. 200.

23. Laing FC: Commonly encountered artifacts in clinical ultrasound. Semin Ultrasound 4:27, 1983.

24. Cartee RE, Hudson JA, Finn-Bodner S: Ultrasonography. Vet Clin North Am Small Anim Pract 23:345, 1993.

25. French DA, Pharr JW, Fretz PB: Removal of a retropharyngeal foreign body in a horse, with the aid of ultrasonography during surgery. J Am Vet Med Assoc 194:1315, 1989.

26. McNeel SV: *The small bowel.* In *Textbook of Veterinary Radiology.* Edited by DE Thrall. Philadelphia: WB Saunders, 1986, pp. 493–510.

27. O'Brien TR: *Radiographic Diagnosis of Abdominal Disorders in the Dog and Cat.* Davis, CA, Covell Park Vet Co., 1981, pp. 302–311.

28. Bernard WV, et al: Ultrasonographic diagnosis of small-intestinal intussusception in three foals. J Am Vet Med Assoc 194:395, 1989.

29. Restrepo R, Merritt CRB: The pediatric abdomen: Intussusception. Applied Radiol 19:26, 1990.

30. Skaane P, Skjennald A: Ultrasonic features of ileocecal intussusception. JCU 17:590, 1989.

31. Chiapella AM: *Diseases of the small intestine: Mycotic diseases.* In Morgan RV. *Handbook of Small Animal Practice.* Edited by RV Morgan. New York: Churchill Livingstone, 1988, pp. 402–403.

32. Wallace KD, Selcer BA, Becht JL: Technique for transrectal ultrasonography of the cranial mesenteric artery of the horse. Am J Vet Res 50:1695, 1989.

33. Wallace KD, et al: Transrectal ultrasonography of the cranial mesenteric artery of the horse. Am J Vet Res 50:1699, 1989.

34. Matre K, Odegaard S, Hausken T: Endoscopic ultrasound Doppler probes for velocity measurements in vessels in the upper gastrointestinal tract using a multifrequency pulsed Doppler meter. Endoscopy 22:268, 1990.

35. Lamb CR, Mason GD, Wallace MK: Ultrasonographic diagnosis of peritoneopericardial diaphragmatic hernia in a Persian cat. Vet Rec 125:186, 1989.

36. Cowan WD, Feeney DA, Walter PA: What is your diagnosis? Peritoneopericardial diaphragmatic hernia. J Am Vet Med Assoc 194:1331, 1989.

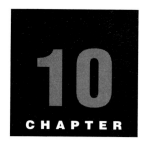

THE SPLEEN

Judith A. Hudson

CHAPTER 10

INDICATIONS

Indications for sonographic examination include splenomegaly, splenic mass, and hemo-peritoneum.[1] Focal lesions include primary or secondary neoplasia or hematomas. Abscesses, infarcts, or hyperplastic nodules are less common.[1] Sonography can be used to search for metastasis after identification of neoplasia.[1] This technique is less helpful in cases of diffuse involvement of the spleen without parenchymal abnormalities, but some diseases can be ruled out. Ultrasound can be used to guide needle placement for percutaneous biopsy for both diffuse and focal lesions. Serial sonography can be used to evaluate the response to therapy.[2] Additionally, full examination of the spleen should be made as part of abdominal sonography for diseases of other organs. Significant splenic disease can exist without disease related to the spleen (Fig. 10–1).

Figure 10–1

Full abdominal sonogram of a dog with cystitis revealed a large mass in the tail of the spleen. The mass measured 23.0 mm between the "+" caliper marks and 26.1 mm between the "x" caliper marks. Subsequent thoracic radiography revealed extensive pulmonary metastasis.

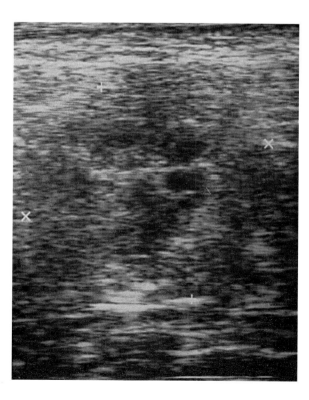

TECHNIQUE

In small animals, a 7.5-mHz probe is usually optimal for evaluation of the spleen because of its high resolution of structures to a depth of 6 to 8 cm. A 5.0-mHz probe is needed for structures at greater depths.[1] Depth and gain of the ultrasound machine should be set to optimize near field evaluation because the spleen is located close to the abdominal wall.[3] In horses, a low frequency (3.0-mHz) probe can be used for transabdominal evaluation; a 5.0-mHz probe can be used for foals.[4] Transrectal abdominal evaluation of horses can be made using a 5.0-mHz probe.[5]

The spleen is a tongue-shaped organ lying in the left hypogastric region, roughly parallel to the greater curvature of the stomach. The head or dorsal extremity is relatively fixed in position between the gastric fundus and the left kidney (Fig. 10–2). The tail or ventral extremity is variable in position, depending on the fullness of the stomach. The tail may cross the ventral midline to the right side and may extend caudally to the level of the second to fourth lumbar vertebra.[6] The spleen can be examined in the area cranial to the left kidney or from the costal arch with the animal in right lateral recumbency.[1] In one study, dorsal and transverse images were made at and caudoventral to the eleventh intercostal space with the probe perpendicular to the left thoracic and abdominal wall. For sagittal images, the probe was placed parallel to the left lateral abdominal wall and pushed under the costal arch with the probe's contact surface directed craniad.[7] Examination of the body and tail of the spleen can be made with the patient in ventrodorsal (Fig. 10–3) or left lateral recumbency. Visualization of the well-defined echogenic splenic capsule can determine whether the spleen is in contact with a mass or continuous with it. Lesions should be classified as focal or diffuse.[1]

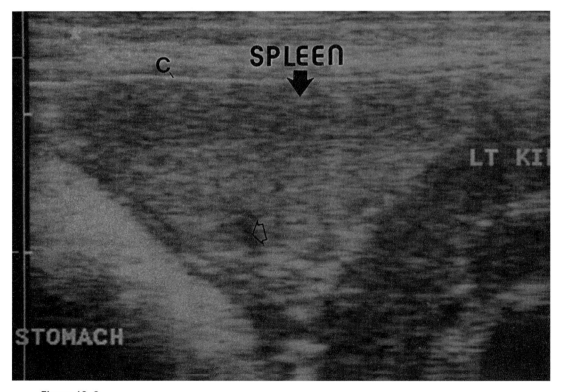

Figure 10–2

Sonogram of the spleen of a normal dog shows the position of the head of the spleen (solid arrow) between the left kidney and stomach. The dog was in right lateral recumbency during scanning of the left abdomen. The band of decreased echogenicity in the near portion of the spleen is caused by a near field artifact in the transducer. A stand-off pad can be used to avoid such artifacts, if necessary. C, capsule of the spleen; open arrow, splenic vein.

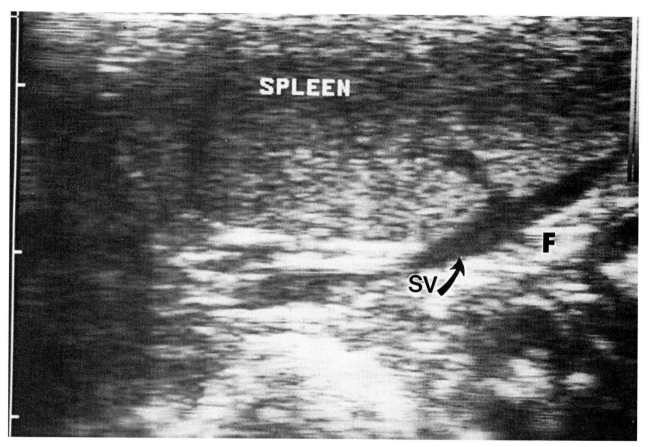

Figure 10-3

Sonogram of the spleen of a normal dog shows the body of the spleen caudal to the stomach. The dog was in dorsal recumbency during scanning of the midabdomen. SV, splenic venous branch at the splenic hilus; F, fat.

Focal lesions of the spleen are easier to recognize than diffuse lesions. The normal spleen has a hyperechoic, uniform echo pattern and is normally compared to the liver and kidney for evaluation of echo density. It should be understood, however, that tissue texture is not a true image of histologic structure, but it is based on an interference pattern determined by beam characteristics. Factors such as depth, transducer frequency and bandwidth, and processing by the electronic system influence the texture or speckle pattern.[8] Also, when comparison is made between organs, it is assumed that the organs used for comparison are normal (Fig. 10-4). For example, an enlarged spleen with echogenicity similar to that of the liver may actually have normal echogenicity if hepatocellular disease has decreased hepatic echogenicity.[9]

The location of the focal point is important when using a focused transducer. Because fluid-filled cysts have acoustic enhancement of the far wall and deeper structures, the focal point should be superficial to the far wall when scanning cystic structures. Solid masses have central echoes resulting in poor accentuation of deeper structures. The focal point should be placed deep to the lesion with solid masses.[4]

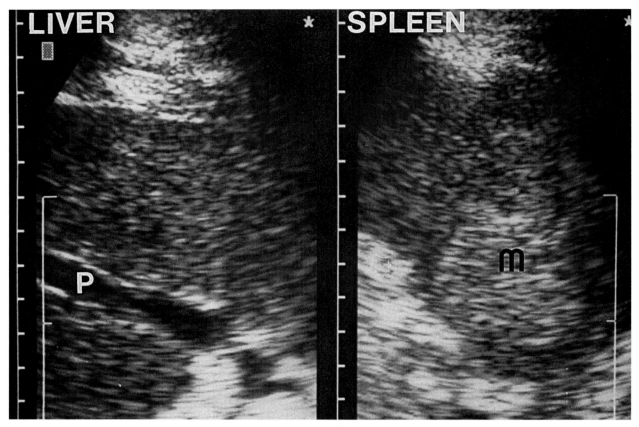

Figure 10–4

Sonogram of the liver and spleen of a horse. The liver and spleen have similar echogenicity but neither is normal. A mass (m) is visible in the spleen. Concurrent hepatic disease explained the increased echogenicity. P, portal vein.

In horses, the cranial portion of the abdomen is ventral to the caudal thorax. The spleen is found on the left side, medial or (occasionally) lateral to the liver, one or two intercostal spaces caudal to the diaphragmatic cupola. More caudally, the spleen can be seen ventral to the left lung border and lateral to the left kidney. The spleen may reach the mid-ventral abdomen in normal horses and is larger in tranquilized horses. The thick mid-body of the spleen (up to 15 cm) may interfere with transabdominal imaging of the left kidney.[10] Only the caudal aspect of the spleen can be seen with transrectal sonography.[5]

NORMAL ANATOMY

Correlation was made between the sonographic appearance and normal anatomy of the canine spleen using 27 dogs. Dorsal, transverse, and sagittal scans were made in eight anesthetized dogs. The splenic capsule was a fine echogenic line when visualized incident to the ultrasonic beam.[7] The spleen has smooth borders and a uniform echo pattern that is slightly more echogenic than the liver (see Figs. 10–2 and 10–3). Fat adjacent to the vessels and the hilus of the spleen is hyperechoic.[7] Volume averaging can cause the appearance of artifactual hyperechoic "masses" adjacent to parenchymal vessels.

Dissection of 23 embalmed canine spleens showed two to five venous rami in the hilus of the dorsal extremity and four to nine venous rami in the hilus of the ventral extremity.[7] Additional rami exited the hilus at the midportion of the spleen. These rami emptied blood into dorsal and ventral "polar" veins that traveled in the gastrosplenic ligament and united to form the splenic vein.[7] Sonographically, the venous rami of the splenic veins can be seen at the splenic hilus (Fig. 10–5).[3,7,11–13] Venous rami within the parenchyma appear hyperechoic when viewed at right angles to the ultrasound probe and hypoechoic when viewed at an oblique angle. Arterial rami can be detected at the hilus, but currently their identification within the splenic parenchyma[7] is not possible without color flow Doppler imaging. In cadaver specimens, splenic arterial rami have smaller lumens and more hyperechoic walls compared to venous rami.[7] Echogenic flow can be detected normally in larger vessels with only gray scale imaging. The appearance of echogenic flowing foci does not indicate the presence of thrombi.

In horses, the spleen can be differentiated from the liver because it is more echogenic and has fewer vessels.[5,10] The capsule is echogenic.[5]

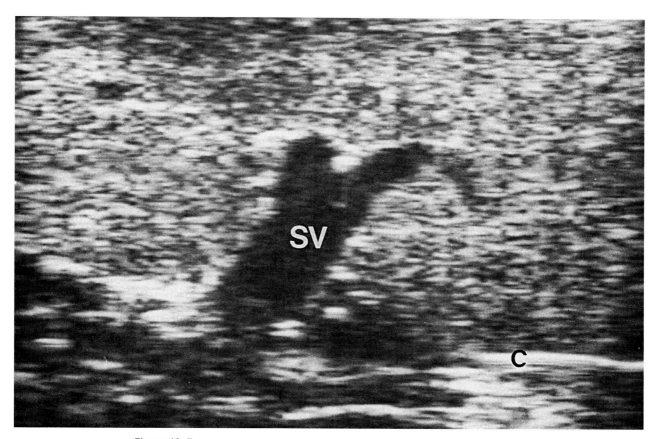

Figure 10–5

Sonogram of a canine spleen shows a venous branch entering at the splenic hilus and dividing. SV, splenic venous branch; C, capsule.

DISEASE PROCESSES

General Characteristics

Lesions of the spleen should be classified according to echogenicity, margination, size, and location.[12] The spleen is usually more hyperechoic than liver. Lesions containing nonviscous fluids are usually anechoic with smooth, well-defined borders and acoustic enhancement of the far wall and deeper structures. Abscesses, other cystic structures containing viscous fluid, hematomas, or neoplasms can be hypoechoic, although hematomas and granulomas can be hyperechoic. Neoplasms are often hyperechoic or complex. Complex lesions contain both hyperechoic and hypoechoic areas, resulting from pathologic processes such as necrotic or fluid-filled cystic areas. Abscesses, granulomas, and neoplasms usually have irregular, ill-defined borders.[14]

Diffuse pathologic change, such as lymphosarcoma, tends to decrease echogenicity. Although venous congestion causes a similar appearance, differentiation is possible because congestion is accompanied by enlarged veins at the hilus. Complete vascular compromise, occurring with torsion or thrombosis of the splenic veins, results in splenic necrosis that causes the spleen to appear coarse, lacy, and profoundly hypoechoic.[1]

Neoplasia

Please recognize that sonographic appearance is *not* specific for cell type.[15]

Hemangiosarcoma

In one study, hemangiosarcoma appeared as a large, complex lesion with multiple small cystic areas (Fig. 10–6).[12] Two other dogs with splenic hemangiosarcoma had similar

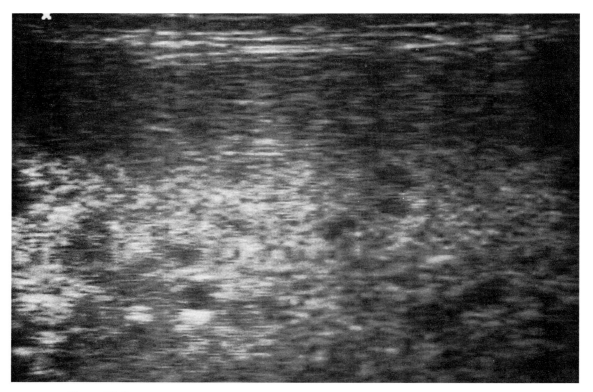

Figure 10–6

Sonogram of the spleen of an 11-year-old castrated male dog with hemangiosarcoma. The spleen was dramatically enlarged, filling most of the midabdomen and containing multiple masses. This scan reveals a complex mass with hyperechoic, hypoechoic, and anechoic areas.

sonographic findings. One had 1.0- to 6.0-cm masses with a mixed echo pattern in the spleen and 1.0- to 3.0-cm hypoechoic masses in the liver. The other had a complex mass (15 × 20 cm) in the spleen; the liver was not scanned.[15] Similar large complex masses were seen with anaplastic sarcoma and undifferentiated sarcoma in two other dogs, emphasizing that sonographic appearance is nonspecific for cell type.[15]

In a retrospective study of 18 dogs with hemangiosarcoma, all dogs had a mass within or protruding from the splenic surface (Fig. 10–7). Most dogs (17 of 18) had complex masses with echogenicity ranging from anechoic to hyperechoic. Anechoic to hypoechoic areas usually had well-defined borders without a capsule. Acoustic enhancement was deep to anechoic areas in five dogs. Hyperechoic or normal parenchyma was found between areas of decreased echogenicity. Only one dog had a mass that was primarily hypoechoic (Fig. 10–8). Hepatic masses were seen in eight dogs. Metastatic hemangiosarcoma was confirmed after biopsy or necropsy in seven of these dogs. Hepatic masses varied from large (9 cm in diameter) masses similar to the splenic masses to small (1 cm in diameter) anechoic lesions surrounded by ill-defined areas of coarse, hypoechoic, hepatic parenchyma. Nine dogs had sonographic evidence of peritoneal effusion (Fig. 10–9); six had hyperechoic peritoneal nodules suggestive of metastasis.[16] Regional lymph nodes may be enlarged (Fig. 10–10).

Histopathologic examination of these tumors reveals endothelial cells lining vascular spaces. Hemorrhage, necrosis, and cyst formation are frequent findings.[17] Areas with reduced echogenicity may represent vascular spaces, chronic hematomas, cysts, abscesses, or areas of liquefactive necrosis. Hyperechoic areas may represent fibrosis, mineralization, or recent hematomas (see Fig. 10–9).[16]

Figure 10–7

Sonogram of the spleen of a 7-year-old mixed breed dog with hemangiosarcoma. Arrows indicate a portion of a large (3.8 × 3.9 cm) mass protruding from the tail of the spleen. The internal architecture is complex with multiple, cystic areas. Note also a large (8.4 × 8 cm) pedunculated mass extending from the right medial liver lobe. Postmortem diagnosis was severe hemangiosarcoma involving liver, spleen, omentum, and serosa.

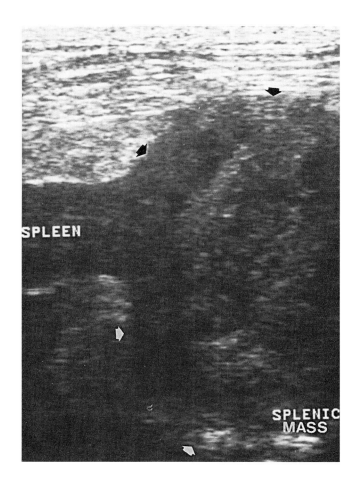

Figure 10–8

Sonogram of the spleen of a 9-year-old Rottweiler with hemangiosarcoma. Although splenic hemangiosarcoma frequently manifests as a complex mass, occasionally the spleen is primarily hypoechoic. This spleen is enlarged with ill-defined hypoechoic areas. The dog had a 1-month history of anemia and weight loss. Hemoperitoneum and pancreatic involvement was also present. The diagnosis of hemangiosarcoma was rendered on the basis of the histopathologic analysis after total splenectomy. Arrows indicate some of the ill-defined hypoechoic areas.

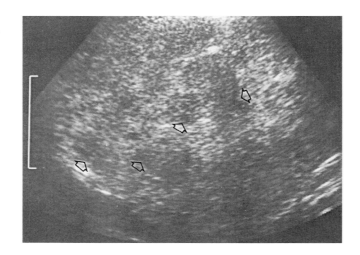

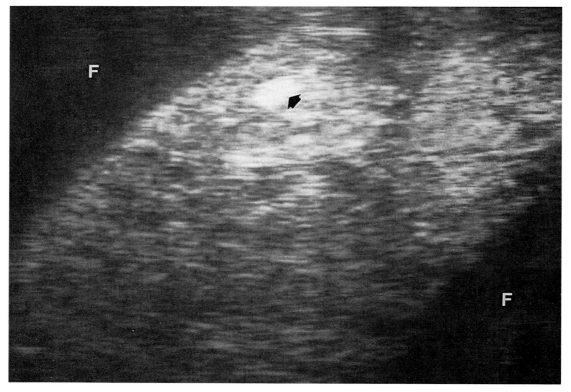

Figure 10–9

Sonogram of the spleen of the same dog with splenic hemangiosarcoma as in Figure 10–6. Note the intermixing of hyperechoic and hypoechoic regions. The arrow indicates one distinctive hyperechoic area that might represent fibrosis, mineralization, or recent hematoma. Free peritoneal fluid (F) seen on both sides of the spleen was blood, resulting from splenic rupture.

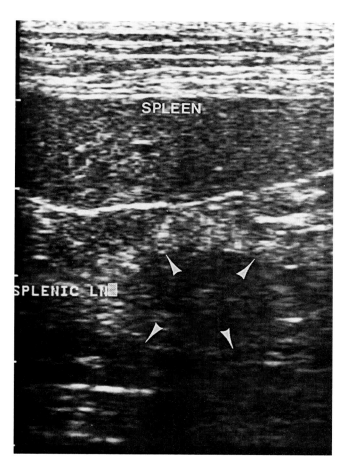

Figure 10–10

Sonogram of the spleen and splenic lymph node of the same dog with splenic hemangiosarcoma as in Figure 10–7. This portion of the spleen appeared normal. The splenic lymph node (arrowheads) is enlarged.

Lymphosarcoma

One author described lymphoma as being associated with focal areas of decreased echogenicity.[12] In a retrospective study of hepatic and splenic masses, a "Swiss cheese" appearance (Figs. 10–11 and 10–12) was found in the spleen of a dog with multiple hypoechoic, 1.0- to 9.0-cm masses.[15] In another study, lymphosarcoma in 12 dogs caused nonhomogeneous echo patterns with poorly marginated hypoechoic to anechoic nodules (4 mm to 3 cm) in all dogs and no acoustic shadowing or enhancement of the underlying tissues. The echo intensity of the splenic parenchyma between the nodules was hypoechoic in 10 dogs and normal in 2 dogs. Three dogs had a well-circumscribed focal splenic mass measuring between 5 and 9 cm. These masses (one hyperplastic nodule and two old hematomas) had a mixed echo pattern varying from anechoic, irregularly shaped fluid accumulations to patchy hyperechoic tissue. The shape of the spleen was distorted. The degree of splenic necrosis and degeneration was variable and all masses were found in areas affected by lymphosarcoma.[18] Figures 10–12 and 10–13 illustrate two cases in which masses were found in spleens affected by lymphosarcoma.

Other organs should be examined for evidence of involvement. In the last study described in the previous paragraph, focal hypoechoic hepatic lesions were present in three dogs, patchy areas of coarsened hypoechoic parenchyma were seen in six, and echo intensity was reduced in two. Lymph nodes should also be examined (Fig. 10–14).[18]

Sonography may be more reliable for identification of lymphosarcoma in the spleen than in the liver. In a study of 10 dogs and 5 cats, sonography had a sensitivity of 83% for detection of splenic lymphosarcoma but only 21% for detection of hepatic lymphosar-

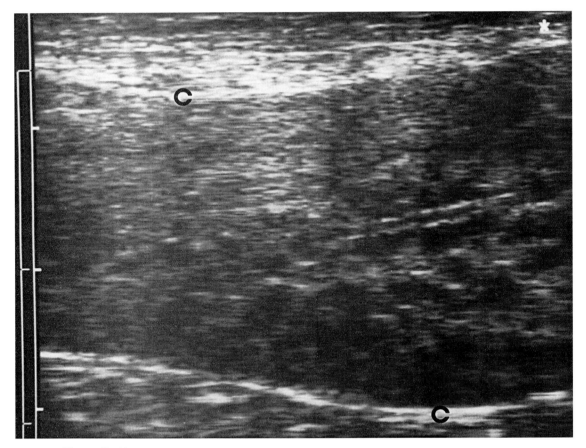

Figure 10-11

Sonogram of the spleen of a 12-year-old Scottish terrier with lymphosarcoma demonstrates the typical motheaten or "Swiss cheese" appearance of splenic lymphosarcoma. C, capsule of the spleen.

Figure 10-12

Sonogram of the spleen of a 6-year-old Beagle with splenic lymphosarcoma. The spleen had a typical "Swiss cheese" appearance and contained a sharply marginated hypoechoic mass. Calipers measure the mass, which was 2.01 × 2.25 cm.

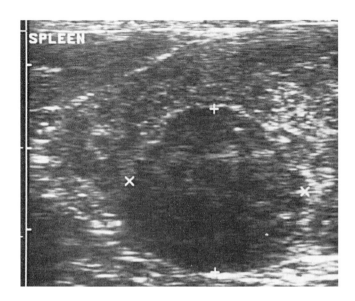

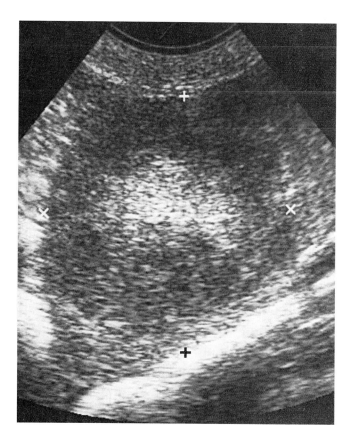

Figure 10–13

Sonogram of an 11-year-old female Boxer with lymphosarcoma. The spleen was diffusely hypoechoic and contained a complex, well-circumscribed mass. Calipers measure the mass, which was 47.5 mm between the "+" caliper marks and 47.1 mm between the "x" caliper marks.

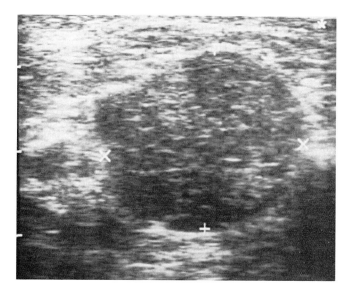

Figure 10–14

Sonogram of an enlarged sublumbar lymph node in the same dog with lymphosarcoma as in Figure 10–12. The dog had multicentric lymphosarcoma with peripheral and internal lymphadenopathy and splenomegaly. Normal sublumbar lymph nodes are oval and usually measure less than 1 cm in length. This lymph node measured 21.4 mm between the "+" caliper marks and 24.9 mm between the "x" caliper marks.

coma. In 6 animals with splenic lymphosarcoma, abnormalities noted on sonograms of the spleen included diffuse hypoechogenicity (2); multiple hypoechoic foci (1); irregular, bosselated border (1); and a large cavitated mass (1 with histiocytic lymphosarcoma). In animals in which splenic involvement is apparent sonographically, the possibility of hepatic involvement cannot be excluded, even if no hepatic abnormality is visible.[19]

Transrectal examination of the abdomen of a horse with lymphosarcoma revealed multiple round nodules with a complex echo pattern in the spleen. The remainder of the spleen had a mixed echo pattern with normal areas interspersed between poorly defined areas with complex echogenicity. Abnormalities were seen also in the left kidney. Necropsy revealed metastasis from a large mass in the cranial region of the spleen. Histopathologic analysis confirmed splenic lymphosarcoma.[5] Abdominal sonography of a Thoroughbred gelding revealed a mass consisting of many irregular hyperechoic nodules measuring up to 3.0 cm in diameter. Anechoic areas were found between the nodules. Splenic vessels could be traced from normal appearing splenic parenchyma, showing that the mass originated from the spleen.[20]

Mast Cell Tumor

Metastases were found in the liver and spleen during necropsy of a cat with mast cell tumor originating in the duodenum. Sonographic assessment, however, revealed no abnormalities in the spleen and hyperechoic 3- and 5-cm masses in the liver.[15] Fine needle aspiration allowed the diagnosis of splenic mastocytosis in two dogs with splenomegaly.[21] In our experience, splenic mastocytosis usually causes decreased echogenicity, which may be generalized or patchy (Figs. 10–15 and 10–16). Differential

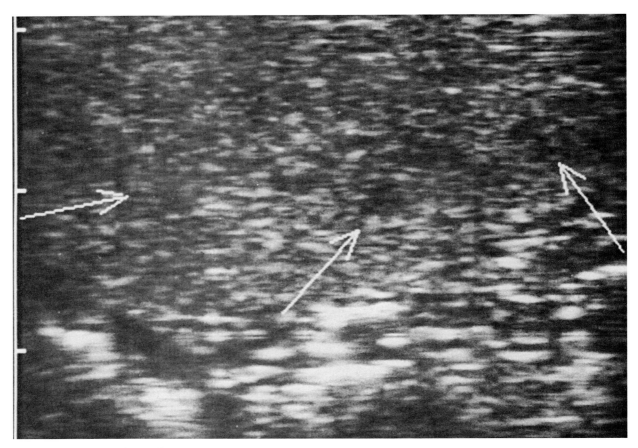

Figure 10–15

Sonogram of the spleen of a 10-year-old spayed female dog with systemic mastocytosis. The spleen was enlarged with irregular, poorly defined hypoechoic areas (arrows). Fine needle aspiration confirmed the presence of splenic mast cell tumor.

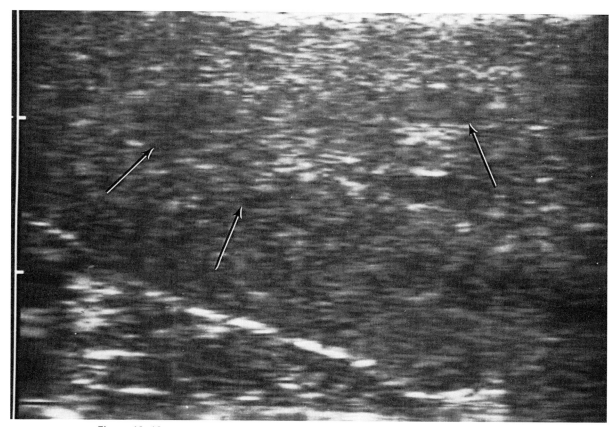

Figure 10–16

Sonogram of the spleen of an 11-year-old Golden Retriever with mastocytosis involving the oral cavity and bone marrow. Histopathologic analysis confirmed diffuse mast cell sarcoma after splenectomy. Arrows indicate irregular, poorly defined hypoechoic areas similar to those in the spleen of the dog in Figure 10–15.

diagnoses associated with splenomegaly are numerous and include congestive splenomegaly (e.g., right-sided heart failure), other infiltrative processes (e.g., lymphosarcoma, extramedullary hematopoiesis), and peripheral vasodilation caused by drugs such as acepromazine or barbiturates.[21] Free peritoneal fluid may be present (Fig. 10–17).

Metastatic Disease

Metastatic disease in the spleen and liver from a duodenal mast cell tumor in the cat has been described, as noted previously.[15] In horses, carcinomatosis associated with gastrointestinal squamous cell carcinoma has been reported. Sonography was used to evaluate multiple neoplastic implants measuring up to several centimeters on the serosal surfaces of the omentum, intestines, liver, peritoneum, and spleen.[5] Transrectal sonography revealed numerous hyperechoic nodules, between 3 and 20 mm in diameter, involving the uterus, broad ligaments, peritoneal surfaces, and serosal surfaces of the large colon in an 11-year-old Arabian mare with endometrial adenocarcinoma.[22]

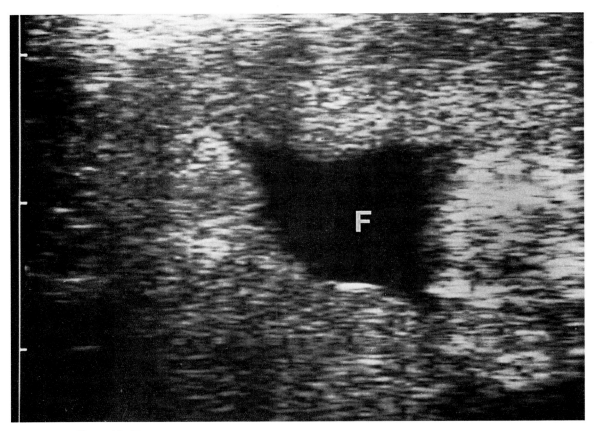

Figure 10-17

Sonogram of the spleen of a 12-year-old spayed female cat with systemic mastocytosis and a palpable abdominal mass revealed free peritoneal fluid (F) and an enlarged spleen that is bent around the free fluid. Chemotherapy was initiated after the spleen was removed to reduce the tumor burden. Cytologic analysis revealed the free fluid was a nonseptic, noninflammatory effusion without any mast cells.

Benign Neoplasia

Not all splenic lesions are neoplastic nor is all splenic neoplasia malignant. Unfortunately, hemangioma (Fig. 10–18) and hematomas cannot be differentiated from hemangiosarcoma on the basis of findings of either fine needle aspiration or sonography. Lesions detected in the liver using sonography or pulmonary nodules identified using thoracic radiography can help to differentiate malignant from benign lesions. Partial or complete splenectomy may be necessary to allow definitive histopathologic identification.[1]

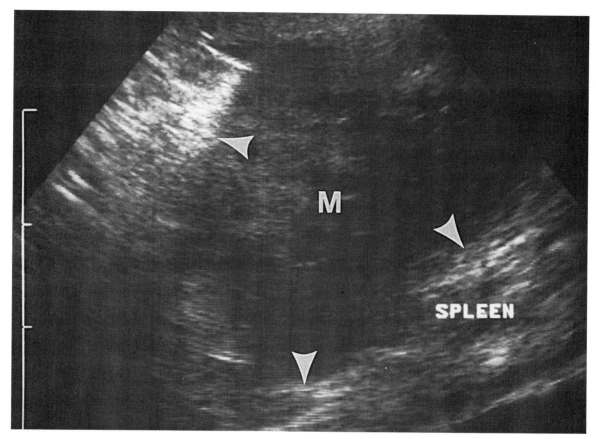

Figure 10–18

Sonogram of the spleen of a 10-year-old male Golden Retriever with a final diagnosis of chronic degenera-
tive splenic hemangioma shows a large, primarily hypoechoic mass in the tail of the spleen. Arrowheads
indicate the borders of the mass (M). The sonographic appearance suggests hemangiosarcoma or other
neoplasia. Splenectomy, however, revealed a large focal area of degenerated blood and splenic tissue
surrounded by a thick zone of fibrous connective tissue and numerous hemosiderin-laden macrophages.
The capsule was thickened.

Passive Congestion

Administration of anesthetic agents, chronic liver disease, and right-sided heart failure
can cause passive congestion of the spleen resulting in splenomegaly (Fig. 10–19).
Echogenicity is usually normal or decreased, although chronic congestion can lead to
increased echogenicity in man. Enlargement of the hepatic veins may be indicative of
hepatic involvement.[3]

Myeloproliferative Disease

Myeloproliferative disease in one cat caused the appearance of a hypoechoic, 3.0- to 4.0-
cm mass in the spleen and a diffuse, hypoechoic pattern in the liver.[15] Review of the literature indicated that myeloproliferative disease in man causes an enlarged spleen with
normal or increased echogenicity.[15,18]

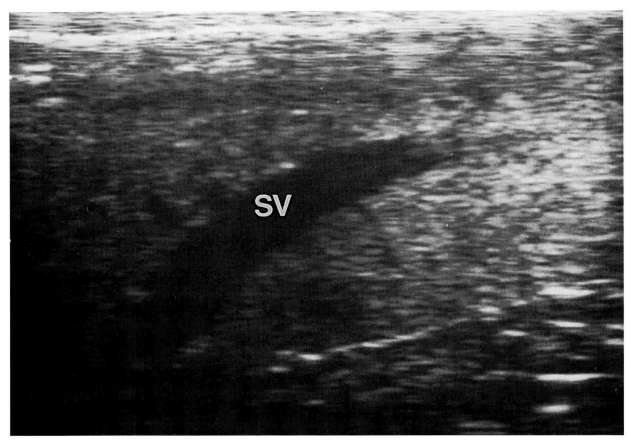

Figure 10–19

Sonogram of a canine spleen illustrating passive congestion. A dilated branch of the splenic vein (SV) is apparent within the splenic parenchyma.

Extramedullary Hematopoiesis

Extramedullary hematopoiesis was the most common cytologic diagnosis in a series of 28 dogs and 5 cats with splenomegaly. The condition occurs when the bone marrow is unable to meet a demand for hematopoiesis, but it has also been noted in animals without obvious hematologic abnormalities.[21] Nodular extramedullary hematopoiesis can result in the presence of a non-neoplastic splenic mass.[21] Figure 10–20 shows a canine spleen containing a hypoechoic, ill-defined lesion identified as extramedullary hematopoiesis after fine-needle aspiration.

Hematoma

Hematomas cannot be differentiated from hemangiosarcoma sonographically. Both can be hypoechoic or complex. Hematomas may resemble a benign lesion (Fig. 10–21) or may be present within a neoplastic mass. The appearance of hematomas varies with the stage of hemorrhage. Initial hemorrhage is anechoic to hypoechoic. As clotting occurs, acute hemorrhage appears as a solid hyperechoic lesion because of multiple acoustic interfaces formed by red cell aggregates held within a fibrin mesh. Clot hemolysis occurs after approximately 96 hours, causing the development of a hypoechoic or anechoic appearance. Increased echogenicity reappears with the reorganization and eventual calcification of the hematoma. Hematoma is difficult to differentiate from hemangioma and hemangiosarcoma on the basis of findings from fine needle aspiration.[1]

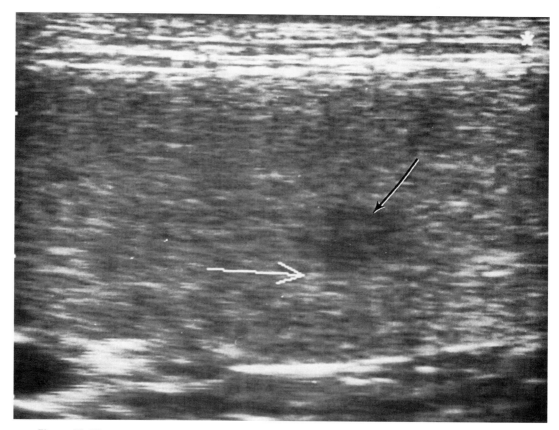

Figure 10–20

Sonogram of the spleen of an 11-year-old mixed breed male dog with oral squamous cell carcinoma and cutaneous malignant melanoma. Arrows indicate a hypoechoic, ill-defined lesion that was determined on fine needle aspiration to represent extramedullary hematopoiesis.

Splenitis

The veterinary literature has little reference to inflammatory conditions of the spleen. In man, reactive hyperplasia related to acute and chronic infection or splenitis associated with granulomatous disease causes a diffusely hypoechoic spleen.[23] One dog (Fig. 10–22) with a histopathologic diagnosis of diffuse, subacute, moderate splenitis had a spleen that appeared sonographically to be folded on itself and contained multiple hypoechoic nodules of varying size. Although infectious or inflammatory conditions may have other sonographic presentations, it is important to remember that these conditions cannot be differentiated from neoplasia on the basis of the sonographic examination.

Abscesses

Abscesses are uncommon but usually are hypoechoic or, occasionally, complex with variable encapsulation.[1] In a study in dogs of intra-abdominal abscesses involving the spleen (1), liver (3), kidney (2), uterine stump (1), and mesentery (1), all abscesses had an irregular border but wall thickening was seen only in the single splenic abscess and one hepatic abscess. Walls were not visible in the other abscesses. Minimal to no through transmission was seen in tissues deep to the abscesses. The splenic abscess was hypoechoic with low level echoes mixed with anechoic regions. Through transmission was mild.[24] Differential diagnoses include hematoma, hyperplastic nodules, lymphosarcoma, cystadenocarcinoma, primary or metastatic neoplasia with necrosis or hemorrhage, and complex cysts with cellular debris or hemorrhage.[1,24]

Figure 10–21

Sonogram of the spleen of a 10-year-old spayed female dog with a splenic hematoma. The patient was examined because of a palpable splenic mass. Sonography revealed a large (5.0 cm maximum diameter) complex splenic mass with multiple cysts and some hyperechoic areas in the head of the spleen. The mass had poor vascularity; most large vessels were peripheral to the mass. The patient underwent exploratory laparotomy and splenectomy. Histopathologic analysis showed that the mass consisted of clotted blood. Normal splenic tissue surrounded the mass. Arrows indicate the borders of the mass. C, cystic area within the mass. Caliper marks measure the cystic area.

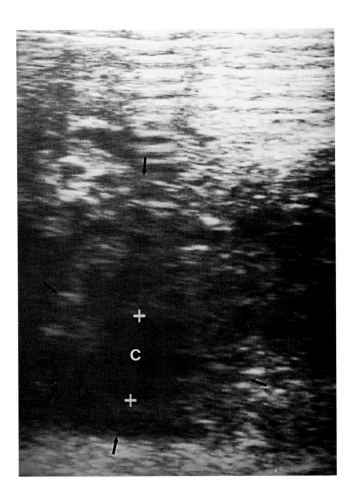

Figure 10–22

Sonogram of the spleen of a 12-year-old castrated male Tibetan terrier with anemia and weight loss. The spleen appeared folded on itself and contained multiple hypoechoic nodules of various sizes. Arrows denote some of the nodules. Histopathologic analysis showed dispersed accumulations of neutrophils and plasma cells in the red pulp. Dense accumulations of cells with a small amount of amphophilic cytoplasm and pale basophilic nuclei with prominent nucleoli were seen in lymphoid follicles. The histopathologic diagnosis was splenitis.

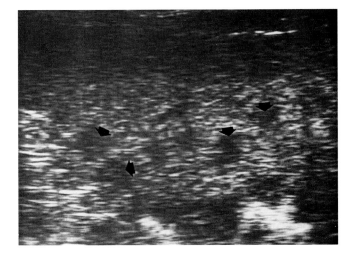

Nodular Hyperplasia

Nodular hyperplasia is common in spleens of old dogs. Nodules usually project from the surface and vary up to 2 cm in diameter. Rarely, hyperplastic nodules become 5 cm or greater in diameter.[25] Nodular hyperplasia can appear similar to hemangiosarcoma on a sonogram. Nodules may become necrotic or intrasplenic hematomas may develop, as occurs in spleens affected by hemangiosarcoma. Peritoneal effusion or evidence of metastatic disease in the liver or other organs makes the diagnosis of nodular hyperplasia less likely than that of hemangiosarcoma.[26] In a retrospective study of 12 dogs with lymphosarcoma, three dogs had a well-circumscribed complex mass measuring between 5 and 9 cm in diameter and located within an affected area of the spleen. Two masses were old hematomas, but the third was a hyperplastic nodule. Echogenicity of the masses varied from anechoic, irregular fluid accumulations to patchy hyperechoic areas. The masses deformed the borders of the spleen unlike other areas affected by lymphosarcoma.[18]

Infarction/Necrosis

Splenic infarcts can occur in association with valvular endocarditis, neoplasia, trauma, and splenic torsion.[3,27] A variation in appearance of splenic infarcts from anechoic (occasionally, cyst-like) or hypoechoic round lesions to hyperechoic wedge-shaped lesions with the apex toward the hilus has been reported in both man and dogs.[1,3,27,28] Edema, inflammation, and necrosis appear to account for early low echogenicity, whereas fibrosis and shrinkage cause progressively increased echogenicity and decreased size.[3,27,28]

Two additional patterns of infarction have been described in dogs. In one pattern, round hypoechoic or isoechoic, well-marginated nodules deform the splenic border. Differential diagnoses for this pattern include nodular hyperplasia, neoplasia, hematoma, cyst, and abscess formation.[28] The other pattern consisted of a heteroechoic or hypoechoic, diffuse, coarse/"lacy" appearance in the affected area of the spleen without deformation of the splenic border. The latter pattern correlated to areas of splenic necrosis noted on histopathologic analysis. Splenic necrosis was believed to be secondary to infarction.[27] Gas may be present in the area of infarction/necrosis, caused by gas-forming anaerobes (such as Clostridium) or by release of oxyhemoglobin during the development of pathology.[27]

Splenic Torsion

Splenic torsion occurs when the spleen rotates on its vascular pedicle, occluding vessels at the hilus. The condition usually affects large or giant breed dogs and frequently, but not always, is associated with gastric dilatation-volvulus. Complete occlusion of the thin-walled splenic vein and partial occlusion of the thicker walled artery allows blood to enter but not leave the spleen, resulting in splenic congestion and splenomegaly. Splenic vein thrombosis may occur if torsion persists. Infarction may follow occlusion of the arterial blood supply.[29]

Sonographic assessment of a torsed spleen reveals splenomegaly and distention of the splenic veins.[3,30,31] A diffusely hypoechoic spleen with linear echo densities separating large, anechoic areas was described in two reports of three dogs with splenic torsion.[30,31] Two of these dogs had splenic necrosis, and a third had hemorrhage and loss of normal architecture. The sonographic pattern in these three dogs is similar to the "coarse/lacy heteroechoic pattern" described in three other dogs with splenic infarction and necrosis. One of these dogs had splenic torsion with secondary infarction/necrosis.[27] Thus, splenomegaly accompanied by distended splenic veins and this unique echo pattern may suggest splenic torsion with secondary infarction/necrosis. If Doppler sonography or color flow imaging is available, examination of the splenic vessels may aid in the evaluation of the splenic blood supply (Fig. 10–23). Apparent enlargement of vessels may be caused by thrombosis.[27]

Splenic Rupture

Splenic rupture may be caused by trauma, but it can occur as a result of pathologic change. Hematoma formation or free peritoneal fluid may be seen along with parenchymal splenic lesions (Figs. 10–9 and 10–24). Rupture of a neoplasm, especially a hemangiosarcoma, should be considered in older dogs (see Fig. 10–9).[3]

Figure 10-23

Sonogram of the spleen of a 5-year-old German Shepherd with splenic torsion revealed dilated cyst-like areas, suggestive of congestion with dilated sinusoids. The spleen was abnormally located in the right cranial abdominal quadrant and extended ventrally. The splenic veins could not be followed reliably into the portal vein. Color flow Doppler imaging was used to interrogate the outlined in white. No detectable flow was present.

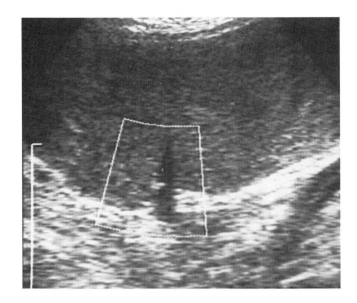

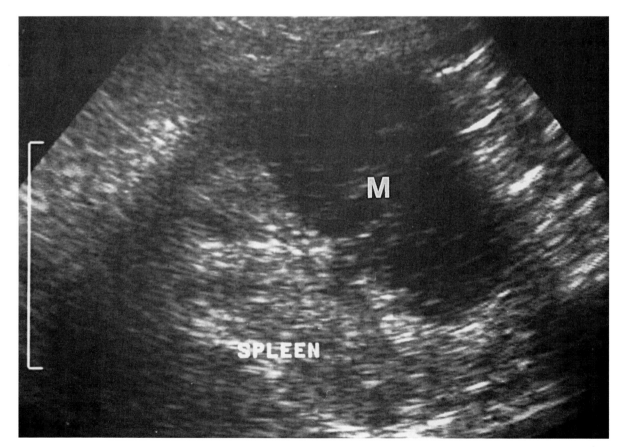

Figure 10-24

Sonogram of the spleen of an 11-year-old castrated male Airedale terrier with a palpable abdominal mass revealed an enlarged spleen with multiple, complex, lobulated mass-like areas. After splenectomy, histopathologic analysis showed that these areas comprised a large amount of hematopoietic tissue. Splenic tissue found in surrounding adipose tissue indicated previous splenic rupture. M, large mass-like area.

REFERENCES

1. Lamb CR: Abdominal ultrasonography in small animals: Examination of the liver, spleen and pancreas. J Small Anim Pract *31:*6, 1990.
2. Nyland TG, Hager DA, Herring DS: Sonography of the liver, gallbladder, and spleen. Semin Vet Med Surg (Small Anim) *4:*13, 1989.
3. Nyland TG, Hager DA: Sonography of the liver, gall bladder and spleen. Vet Clin North Am Small Anim Pract *15:*1123, 1985.
4. Rantanen NW, Ewing RL III: Principles of ultrasound application in animals. Vet Radiol *22:*196, 1981.
5. Schmidt AR: Transrectal ultrasonography of the caudal portion of abdominal and pelvic cavities in horses. J Am Vet Med Assoc *194:*365, 1989.
6. Bezuidenhout AJ: *The lymphatic system. The spleen.* In *Miller's Anatomy of the Dog,* 3rd Ed. Edited by HE Evans. Philadelphia: WB Saunders, 1993, pp. 749–753.
7. Wood AK, McCarthy PH, Angles JM: Ultrasonographic-anatomic correlation and imaging protocol for the spleen in anesthetized dogs. Am J Vet Res *51:*1433, 1990.
8. Thijssen JM, Oosterveld BJ: Texture in tissue echograms. Speckle or information? J Ultrasound Med *9:*215, 1990.
9. Mittelstaedt CA, Parfain CL: Ultrasonic-pathologic classification of splenic abnormalities: Gray scale patterns. Radiology *134:*697, 1980.
10. Rantanen NW: *Diseases of the abdomen.* Vet Clin North Am Equine Pract *2:*67, 1986.
11. Cartee RE, Hudson JA, Finn-Bodner S: Ultrasonography. Vet Clin North Am Small Anim Pract *23:*345, 1993.
12. Herring DS: Abdominal ultrasound: Theory and practice. Semin Vet Med Surg (Small Anim) *1:*102, 1986.
13. Barr F: Diagnostic ultrasound in small animals. In Practice, January 17–25, 1988.
14. Park RD, et al: B-mode gray-scale ultrasound: Imaging artifacts and interpretation principles. Vet Radiol *22:*204, 1981.
15. Feeney DA, Johnston GR, Hardy RM: Two-dimensional, gray-scale ultrasonography for assessment of hepatic and splenic neoplasia in the dog and cat. J Am Vet Med Assoc *184:*68, 1984.
16. Wrigley RH, et al: Ultrasonographic feature of splenic hemangiosarcoma in dogs: 18 cases (1980–1986). J Am Vet Med Assoc *192:*1113, 1988.
17. Jubb KVF, Kennedy PC, Palmer N: *Pathology of Domestic Animals.* 4th Ed. San Diego: Academic Press, 1992, pp. 99, 233.
18. Wrigley RH, et al: Ultrasonographic features of splenic lymphosarcoma in dogs: 12 cases (1980–1986). J Am Vet Med Assoc *12:*1565, 1988.
19. Lamb CR, et al: Ultrasonic findings in hepatic and splenic lymphosarcoma in dogs and cats. Vet Radiol *32:*117, 1991.
20. Marr CM, Love S, Pirie HM: Clinical, ultrasonographic and pathological findings in a horse with splenic lymphosarcoma and pseudohyperparathyroidism. Equine Vet J *21:*221, 1989.
21. O'Keefe DA, Cuoto CG: Fine-needle aspiration of the spleen as an aid in the diagnosis of splenomegaly. J Vet Intern Med *1:*102, 1987.
22. Chaffin MK, et al: Endometrial adenocarcinoma in a mare. Cornell Vet *80:*65, 1990.
23. Mittelstaedt CA: *Spleen.* In *General Ultrasound.* Edited by CA Mittelstaedt. New York: Churchill Livingstone, 1992, p. 682.
24. Konde LJ, et al: Sonographic application in the diagnosis of intraabdominal abscess in the dog. Vet Radiol *27:*151, 1986.
25. Jubb KVF, Kennedy PC, Palmer N: *Pathology of Domestic Animals.* 4t¹ Ed. San Diego: Academic Press, 1992, pp. 234–235.
26. Wrigley RH: Ultrasonography of the spleen. Probl Vet Med *3:*574, 1991.
27. Schelling CG, Wortman JA, Saunders M: Ultrasonic detection of splenic necrosis in the dog. Three case reports of splenic necrosis secondary to infarction. Vet Radiol *29:*227, 1988.
28. Maresca G, et al: Sonographic patterns in splenic infarct. JCU *14:*23, 1986.
29. Lipowitz AJ, Blue J, Perman V: *The spleen. Torsion of the spleen.* In *Textbook of Small Animal Surgery.* Edited by DH Slatter. Philadelphia: WB Saunders, 1985, pp. 1211–1213.
30. Konde LJ, et al: Sonographic and radiographic changes associated with splenic torsion in the dog. Vet Radiol *30:*41, 1989.
31. Thomas WB, Hudson JA, Cartee RE: Splenic torsion in a dog. Vet Radiol *32:*227, 1991.

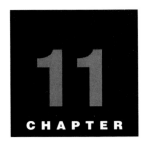

THE KIDNEYS

Susan T. Finn-Bodner

Technical improvements in resolution in ultrasound machines, decreased equipment costs, and availability of reasonable financing has made sonography an increasingly powerful tool for veterinary practice. The ability to combine detailed imaging with ultrasound-guided percutaneous biopsy and centesis has allowed sonography to replace traditional radiography and contrast radiography in many instances. To use this powerful diagnostic tool, the veterinary sonographer must be familiar with its abilities and limitations. The focus of this chapter is on the sonographic appearance of the normal anatomy and commonly encountered disease processes of the upper urinary system.

INDICATIONS FOR SONOGRAPHY

Indications for nephrosonography include abnormal kidney size, shape, or position; uremia; hematuria; flank pain; inability to palpate kidneys or to visualize them radiographically; enlargement, loss of detail, or abnormal opacities in the retroperitoneal space; and as part of routine abdominal sonography.[1] Sonography is more sensitive than radiography for small parenchymal masses and changes in internal architecture of the kidney.[2] Nephrosonography can differentiate solid from cystic masses, pinpoint lesion location, and evaluate adjacent organs when a renal mass is suspected. It is more specific and sensitive in detecting and localizing mineralization or calculi to the renal pelvis, pelvic diverticula, or cortex.[3,4] Sonography is a sensitive indicator of renal pelvic or ureteral disease if dilatation is present, but research to date indicates that excretory urography may be slightly more sensitive in detecting scarring and deformity of the pelvic diverticula in chronic pyelonephritis.[3,4]

Excretory urography is traditionally the recommended technique for complete evaluation of the upper urinary tract, although it is time consuming, expensive, invasive, and exposes the patient and handlers to ionizing radiation. Additionally, this technique may require sedation or anesthesia, placement of an intravenous catheter, and adequate renal function for a diagnostic examination. Reported risks of excretory urography usually involve adverse reaction to contrast medium, including nausea, vomiting, urticaria, and contrast medium-induced renal failure.[5–8]

Sonography involves no radiation and does not require intravenous or bladder catheterization. It is easy and rapid, with good acceptance in the nonsedated patient, and has no reported complications. Hypovolemia or decreased renal blood flow does not affect image quality, although subcutaneous fat appears more echogenic and may transmit sound less readily in the dehydrated patient. Poor radiographic contrast, because of emaciation or abdominal fluid, and previous positive contrast radiographic procedures does not affect the quality of sonography.[3,4] Additionally, simultaneous ultrasound-guided biopsy and aspiration of detected lesions can be obtained. Sonography should be considered the initial step in diagnostic imaging to evaluate the upper urinary tract along with associated lymph nodes and organs. Additional information or confirmation of pathology should be pursued with excretory urography.[1,2]

TECHNIQUES

The kidney is scanned in three planes; midsagittal, midtransverse, and mid-dorsal (coronal). The image plane of the kidney relative to the patient's body wall depends on the position of the patient and the resulting position of the mobile kidney. While scanning the patient in dorsal recumbency, positioning the probe along the ventral body wall results in the best midsagittal images. Access to the right kidney is more difficult but can be obtained from the right costospinal angle. The transducer can be placed ventrally over the caudal extremity of the kidney and angled cranially if the kidneys are located deep to the ribs. Occasionally, the transducer must be placed in the intercostal space to visualize the right kidney. A good midsagittal image of the kidney shows the dorsal and ventral diverging branches of the renal diverticula and associated renal vessels in cross section as two bright parallel bars (Fig. 11–1).[9–11] Sliding the transducer medially from this point allows visualization of the renal hilus and the tips of the cranial and caudal pole cortices and medullary areas (Fig. 11–2). Moving the transducer laterally from the midsagittal image point shows the lateral cortex surrounding the nearly circular bases of the medullary pyramids, which are subdivided by echogenic diverticula (Fig. 11–3).[11] The pyramids are fused in the cranial and caudal extremities but not in the middle of the kidney.[9,12]

A transverse image of the right kidney is obtained by placing the probe in one of the last two intercostal spaces. The left kidney is imaged transversely from within or caudal to the last intercostal space. In a good midtransverse image of the kidney, the echogenic renal sinus with central interlobar arteries and veins forms a "C-sign" around the renal crest (the fused papilla of the medullary pyramids) (Fig. 11–4).[10] The hilar area, containing renal vessels, adipose tissue, and ureter, is seen extending dorsomedial toward the caudal vena cava and aorta. Distinct medullary papillae and vessels are described only in the dog,[3,12] although similar, less well-defined structures are present in the cat kidney.

A good mid-dorsal image of the kidney is obtained by placing the patient in lateral recumbency and placing the probe in the costospinal angle parallel to the spine. The surface of the transducer is placed along the lateral border of the kidney and directed toward the hilus along the long axis of the kidney (Fig. 11–5). This image of the kidney looks remarkably like its appearance at necropsy when the organ is split longitudinally, like a bean, starting at the hilus. In this scan plane, the renal hilus and hilar vessels are directed dorsomedial as in excretory urograms. In this scan plane, the interlobar vessels are oriented parallel to the sound beam for good Doppler evaluation of blood flow.

Survey radiographs to evaluate renal size can be inaccurate because of radiographic magnification and incomplete visualization of the kidneys in about 50% of radiographs.[9,13] Excretory urography improves visualization of the kidneys, but hypertonic iodinated urographic contrast medium transiently increases kidney size.[13–15] Sonographic size determinations are more accurate than radiographic determinations. Obtaining a true midsagittal, mid-dorsal, and midtransverse image is important to provide accurate renal length, height, and width measurements to calculate volume. Care is needed to avoid oblique image planes that alter linear measurements. Noninvasive calculation of kidney volume using sonography is sufficiently accurate to be clinically useful, particularly if used serially on the same patient to detect disease progression.[16] The sonographically derived measurements of length, width, and height can be used along with the formula for a prolate ellipsoid (Volume = L × W × H × 0.523) to calculate

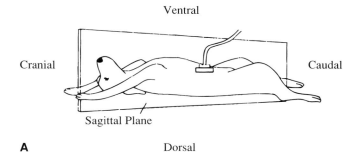

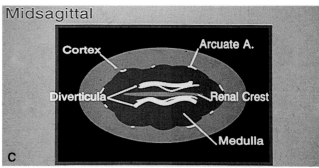

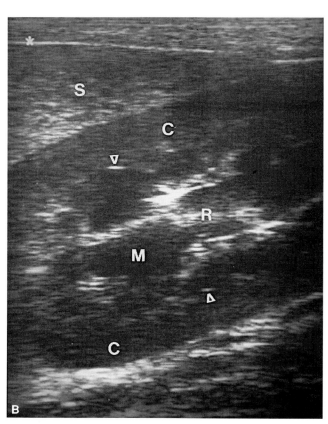

Figure 11–1

A. Probe placement for a midsagittal image of the kidney. The probe is placed on the ventral body wall parallel to the sagittal plane of the body. Minute changes in probe angulation are necessary to obtain the maximum renal length and to obtain this image with individual variations in body habitus. Images are improved by complete hair removal, massaging ultrasound coupling gel into the skin before examination, and examining the abdomen as early in the day as possible to avoid build-up of gastrointestinal gas. Patients can be in dorsal or lateral recumbency during scanning. Midsagittal sonogram **(B)** and schematic **(C)** of the normal left kidney of a dog demonstrate the parallel echogenic lines of the dorsal and ventral diverging branches of the renal diverticula. The cortex (C) is more echogenic than the medulla (M). The renal crest (R) is as echogenic as the cortex. Brightly echogenic "dots," the arcuate arteries (arrowheads), are seen at the corticomedullary junction. Note that the kidney is hypoechoic relative to spleen (S) and perirenal fat.

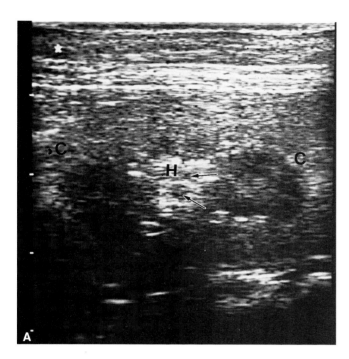

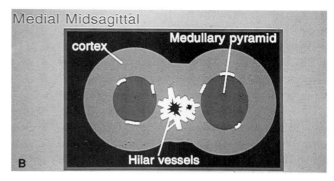

Figure 11-2

Medial parasagittal sonogram **(A)** and schematic **(B)** of a normal kidney of a cat obtained by sliding the probe slightly medial to the midsagittal plane of the kidney illustrated in Figure 11-1. Note the hyperechoic renal hilus (H) with cross section of renal vessels (arrows) and the cranial and caudal pole cortices (C).

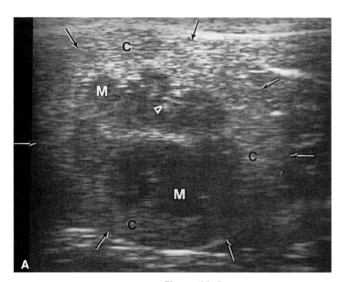

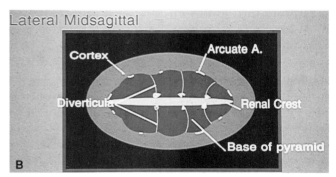

Figure 11-3

Lateral parasagittal sonogram **(A)** and schematic **(B)** of a normal kidney (arrows) of a cat obtained by sliding the probe slightly lateral to the midsagittal plane shown in Figure 11-1. The base of the medullary pyramids (M) are nearly circular and hypoechoic relative to the renal cortex (C). Echogenic renal diverticula (arrowhead) and vessels subdivide the pyramids. The cortex of this cat is fairly hyperechoic because of fat in the renal tubules. The medulla is relatively hypoechoic and corticomedullary distinction is good, allowing differentiation of this normal variation in sonographic renal appearance from that associated with pathologic change.

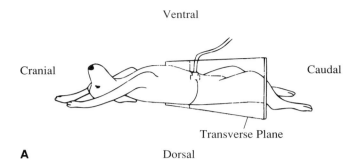

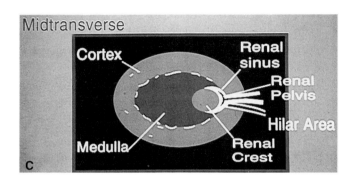

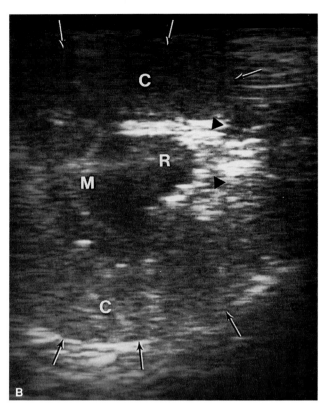

Figure 11–4

A, Probe placement for a midtransverse image of the kidney. The probe is rotated 90° from the position in Figure 11–1**A.** In a midtransverse sonogram **(B)** and schematic **(C)** of a normal kidney (arrows) of a cat, note the echogenic reversed "C" or "Y" formed by the renal pelvis (arrowheads) with the base of the Y composed of the renal hilus containing the large renal vessels and ureter. The "arms" of the Y are composed of the dorsal and ventral diverging branches of the diverticula. The echogenicity of the ridge-like renal crest (R) is slightly increased when compared to that of the medulla (M). The echogenic renal cortex (C) encircles the kidney. The gain has been decreased in the near field, creating an artifactual decrease in cortical echoes.

renal volume.[16,17] The use of a linear correction factor and measurement of width and height at three levels is more time consuming but can provide additional accuracy.[16] An accurate and easier method for volume evaluation involves the use of longitudinal area and length of the kidney in a dorsal or midsagittal image to calculate renal volume (Volume = [Area^2 × 0.85] / Length) if the ultrasound system used has area measurement capabilities.[18] Sonography consistently underestimates actual renal volume by an acceptably small amount.

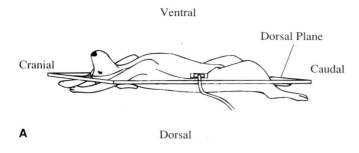

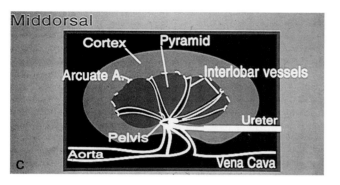

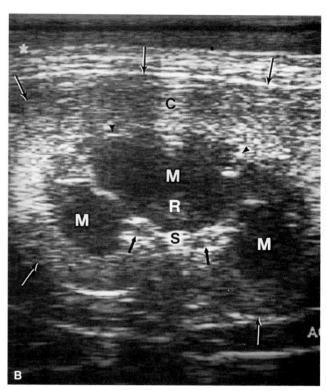

Figure 11–5

A, For a mid-dorsal image of the kidney, the probe is placed along the lateral body wall, just ventral to the transverse processes of the spine and directed toward midline by small angular increments. In a mid-dorsal sonogram **(B)** and schematic **(C)** of a normal kidney (arrows) of a cat, homogeneous echogenic renal cortex (C) surrounds the hypoechoic medullary pyramids (M), which are fused at the tip into the renal crest (R). Hyperechoic diverging branches of the renal pelvic diverticula are not visualized because this plane is located between them. Hyperechoic semicircle of the renal sinus (S) contains the potential space of the renal pelvis. Anechoic fluid separation of the pelvis is not seen normally, unless diuresis is present. Branches of the main renal artery and vein (arrows) are parallel-walled hypoechoic structures extending from the renal pelvis. Arcuate arteries (arrowheads) are bright "dots" at the corticomedullary junction. Aorta (AO) is seen dorsal and medial to the hilus.

Surrounding landmarks can be used to locate and identify the kidney when pathology in the abdomen or kidney, displacement of the kidney, or patient conformation makes identification of the kidney difficult. Structures adjacent to the right kidney are as follows: dorsally, diaphragmatic crus and psoas muscles; medially, caudal vena cava; ventrally, duodenum and pancreas; cranioventrally, colon and a distended stomach; cranially, renal fossa of caudate liver lobe; and laterally, abdominal wall. The left kidney is surrounded laterally by spleen and abdominal wall, cranially by pancreas and stomach, craniomedially by colon, and medially by aorta. The aorta and vena cava are the most reliable landmarks to locate and follow the renal vein and artery to the kidneys (Fig. 11–6).

Figure 11–6

Dorsal oblique sonogram of the left perirenal area of a dog. The renal artery (A) makes a U turn as it leaves the aorta (AO) and approaches the left renal hilus (H). These vascular landmarks can be used to identify an abnormal appearing kidney or to locate the left adrenal gland, which usually is close to the U turn in the renal artery. The left adrenal gland of this dog contained a carcinoma.

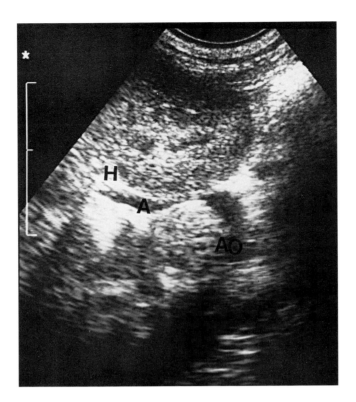

NORMAL RENAL ANATOMY

The kidney is composed of 12 to 16 radially arranged, poorly defined lobes of caplike cortex enclosing the bases of pyramid-shaped medulla. The apices of the pyramids fuse to form a ridge-like common papilla, the renal crest. The renal crest projects into the pelvis, which has several recesses (diverticula) containing grooves for interlobar vessels.[9] The sonographic architecture of the kidney is complex, containing a mixture of hyperechoic, hypoechoic, and anechoic patterns. In comparison, most of the other organs in the abdomen are relatively homogeneous. Intra-abdominal pathology, such as neoplastic masses, often create echo complex lesions. The repetitiveness of the echo complex pattern of the kidney allows one to distinguish between it and a pathologic mass.

The major regions of the kidney include the echogenic cortex, the less echogenic medullary pyramids, the hyperechoic radiating striations of the diverticula and vasculature, and the extremely hyperechoic fat and fibrous tissue of the renal sinus (see Fig. 11–5). Areas of the kidney have been ranked from most to least echogenic as follows: capsule > diverticula and vasculature > renal sinus > cortex = area cribrosa of renal crest > medulla.[3,10] The capsule appears to be echogenic, mostly with lower frequency transducers (3.5 and 5.0 mHz). Echogenicity of the capsule is variable and depends on the angle of the ultrasound beam as it reflects off of the renal surface (anisotropism). The capsule is seen as a bright linear echo when the ultrasound beam is perpendicular to the surface of the kidney or when the kidney is scanned in vitro (Fig. 11–7). The echogenic band that surrounds the renal cortex is a combination of fibrous capsule and perirenal fat. At the cranial and caudal poles, the capsule of the kidney is less easy to define because of off-incidence artifact of the ultrasound beam.

The renal cortex is a coarsely homogeneous echogenic rim, the echogenicity of which is created by renal corpuscles (glomerulus, glomerular capsule, and convoluted tubules) and resulting collagen interfaces.[11] Traditionally, the cortex has been deemed

Figure 11–7

In vitro transverse sonogram of a normal kidney of a dog. The renal capsule (arrows) is echogenic because of the difference in acoustic impedance between the surrounding fluid and renal parenchyma and in part because of an increase in collagen in the capsule. In vivo, the renal capsule is difficult to detect.

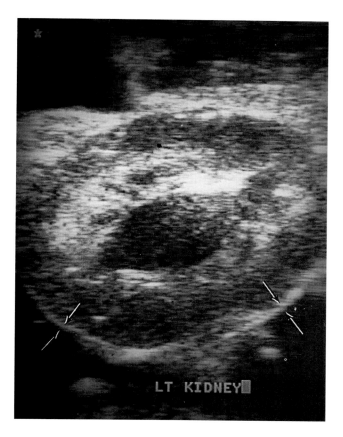

sonographically normal when it is relatively less echogenic than the liver and spleen. Several pitfalls exist with this method of comparative organ ultrasonology. The sonographer must assume that the control organ is normal and it must be at the same depth as the organ being evaluated. Intervening organs or superficial tissue changes can impede the sound beam and change the relative echogenicity of two adjacent organs. The echogenicity of the renal cortex depends on the direction and angle of the sound beam. Therefore, the kidneys may be scanned from different transducer positions to more clearly assess suspected changes in renal echogenicity. Additionally, the amount of fat in vacuoles in renal cortical tubular epithelium of cats correlates with increases in renal size and cortical echogenicity, which can emphasize differences in echogenicity between cortex and medulla but makes cortex appear more like renal sinus.[19] Age may affect the relative echogenicity of the cortex and medulla, with the renal medulla of neonates and infants appearing nearly anechoic.

Normal renal cortex can appear isoechoic, hypoechoic, or hyperechoic relative to liver parenchyma depending on the frequency of the transducer being used (Fig. 11-8). In a study of 34 dogs with histologically normal kidneys, most renal cortices were isoechoic or hypoechoic relative to the liver when imaged with a 5-mHz transducer.[20] In contrast, nearly one half of the renal cortices were hyperechoic to the liver when imaged with a 7.5-mHz transducer. Therefore, comparing renal echogenicity to liver and spleen parenchyma may not be diagnostic unless the relative echogenicities are dramatically different. Normal renal cortex is always hyperechoic relative to the medulla, however, and this internal comparison may be more reliable in detecting diffuse changes in renal echogenicity with infiltrative disease.[19] An ultrasound-guided biopsy is beneficial in diagnosing diffuse infiltrative renal disease.

In the mid-dorsal image, five or more medullary pyramids are well defined and directed with the apex toward the renal sinus. The renal medulla has been described as "an-

Figure 11–8

Enlarged lateral parasagittal sonogram of the cranial pole of the right kidney of a dog within the renal fossa of the caudate liver lobe (L). Similar echogenicity between liver and renal cortex (C) would make boundary detection difficult if not for the presence of hyperechoic perirenal fat (arrow) and a small amount of anechoic abdominal fluid in this patient (F).

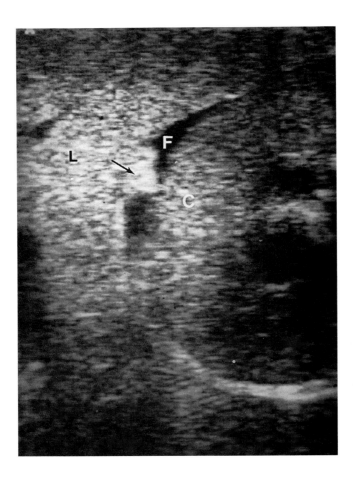

echoic" or hypoechoic. The term anechoic should be reserved for structures that, unlike the medulla, have no internal echoes. Adequate sonographic resolution is needed to detect the subtle internal echoes of medullary tissue. The paucity of echoes from the medulla is because of the presence of predominantly thin-walled straight tubular loops and collecting ducts. Subtle increases in echoes are detected at the corticomedullary junction and renal crest (see Fig. 11–5). A 1- to 3-mm thick hyperechoic band, located several millimeters inside and paralleling the corticomedullary junction, has been positively associated with a band of mineral deposition in medullary tubules of histologically normal cats.[19] The cortex to medullary ratio should be approximately 1 to 1,[12] measured on lateral sagittal images across the cortex and base of a medullary pyramid (Fig. 11–3). The average medullary base diameter is 8 mm and varies from 5 to 12 mm.[21] An increase in the size of the medulla during diuresis has been reported.[22,23] This change may be less detectable in cats undergoing diuresis.[10]

The renal pelvis is the proximal expansion of the ureter, and the renal sinus is the cavity in the kidney that contains the pelvis, vessels, nerves, and fat. The potential cavity of the renal pelvis typically is not visualized with ultrasound.[3,10,12,23,24] Visualization of an anechoic lumen in the renal pelvis of dogs and cats with lower frequency transducers has been described as consistent with hydronephrosis or pyelonephritis,[3,4] although visualization of the renal pelvis depends on the resolution of the ultrasound instrument used.

With high resolution sonography (≥7.5 mHz), renal pelvic distention (pyelectasis) can be detected in normal dogs undergoing supraphysiologic diuresis, creating a small anechoic zone between the hyperechoic lines of the renal sinus (Fig. 11–9).[25] Renal pelvis dilatation greater than 3 to 4 mm may be indicative of pathologic change.[9] This

Figure 11–9

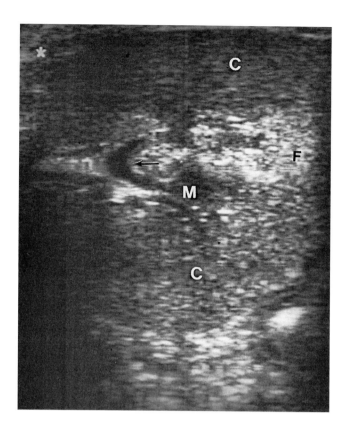

Transverse sonogram of the right kidney in a 12-year-old cat undergoing supraphysiologic intravenous fluid diuresis for chronic interstitial nephritis. Note the anechoic fluid separating the walls of the renal pelvis (arrow) secondary to diuresis in the absence of hydronephrosis or pyelonephritis. Note also the generalized increase in renal echogenicity, increased cortical thickness, and decreased difference in echogenicity between the cortex (C) and medulla (M), making their boundaries indistinct. The triangular hyperechoic foci (F) in the cortex is an infarct.

observation has not yet been reported in cats, possibly because of an inability to resolve the small degree of pelvic separation. Mild pyelectasis has been detected in normal humans with distended bladders because of altered ureteral peristalsis and changes at the ureterovesicular junction resulting from back pressure.[26] This effect has not yet been documented in dogs and cats. First order branches of the renal vessels can be differentiated from mild dilatation of the renal pelvis using color flow Doppler (Fig. 11–10). If color flow Doppler is not available, the bright continuous parallel walls of renal vessels can be differentiated from the noncontinuous and nonparallel borders of the dilated renal pelvis.

The sonographic size of the cat kidney is 3.8 to 4.4 cm long, 2.7 to 3.1 cm wide, and 2.0 to 3.5 cm high with a 2- to 5-mm thick renal cortex.[9,13,24] Absolute renal measurements in the dog are less valuable because of extreme variation in the size of various breeds. A significant correlation exists between sonographic renal length, calculated renal volume, and body weight in dogs (Table 11–1).[17,18] Cortical width in the dog is 3 to 9 mm.[21,24] The dimensions of the left and right kidneys are considered similar, as are the dimensions of the kidney in dogs of either sex.[16]

The kidney of the normal dog is radiographically 2.5 to 3.5 times the length of the second lumbar vertebrae.[27] Similarly, the sonographically measured length of the kidney may be compared to the length of the second lumbar vertebrae as seen on an abdominal radiograph.[9] Magnification of structures does not occur during sonography, however, as it does during radiography. Therefore, the sonographically measured kidney would seem relatively small when compared to radiographically magnified vertebrae. An additional problem with this technique is that a radiograph must be taken for comparison. The length of the lumbar vertebral bodies is visible sonographically and could be compared to renal size determined sonographically to normalize renal size in the various canine breeds (Fig. 11–11).

The ureters typically parallel the psoas muscles and are retroperitoneal. The ureters tunnel through the dorsal bladder wall and empty at a ureteral orifice onto converging

Figure 11–10

Mid-dorsal sonogram of the caudal pole of the left kidney of a dog with hypercalcemic nephropathy undergoing fluid diuresis. The dilated renal pelvis is seen as a triangular anechoic area (P) separating the renal sinus. Renal arterial (red) and venous (blue) flow is indicated by color-tagging directional blood flow with color Doppler. Absence of Doppler-detected flow at these settings confirms that this structure is not a hilar blood vessel. Note the undulant hyperechoic line parallel to the corticomedullary junction, the "medullary rim sign" (arrows), associated with pathologic calcium deposition. The cranial pole is not visualized because of loss of contact of the probe at the skin surface creating reverberation artifact (R).

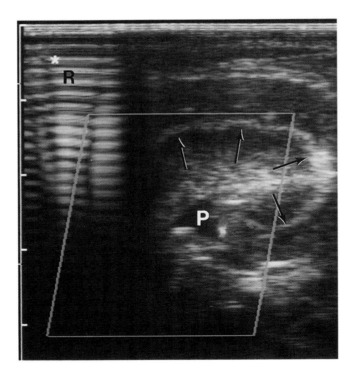

TABLE 11–1

Weight	Renal Length (cm)			Renal Volume (ml)		
	Range	Mean	SD	Range	Mean	SD
0–4	3.2–3.3	3.2	0.09	3.3–3.7	3.5	.24
5–9	3.2–5.2	4.4	0.50	6.6–18.0	12.7	3.32
10–14	4.8–6.4	5.6	0.60	14.1–39.6	24.7	8.49
15–19	5.0–6.7	6.0	0.40	19.0–40.1	30.5	5.68
20–24	5.2–8.0	6.5	0.72	26.2–5.13	39.8	7.43
25–29	5.3–7.8	6.9	0.58	25.2–64.0	44.5	8.80
30–34	6.1–8.7	7.2	0.60	30.5–75.5	53.1	12.14
35–39	6.6–9.3	7.6	0.72	44.4–102.1	60.7	14.82
40–44	6.3–8.4	7.6	0.54	41.2–87.7	63.0	12.83
45–49	7.6–9.1	8.5	0.46	58.2–98.6	83.6	13.60
50–59	7.5–10.6	9.1	1.27	56.7–120.9	94.8	26.85
60–69	8.3–9.8	9.0	0.63	80.0–124.9	102.6	20.19

ridges that sometimes are seen as focal thickenings in the dorsal wall of the bladder trigone (Fig. 11–12).[28] Ureters are typically not identified sonographically if they are normal. Peristaltic emptying of urine from the ureteral orifice into the bladder, "ureteral jets," can be detected with color flow Doppler.[28] Administration of furosemide before sonographic evaluation changes the relative physical density between urine emptying from ureters and urine within the bladder, improving sonographic visualization of ureteral jets. The increased velocity, volume, and frequency of the jets after administration of the diuretic also assists visualization.[28] In some animals, ureteral jets can be detected during gray scale imaging without Doppler evaluation, possibly because of protein, fat droplets, or cells within the urine.

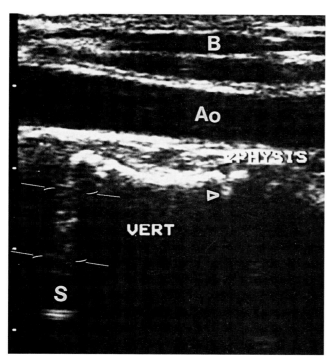

Figure 11–11

Sagittal sonogram of the caudal vertebral column of a dog. The sound beam is completely attenuated and reflected at the hyperechoic curvilinear surface of the ventral vertebral body (VERT). The beam penetrates the intervertebral disk space (arrows) and reveals the spinal cord (S) dorsal to the disk. The cartilaginous physis (arrowhead) of the vertebral end plate is partly penetrated by the sound beam. The vertebral body length can be compared to kidney length to evaluate renal size in animals of differing size. Note the sagittal view of the bright-walled anechoic aorta (Ao) and small intestine (B) ventral to the vertebral body.

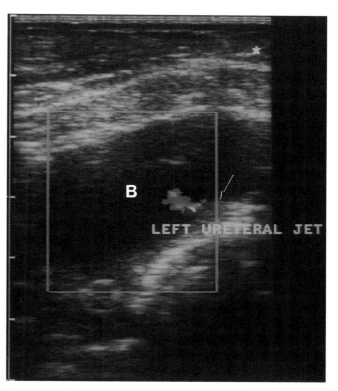

Figure 11–12

Transverse sonogram of the urinary bladder (B) in an incontinent female dog shows a prominent conical ureteral papilla (arrow). When visualized, this normal structure can be differentiated from mucosal masses by location and the presence of ureteral "jets" of urine emptying from them. The color Doppler signal identifies a ureteral jet of urine emptying into the bladder from the left ureteral papillae. A jet from the right ureter could not be identified. The ureter was confirmed as ectopic during surgery.

The main branches of the renal artery and vein and interlobar arteries and veins are best seen on mid-dorsal images as parallel hyperechoic linear structures with anechoic lumina in the renal pelvis and pelvic diverticula, respectively (Fig. 11–13). Thirteen to 20% of dogs have multiple arteries entering the renal hilus, especially to the left kidney.[9] The renal vein is more compressible and the vascular diameter is often greater than the adjacent renal artery. The intima of the renal vein is reportedly slightly less reflective than the intima of the artery, but this difference is difficult to detect. Doppler evaluation of blood flow direction and characteristics is the best way to differentiate renal vein and artery. The renal vein may appear to pulsate because of proximity to the artery.[9] The renal artery and vein exit the hilar area of the kidney, travel caudodorsomedial, and can be followed back to the aorta and vena cava, respectively. Approximately 5 mm from the hilus, the main renal artery and vein divide into interlobar vessels that are contained within the renal diverticula. Interlobar arteries and veins can be visualized as parallel echogenic lines with anechoic lumen within the renal diverticula between medullary pyramids (Fig. 11–14). The interlobar vessels branch into arcuate arteries at the corticomedullary junction. Cross-sectional views of the arcuate arteries are seen at the corticomedullary junction as focal hyperechoic dots (Fig. 11–15).[11] Arcuate vessels branch into interlobular vessels in cortical parenchyma and can be seen, in some instances, as echogenic lines in the cortex.[11]

Color Doppler imaging allows excellent visualization of the renal vasculature. Placement of a sample volume within the lumen of a vessel and correction of the Doppler angle to match the linear course of the sample vessel allows analysis of blood flow with pulsed Doppler imaging (Fig. 11–16). The magnitude of the Doppler-detected blood flow velocity is extremely dependent on the angle at which the emitted sound beam contacts the moving blood cells. Various ratios of the blood flow velocities during different phases of the cardiac cycle can be used as mathematic means of eliminating this dependence on Doppler angle. The resistive index (peak systolic velocity - end diastolic velocity/peak systolic velocity) is used commonly in human vascular sonography and indicates the resistance of an organ to perfusion. The normal resistive index in dogs has been established as 0.63 ± 0.05.[29] Renal disease in humans, such as diabetic nephropathy, allograft rejection, arteriosclerosis, edema, and infiltrative disease within the glomerulointerstitial compartment, is associated with an increase in the resistive index.[30] An increase in the resistive index has been found in dogs with acute ureteral obstruction.[29] We have seen elevated resistive indices of 0.74 to 0.89 associated with a hypercalcemic nephropathy, ethylene glycol toxicity, and radiographic contrast media- induced acute renal failure (see Fig. 11–16).[8] More research in the field of veterinary sonography is needed to make the renal blood flow indices clinically useful.

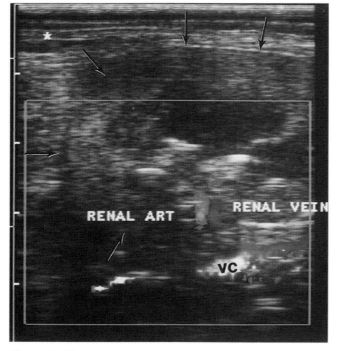

Figure 11–13

Mid-dorsal sonogram of the kidney (arrows) of a cat shows the paired renal artery (red) and vein (blue) entering the renal hilus. Color Doppler "tags" vessels with color according to the direction of blood flow, with red denoting arterial flow toward the probe and blue indicating venous flow away from the probe, as indicated by the color wheel (W). The caudal vena cava (VC) is blue because flow is moving away, at a slight angle, from the probe face located adjacent to the caudolateral renal cortex.

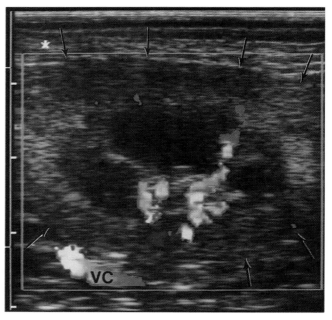

Figure 11–14

Mid-dorsal sonogram of the kidney (arrows) of a normal cat shows red- labeled blood flow in the interlobar arteries moving toward the probe face. Red flow is seen also in the caudal vena cava (VC) because blood flow returning to the heart is moving at a slight angle toward the probe face, which is positioned cranially on the kidney and angled toward the caudal pole.

Figure 11–15

Mid-dorsal sonogram of the kidney (arrows) of a normal cat. The red-coded blood flow at the corticomedullary junction (arrowheads) is within arcuate arteries. Flow is not seen within the interlobar arteries because they are outside the thin scan plane of this image. The arcuate arteries appear as hyperechoic "dots" at the corticomedullary junction when color Doppler is not used. The aorta (Ao) is the parallel-walled anechoic structure deep to the kidney. No Doppler flow is visualized in this vessel because the blood flow is perpendicular to the probe face and is not an effective reflector of the sound beam at this angle.

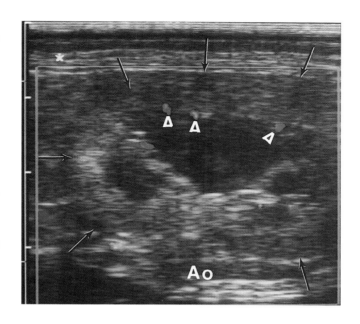

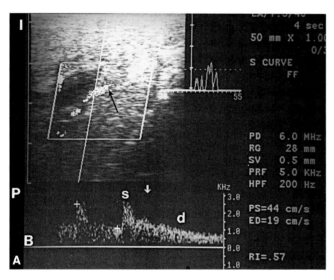

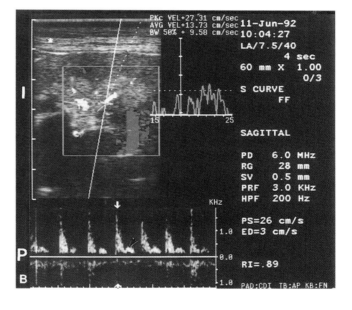

Figure 11–16

A, Mid-dorsal color and pulsed Doppler image (I) of the kidney of a dog with ethylene glycol toxicity. A pulsed Doppler sample volume (arrow) was placed within an interlobar artery to analyze blood flow. On the pulsed Doppler renal spectrum (P), time is registered on the horizontal axis and the Doppler shift frequency, indicating blood flow velocity, is registered on the vertical axis. The biphasic waveforms are above the baseline (B), indicating that blood flow is toward the probe. Although pathologic change is present in this kidney, the pulsed Doppler spectrum is fairly normal, with a steep systolic peak (s) and continuous diastolic blood flow (d), which forms a gradually decreasing slope from the systolic peak. **B,** Mid-dorsal color image (I) and pulsed Doppler spectrum (P) of the left kidney of a dog with contrast-induced renal failure. The pulsed Doppler spectrum from an interlobar artery shows a sharp high velocity peak for systolic flow (arrow) and a lower peak for the "dampened" diastolic flow (arrowhead) in this dog. The normalized ratio between the systolic and diastolic flow, the resistive index (RI = .89), is abnormally high, indicating resistance to perfusion. From Daley CA, Finn-Bodner ST, Lenz SD: Contrast- induced renal failure documented by color Doppler imaging in a dog. J Anim Hosp Assoc *30:*33, 1994.

The sonographic appearance of renal disease has been divided into various classification schemes. In humans, type 1 renal disease is diffuse change in the echogenicity of some part of the kidney such as enhancement of the corticomedullary junction or increased cortical echoes. Type 2 disease disrupts the normal anatomy. The classification scheme to be used in this chapter is: (1) focal or multifocal disease, (2) regional disease, and (3) diffuse disease.

Focal and Multifocal Renal Disease

Sonography is most sensitive in detecting focal and multifocal disease or regional renal disease and least sensitive in detecting diffuse parenchymal disease without architectural change. The sonographic appearance of focal or multifocal renal disease is often nonspecific, however, and cell type or malignancy determinations are usually not possible without biopsy. Focal and multifocal disease of the kidneys includes calculi, neoplasia, infarcts, cysts, abscesses, hematomas, and granulomas.

Calculi

Renal calculi appear as focal, intensely hyperechoic areas associated with the renal pelvis or diverticula (Fig. 11–17). Calculi may not shadow if they are smaller than the active element diameter of the transducer, if thick or heterogeneous tissue intervenes between the transducer and calculus, or if the calculus is outside of the focal zone of the transducer, especially if in the far field.[24] Dystrophic mineralization or fibrosis near the pelvis can be mistaken for small calculi by creating a hyperechoic focus and, sometimes, an acoustic shadow (Fig. 11–18). Small calculi in the diverticula may be obscured by hyperechoic pelvic tissue. Large calculi have been reported to cause reverberation, much like a tissue-air interface, which can fill in an acoustic shadow.[9] This effect can often be controlled by decreasing acoustic power or gain. The chemical composition or radiographic opacity of a calculus does not correlate with acoustic shadowing or echo intensity.[9,12,22] Sonography can be used to monitor dissolution of renoliths because its noninvasive nature permits sequential examinations.

Neoplasia

Most renal tumors, primary and metastatic, are focal or multifocal lesions. The chronicity and growth characteristics of a tumor affect the sonographic appearance. Echogenicity of a tumor varies with the homogeneity of the cells and the presence of hemorrhage and necrosis (hypoechogenic) or fibrosis, high vascularity, and mineralization (hyperechogenic).[3,4,31–33] These variations within the interior of advanced neoplasia often make renal tumors echo complex by the time veterinary patients are presented for sonography.

Most canine renal neoplasms are echo complex, expansile, and anatomically disruptive (87% of carcinomas, 50% of sarcomas) (Fig. 11–19) although some may be focally hyperechoic (13% of carcinomas, 50% of sarcomas).[3,4] Renal adenocarcinomas have been described as heteroechoic, invasive, and poorly demarcated.[3,4,12] Renal carcinomas have been seen with internal mineralization.[9] Occasionally, renal sarcomas and transitional cell papillomas are nearly isoechoic, detectable only by a change in the renal contour](Fig. 11–20).[4]

In contrast, 63% of feline renal neoplasms are poorly defined hypoechoic areas because lymphosarcoma is the most common renal tumor in the cat.[3,4,12,33,34] The hypoechoic masses of lymphosarcoma may mimic feline polycystic disease (Fig. 11–21). Usually, lymphomatous lesions can be differentiated from polycystic change by the presence of minimal to absent through transmission and the absence of clearly defined far and near walls. Solitary neoplastic masses are reportedly uncommon in the cat.[33]

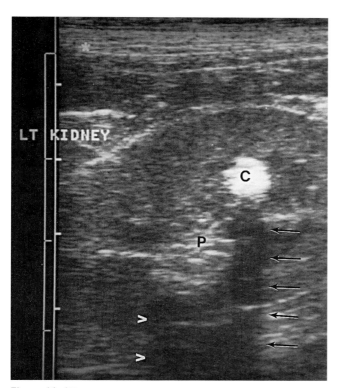

Figure 11–17

Medial parasagittal sonogram of the caudal pole of the left kidney in a dog with renal pain and a chronic urinary tract infection. The brightly hyperechoic curvilinear focus with distal acoustic shadowing (arrows) is a calculus (C) in the diverticula of the renal pelvis (P). Note that although the renal pelvis is echogenic and may cast a weak acoustic shadow (arrowheads), it is not as brightly echo dense or discretely marginated as the calculus.

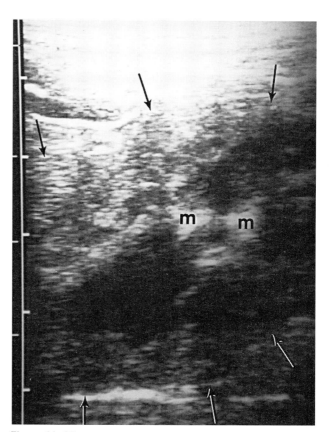

Figure 11–18

Medial parasagittal sonogram of the right kidney (arrows) of a dog with mineralization of the renal pelvis. The hyperechoic foci of mineralization (m) are similar in sonographic appearance to pelvic renoliths. Acoustic shadowing is less dramatic than would be expected in calculi of this size. The appearance may be slightly less discrete than calculi, but often a distinction between a surgical renolith and nonsurgical mineralization cannot be made sonographically.

The ability to detect renal neoplasia increases as the size of the tumor increases.[4,22,32,33] Experimentally implanted tumors have been detected at less than 0.5 to 1 cm, but the implantation site was known.[35] Small renal masses may be difficult to detect if they are isoechoic or subtly hypoechoic.[24] Very large masses may replace renal tissue to the extent that positive identification can be a challenge (Fig. 11–22). Additionally, large renal masses may occupy the abdomen outside of the normal renal boundaries, making geographic orientation difficult.[2] Large masses may have cysts, abscesses, hematomas, or areas of necrosis associated with them, further obscuring their origin from renal tissue (Fig. 11–23).

Alteration of renal architecture was the earliest sonographic abnormality detected in a study of induced carcinomas in rabbit kidneys.[35] These anaplastic tumors altered the renal outline, obliterated the medulla, and created perirenal fluid at 1 to 2 weeks. Internal changes in echogenicity were not seen until 3 to 4 weeks, with the appearance of anechoic and hypoechoic areas of necrosis and hemorrhage.[35] The transducer must be oriented perpendicular to the renal surface to avoid creating artifactual changes in renal outline. Excessive transducer pressure on the surface of the kidney in small or thin animals can deform the shape of the kidney.

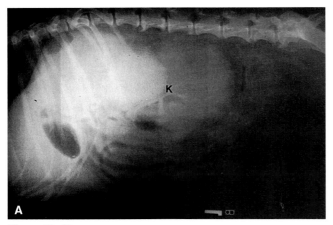

Figure 11–19

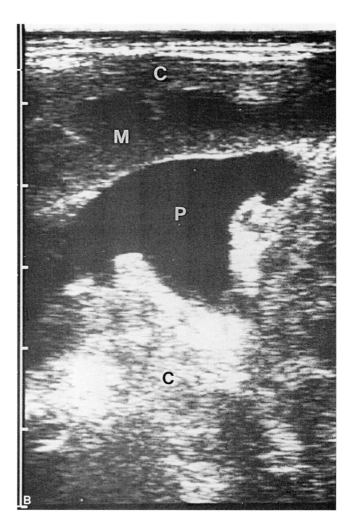

A, Lateral abdominal radiograph of a dog with hematuria shows an enlarged, rounded left kidney (K). Radiographic differentials include neoplasia, hydronephrosis, acute nephritis, acute pyelonephritis, and perirenal pseudocyst. **B,** Mid-dorsal sonogram of the left kidney of the same dog. The entire renal mass is not seen because of the narrow field of view of the linear array probe. A narrowed rind of renal cortex (C) is present in the near field. The near-field medulla (M) is also reduced. The medial portion of the kidney is replaced by a large renal carcinoma (C). Compression by the mass is causing dilatation of the renal pelvis (P).

Figure 11–20

Midsagittal sonogram of the left kidney (arrowheads) of a dog with metastatic carcinoma. The hypoechoic mass (M) is deforming the surface of the cranial pole of the kidney. The hyperechoic renal parenchyma is difficult to distinguish from perirenal fat because of the presence of chronic infiltrative disease. The bright hyperechoic area is part of the renal hilus (H).

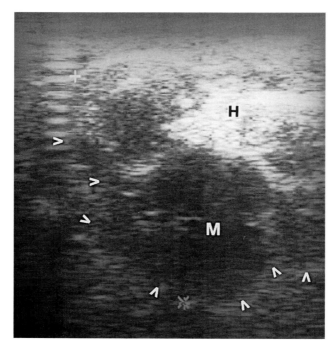

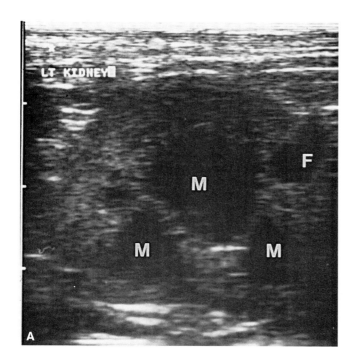

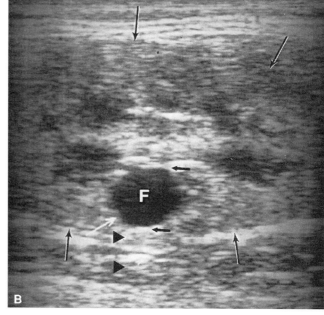

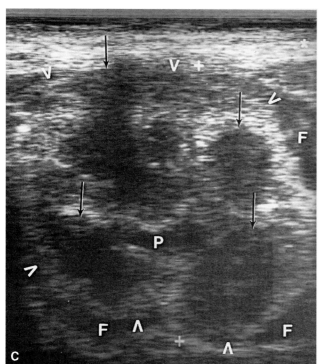

Figure 11–21

A, Mid-dorsal sonogram of the left kidney of a cat with renal lymphoma. Note the irregularly bordered hypoechoic focus (F) within the cortex. Such pathologic foci must be distinguished from normal medulla. **B,** Midsagittal sonogram of the kidney (large black arrows) of a cat with polycystic renal disease. The cortical cyst (white arrow, F) may be differentiated from lymphoma by the smooth circular contour, through transmission (arrowheads), and bright specular near and far wall echoes (small black arrows). Multiple cysts were found in different scan planes through the kidney. **C,** Lateral parasagittal sonogram of the kidney (arrowheads) of an older cat with weight loss, anorexia, and azotemia associated with renal lymphosarcoma. Much of the normal sonographic architecture of the kidney has been replaced by hypoechoic masses (arrows). The renal pelvis (P) is mildly dilated, the kidney (arrows) is enlarged and misshapen, and a small amount of echogenic subcapsular fluid accumulation surrounds the kidney (F).

The ability to correlate sonographic appearance with tumor type or malignancy has not been possible thus far, other than to some degree for lymphosarcoma. Cavitated lesions such as cysts, hematomas, or abscesses may appear solid and mimic neoplastic masses if they contain cellular debris or inspissated material. Frequently, it is necessary to combine sonographic detection of a lesion with guidance for percutaneous fine-needle biopsy.[36] With further investigation, Doppler-detected velocities and resistance of blood flow in renal masses may provide information on malignancy. One study of renal

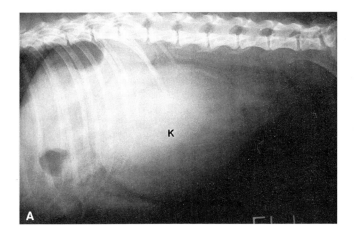

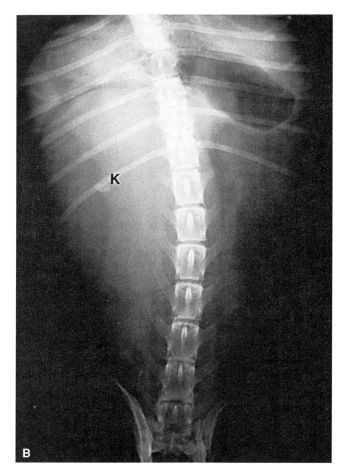

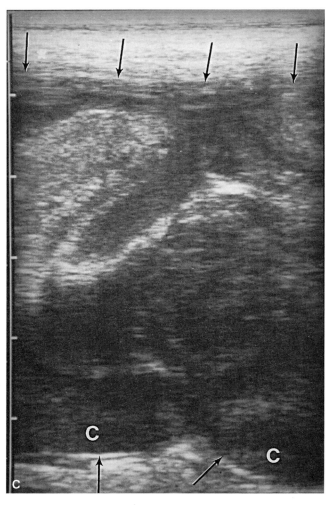

Figure 11–22

Lateral **(A)** and ventrodorsal **(B)** radiographs of a dog with a large mass in the area of the right kidney (K). A mid-dorsal sonogram of the right kidney **(C)** reveals a heteroechoic or echo complex mass has replaced much of the normal architecture of the kidney (arrows). A small portion of renal cortex (C) is visible near the renal hilus.

masses showed that 50% of dogs with renal neoplasia had metastasis to other organs,[32] indicating the importance of examining the entire abdomen during sonographic evaluation.

Infarcts

Renal infarction has a time-dependent sonographic appearance.[37] One study in dogs showed the appearance of hypoechoic renal foci after occlusion of a segmental renal artery for 8 hours.[38] After 24 hours, bulging of the renal outline was associated with these hypoechoic areas of tubular necrosis and interstitial edema (Fig. 11–24). Seven to 10 days

Figure 11–23

Medial parasagittal sonogram of the cranial pole of the kidney (arrowheads) of an older male dog with a previously resected seminoma in a retained testicle. The irregular hypoechoic mass (+) replacing the parenchyma of much of the cranial pole was first perceived to be adjacent to the kidney. Only after rotation of the probe and investigation of the mass in multiple planes was the primary renal origin of the mass appreciated. Note the end-on vessel (arrow) in the echogenic renal hilus.

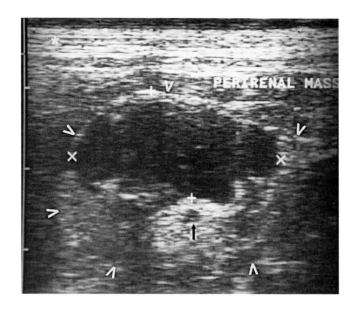

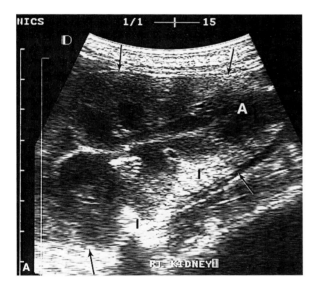

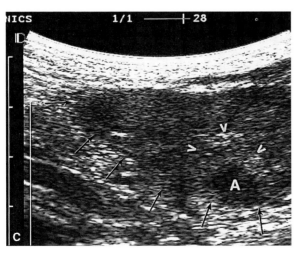

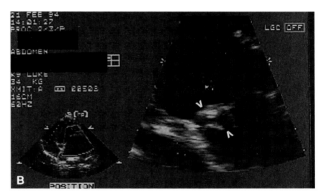

Figure 11–24

A, Lateral parasagittal sonogram of the left kidney (arrows) of a febrile, large-breed male dog. Note the echo complex appearance of the renal cortex with multiple hyperechoic (I) and hypoechoic foci (A). The hyperechoic foci were consistent with chronic infarcts, although differentials for the hypoechoic areas were neoplasia, acute infarcts, and, less likely, abscess. Color Doppler examination confirmed the hypoechoic areas were acute cortical infarcts by the absence of internal vascular flow signals. **B,** Enlargement of the free wall leaflet of the mitral valve (MV) in a left parasternal long axis view of the heart of the same dog. Note the irregular, thickened, hyperechoic appearance of the valve leaflet (arrowheads). Additional lesions were identified in the aortic and tricuspid valves. Staphylococcus and Serratia were cultured repeatedly from the blood of this patient. **C,** Sagittal sonogram of the prostate (arrows) showed multiple slightly irregular hypoechoic areas with minimal through transmission and low level internal echoes. Prostatic abscesses were confirmed at necropsy. Hyperechoic foci (arrowheads) surrounding the hypoechoic area (A) represent parenchymal fibrosis.

later, an increase in the coarse echo pattern was seen as cellular infiltration and fibrosis progressed. Typically, chronic infarcts appear as a well-defined hyperechoic wedge with a broad base at the periphery, tapering to the corticomedullary junction, with thinning of the associated cortex (Fig. 11–25).[37,38] Some infarcts have internal mineralization (Fig. 11–26).[37] Doppler analysis of infarcts show avascularity, which appears as an absence of Doppler signal, differentiating infarction from neoplastic nodules (Fig. 11–27). Complete occlusion of the main renal artery may show no detectable change in the sonographic appearance for up to 10 days.[38] Subcapsular halos created by collateral circulation from capsular vessels may be seen.[38]

Cysts

Renal cysts are focal or multifocal, circular anechoic structures with well-defined near and far walls and through transmission (Fig. 11–28).[22] Some cysts may have low-level internal echoes from hemorrhage or cellular debris. Feline polycystic renal disease, which resembles human neonatal multicystic renal dysplasia, is fairly common and may be seen concurrently with hepatic cysts. One retrospective report on renal sonography found 50% of non-neoplastic feline renal disease to be polycystic disease.[3,12,33] Although common in the cat, renal cysts in the dog are usually small and solitary, and may be incidental.[3,4,12]

Prominent hypoechoic medullary papilla in the neonatal kidney and some forms of lymphosarcoma may mimic polycystic disease (see Fig. 11–28). A variant of feline polycystic renal disease has been described that is characterized by multifocal accumulations of fluid (glomerular filtrate) within renal parenchyma. This disease has been associated with diffuse hyperechoic change in the kidney with no detectable cystic structures.[3,12,33]

Figure 11–25

Lateral parasagittal sonogram of the caudal pole of the kidney (arrowheads) of a dog. Note the classic wedge-shaped, triangular hyperechoic focus of a chronic cortical infarct (I). The hypoechoic areas (M) are oblique images of the bases of the medullary pyramids, as the image plane was near the lateral surface of the kidney.

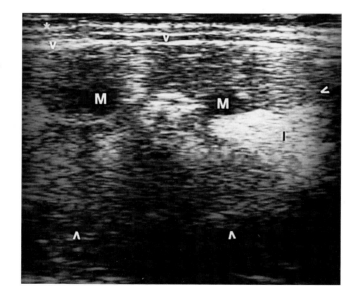

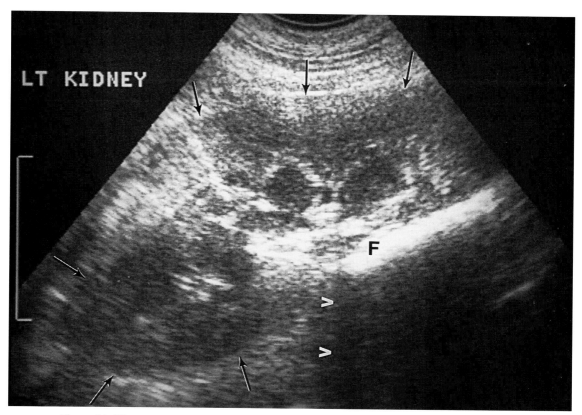

Figure 11-26

Lateral parasagittal sonogram of the kidney (arrows) of a dog obtained after routine abdominal radiographs revealed mineralization in the kidney. Note the linear, brightly hyperechoic focus (F) with distal acoustic shadowing (arrowheads) impeding visualization of the dorsomedial portion of the caudal pole. Final diagnosis was a mineralized chronic cortical infarct. Gas within the descending colon can mimic this lesion, but their distinction is possible with probe rotation.

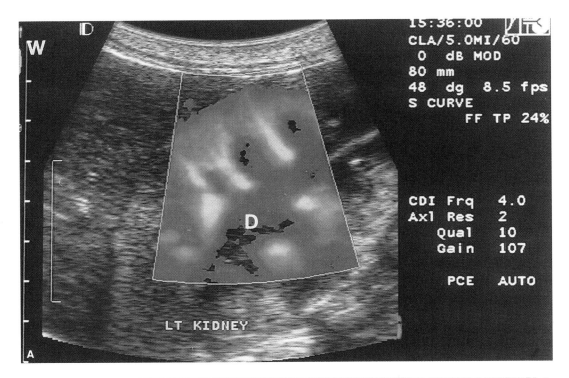

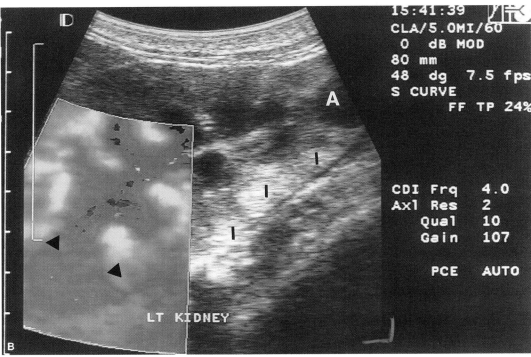

Figure 11-27

Lateral parasagittal sonograms of the left kidney of the dog in Figure 11–24 obtained to evaluate renal perfusion. This new technique (Ultrasound Angio®, Diasonics, Milpitas, CA) allows directionally independent analysis of the intensity of small moving reflectors (red blood cells), providing perfusion information down to the level of very small vessels. High velocity vascular flow in the interlobar arteries is color-tagged yellow and lower velocity flow of parenchymal perfusion is magenta, as indicated by the color wheel (W). **A,** An area of normal cortical blood flow signal. The branching central flow void (D) is the normal, fairly avascular pelvic diverticula and collecting system. **B,** The purple triangular focus (arrowheads) in the cranial cortex represents the vascular flow void of an acute infarct. Note the chronic hyperechoic infarcts (I) in the dorsal cortex and a second large hypoechoic acute infarct (A) in the caudal pole of the same kidney, which was confirmed at necropsy.

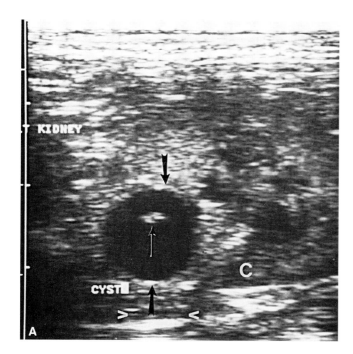

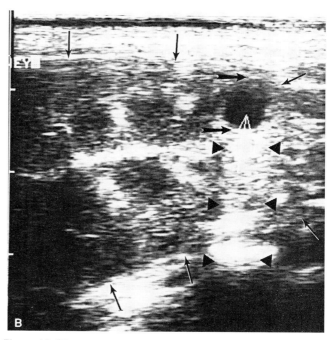

Figure 11–28

Lateral parasagittal sonograms of a cyst in the renal cortex (C) of a cat with polycystic renal disease (**A**) and a dog with a solitary renal cyst (white arrow)(**B**). Both cysts have a smooth circular contour, through transmission (arrowheads), and defined near and far wall echoes (black arrows). The anechoic fluid in the cyst in **A** contains a small echogenic focus (arrow), which may represent cellular debris or hemorrhage. **C**, Mid-dorsal sonogram of the kidney of a normal neonatal dog. The low level echoes of the neonatal medulla (M) are difficult to detect sonographically. They may resemble cystic lesions but do not have the circular shape, through transmission, and defined near and far walls.

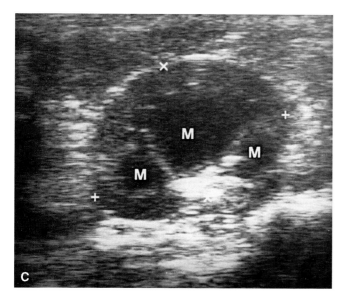

Abscesses

The sonographic appearance of renal abscesses varies from anechoic and cyst-like to an echogenic solid-appearing mass, depending on the character and inspissation of the purulent material (Fig. 11–29). Renal abscesses are reported as uncommon in both the dog and the cat.

Hematomas

The sonographic "life span" of a renal hematoma begins as an anechoic cyst-like structure. With formation of the fibrin clot, the hematoma becomes echogenic. Approximately 96 hours later, with the beginning of hemolysis, the hematoma acquires a complex appearance with anechoic and hyperechoic areas (Fig. 11–30). In chronic hematomas, reorganization and calcification recreates an echogenic appearance with occasional acoustic shadowing.

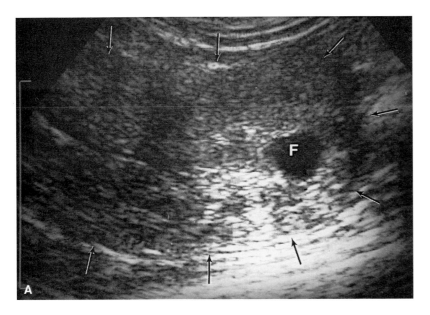

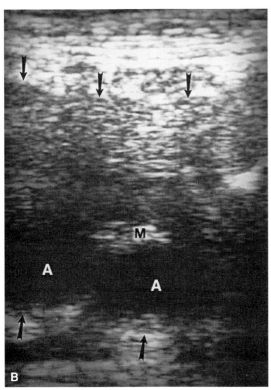

Figure 11–29

Renal abscesses may vary in size and appearance. **A,** Lateral parasagittal sonogram of the lateral cortex of the kidney (arrows) in a dog with abdominal pain, hematuria, and pyuria. Renal medulla is not identified because of the extreme lateral placement of the ultrasound beam. Note the irregular hypoechoic focus (F) of a cortical abscess. The minimal through transmission deep to the abscess indicates a high protein content fluid. Ultrasound-guided aspiration can be used to differentiate abscess from renal cyst and to provide culture information. If the abscess is encapsulated with a thick rind of tissue, a fine-gauge needle is used. The diffuse increase in cortical echogenicity from infiltrative disease in this kidney, a nephritis, makes the cortex difficult to differentiate from perirenal fat. **B,** Enlarged lateral parasagittal sonogram of the right kidney (arrows) of a dog with pain and a draining tract in the right flank. Overall increased echogenicity of the kidney from an acute nephritis makes the medulla difficult to distinguish from the cortex. Fibrosis with collagen deposition causes sound attenuation and an artifactual hypoechogenicity in the deeper portions of the kidney. Note two poorly circumscribed hypo- to anechoic foci (A) in the dorsal cortex with surrounding hyperechoic foci of mineralization (M). Severe chronic renal disease, mineralization, and renal abscessation were confirmed surgically.

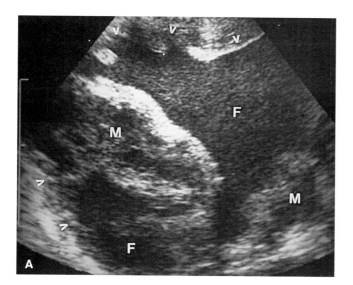

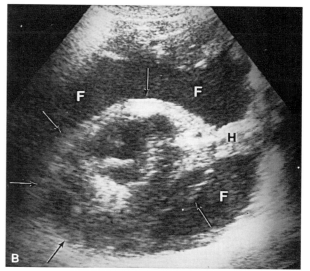

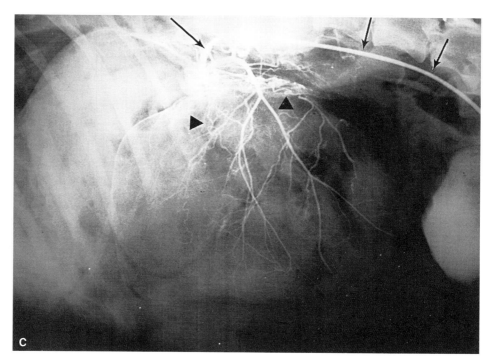

Figure 11–30

A, Sagittal sonogram of the right kidney area of a dog with anemia, a palpable abdominal mass, and acute collapse. A Large encapsulated (arrows) echogenic fluid collection (F) and multiple heteroechoic masses (M) replace the right kidney. During real- time examination, low-level reflectors were seen swirling in the fluid with agitation, indicating cellular material or hemorrhage within the fluid. In another scan plane **(B),** an abnormal appearing kidney (arrows) was seen within the echogenic fluid (F) and attached to the capsule by a stalk-like structure, which appeared to be the renal hilus. Minimal Doppler- detectable blood flow was present within renal parenchyma and vessels in the renal hilus (H). Sonographic differentials included subcapsular hemorrhage with hematomas and renal ischemia or necrosis, complicated perirenal pseudocyst, and neoplasia, such as a nephroblastoma. **C,** A selective renal angiogram (catheter within the aorta to the right renal artery, arrows) showed no evidence of flow in the renal artery but did reveal neovascularization of capsular blood vessels (arrowheads). A ruptured necrotic hydronephrotic kidney with subcapsular hemorrhage and hematomas were found at surgery.

Granulomas

The fibrous connective tissue of granulomas is the cause of their hyperechoic appearance. Renal granulomas are rare.

Regional Renal Disease

Regional disease diffusely affects an anatomic or functional compartment of the kidney and is easier than diffuse renal disease to identify sonographically. The sonographic appearance of some forms of regional disease is nearly pathognomonic. Regional diseases include perirenal pseudocysts and urinomas, nephrocalcinosis and hypercalcemic nephropathy, ethylene glycol toxicity, contrast medium-induced renal failure, pyelonephritis, and hydronephrosis.

Perirenal Pseudocysts

Perirenal pseudocysts are typically encapsulated accumulations of anechoic fluid surrounding the cortex of the kidney (Fig. 11–31) or associated with the ureter in the retroperitoneal space (urinoma or paraureteral pseudocyst).[39,40] Pseudocysts are often elliptic, with sharp borders and marked through transmission. They may have thin septa or low levels of internal echoes or be associated with hydronephrosis and hydroureter.[39] Any accumulation of fluid surrounding the kidney, within the renal capsule, or within the retroperitoneal space can appear as an anechoic zone encircling the renal cortex. Other lesions that must be differentiated from perirenal pseudocysts include ascites (not encapsulated), hematomas, abscesses, true renal cysts, and lymphoceles.

The kidney within the perirenal pseudocyst may have a diffuse increase in echogenicity, poor corticomedullary definition, and pyelectasis (Fig. 11–32).[40] These changes may be associated with chronic compression from the surrounding cyst or, more likely, represent primary renal disease. Care must be taken to control technical gain settings, because normal renal tissue may appear hyperechoic when surrounded by fluid from through-transmission artifact.

Excretory urography may not demonstrate the pseudocyst or extravasation of contrast material adequately because of contrast dilution within the cyst or decreased renal function. Suggested etiologies of perirenal pseudocysts include distal ureteral obstruction, renal or ureteral trauma, renal calculus and secondary rupture, iatrogenic error, tumor erosion, and infection. Urinomas have been seen after accidental ligation and transection of the proximal ureter during ovariohysterectomy. Resulting chronic urine leakage creates a focal peritonitis that stimulates fibroblastic reaction, eventually sealing off the urine into a pseudocyst (Fig. 11–33).[39] Although reported in dogs,[40] most perirenal pseudocysts involve cats and have no conclusive etiology. Ultrasound-guided centesis of pseudocysts can be performed for palliation, to assess renal function after decompression, and for analysis of the fluid. Unfortunately, pseudocysts may refill in 1 to 2 days.

Nephrocalcinosis and Hypercalcemic Nephropathy

Nephropathy may be seen in hypercalcemic animals with paraneoplastic syndromes associated with lymphoma and other neoplasias. Hypercalcemic nephropathy may result in reversible calcification of the loop of Henle, collecting ducts, and distal tubules in the metabolically active outer zone of the medulla.[41,42] Selective calcium accumulation occurs in an echogenic band with no acoustic shadowing, 1 to 3 mm thick, located several millimeters inside and paralleling the corticomedullary junction (Fig. 11–34).[19,41,42] This hyperechoic medullary band, the "medullary rim sign," may represent a poor prognosis.[9] A less echogenic medullary band can be seen in histologically normal kidneys in the normocalcemic feline patient from subclinical calcium deposition.[19] Additionally, the "renal medullary rim sign" has been described in patients with nephrocalcinosis,[9,12] nephritis, feline infectious peritonitis, acute tubular necrosis, and oxalate nephrosis.[42–44]

Nephrocalcinosis has been described as a nonspecific generalized increase in renal echogenicity (Fig. 11–35).[2,9] Additionally, the term nephrocalcinosis has been used to

Figure 11–31

A, Lateral radiograph of a cat with a palpable mid-abdominal mass. Note the enlarged ovate soft tissue opacity creating a mass effect (M) in the area of the right kidney. Ventral, caudal, and left lateral displacement of the gastrointestinal tract is evident. Differentials included renal neoplasia, hydronephrosis, and perirenal pseudocyst. **B,** Lateral parasagittal sonogram of the left kidney shows encapsulated anechoic fluid (C) surrounding the left kidney. Free abdominal fluid was not present elsewhere within the abdomen. The diffuse hyperechogenicity of the kidney within the pseudocyst is attributable to the lack of sound attenuation by the fluid surrounding the kidney and to chronic infiltrative membranous glomerulonephritis. Notice the small, irregularly shaped, and thick hyperechoic cortex. Pseudocyst fluid had been removed for analysis and palliation by ultrasound-guided fine-needle aspiration, but the pseudocyst refilled within 1 day.

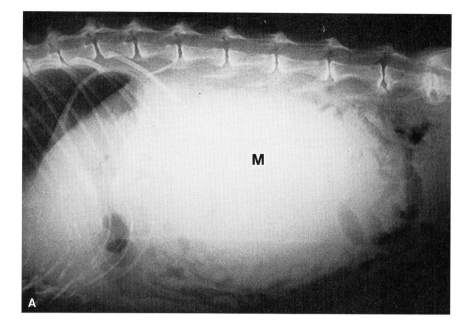

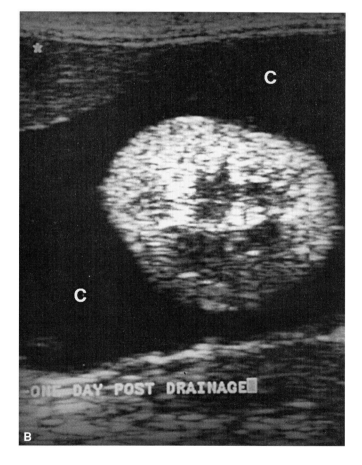

Figure 11–32

An enlarged mid-dorsal view of the left kidney of the same cat as in Figure 11–31 after removal of pseudocyst fluid using ultrasound-guided fine-needle aspiration. Note the poor distinction between cortex (C) and medulla (M) and the diffuse increase in echogenicity of both the thickened cortex and small medulla, indicative of chronic infiltrative renal disease. The mild pyelectasia (dilatation of renal pelvis, arrows) is from fluid diuresis.

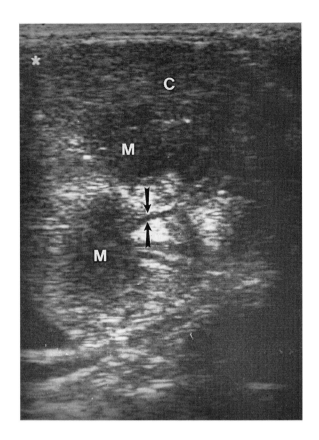

Figure 11–33

Transverse sonogram of the abdomen just caudal to the left kidney of a dog with a history of abdominal trauma and a mass effect in the area of the left kidney. The circular anechoic tube seen in cross section (U) was a dilated ureter, which was followed, sonographically, caudal from the dilated renal pelvis. About halfway to the bladder, the ureter appeared to terminate abruptly and was surrounded by an encapsulated pocket of anechoic fluid, a urinoma (F). Hydronephrosis, tortuous hydroureter, and ureteral stenosis with a surrounding urinoma were found at surgery.

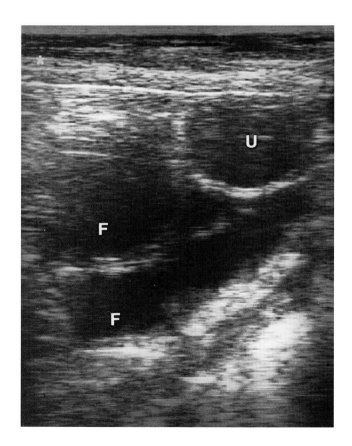

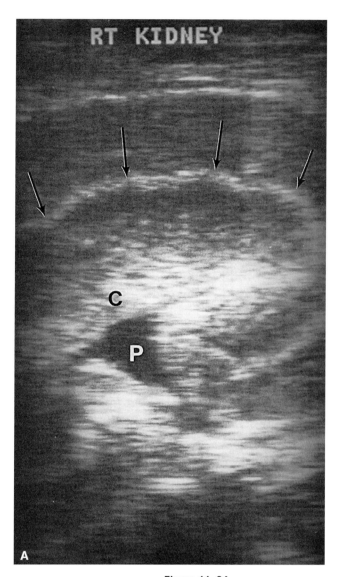

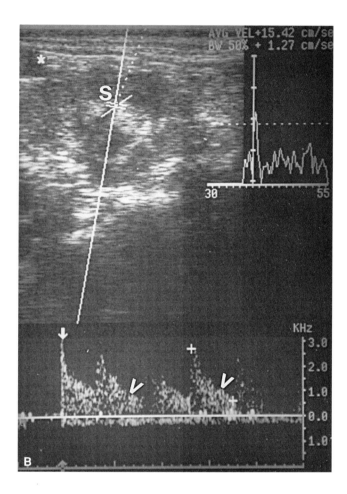

Figure 11–34

A, Mid-dorsal sonogram of the right kidney of a dog with lymphoma and paraneoplastic hypercalcemia. Note the thin, undulant, hyperechoic line paralleling the corticomedullary junction, the medullary rim sign (arrows), caused by hypercalcemic nephropathy and calcium deposition in ducts and tubules in the outer zone of the medulla. Dilation of the renal pelvis (P) is most likely the result of fluid diuresis. The renal crest (C) and peripelvic parenchyma also are increased in echogenicity. **B,** Placement of a pulsed Doppler sample volume (S) within an interlobar artery of the kidney shows a normal resistive index of .78, indicating adequate perfusion. The renal arterial pulsed Doppler spectrum below the image is fairly normal, with a high systolic peak (arrow and +) and gradually decreasing slope of diastolic blood flow (arrowheads).

Figure 11–35

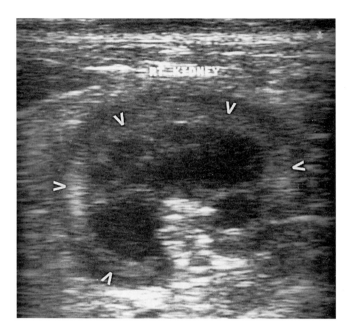

Mid-dorsal sonogram of the right kidney of an older dog. Note the circumferential hyperechoic band in the inner zone of the cortex (arrowheads). Biopsy results showed nephrocalcinosis of the cortex. This sonographic appearance may be seen in patients with and without clinical signs of renal disease.

describe echogenic change, with or without acoustic shadowing, seen in the pelvic diverticula of older, clinically normal dogs (see Fig. 11–18). This echogenic diverticular change may represent mineralization or fibrosis.

Ethylene Glycol Toxicity

Oxalate nephrosis is detected as a mild to dramatic diffuse increase in renal echogenicity that, when detected, warrants a poor prognosis.[43,44] The increase in echogenicity is caused by deposition of intratubular and interstitial refractile crystals. Crystalline deposition in this disease is mostly in the cortex, but an increase in medullary echoes may be present in severe cases (Fig. 11–36). Crystals may accumulate, to a greater degree, in a band-like zone of the medulla just inside the corticomedullary junction, creating a medullary rim sign. Decreased relative crystal deposit in the medulla outside this bright medullary band and a surrounding bright cortex creates alternating hyperechoic and hypoechoic layers, a "halo sign," that has been associated with clinical anuria and a grave prognosis.[43,44] The sonographic appearance of severe forms of ethylene glycol toxicity are nearly pathognomonic, but mild increases in cortical and medullary echogenicity seen in milder intoxications may be indistinguishable from other diseases that create increases in renal echogenicity.

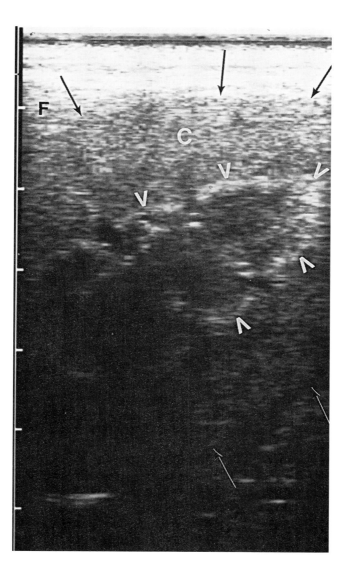

Figure 11–36

Lateral parasagittal sonogram of the caudal pole of the kidney (arrows) of a dog in acute renal failure. The kidney is attenuating the sound beam, making it difficult to penetrate to the far field cortex with a 7.5-mHz probe. The near field cortex (C) is as hyperechoic as perirenal fat (F). The corticomedullary junction is difficult to detect because of the diffuse increase in echogenicity of the medulla. The hyperechoic undulant band (arrowheads) in the medulla parallelling the corticomedullary junction is the medullary rim sign, also called "halo sign" in oxalate nephrosis. Final diagnosis was ethylene glycol toxicity, the increase in echogenicity resulting from oxalate crystal deposition.

Contrast Medium-Induced Renal Failure

Renal disease or renal failure is rarely seen after intravenous administration of contrast media, although some factors such as chronic renal failure, renal insufficiency, diabetes mellitus, multiple myeloma, vascular disease, azotemia, and dehydration have been shown to increase the nephrotoxic effects of these agents.[8] An estimated 1 in 80 intravenous administrations of contrast media results in death.[8] Contrast medium-induced renal failure can be identified radiographically by failure of resolution of the nephrogram phase. Diffuse hyperechoic change without acoustic shadowing has been seen in the medulla, beginning at the corticomedullary junction and extending to the renal papillae (Fig. 11–37). Because vasoconstriction and altered renal hemodynamics appear to be important in the generation of contrast medium-induced renal failure, the use of color Doppler imaging may demonstrate hemodynamic changes such as an increased resistive index.

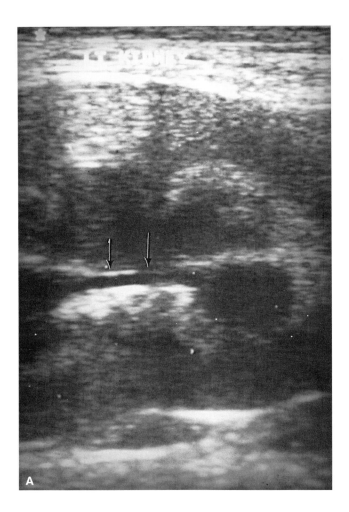

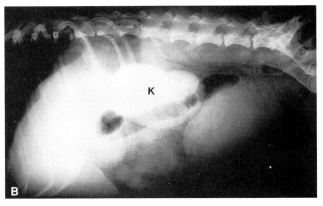

Figure 11-37

A, Mid-dorsal sonogram of the kidney of the dog in Figures 11–16B and 11–29B with signs of acute renal failure after excretory urography. The diffuse hyperechoic change in the medulla extending toward the pelvis was caused by tubular concretions of Tamm-Horsfall protein from radiographic contrast-induced renal failure. Although urine was produced after fluid diuresis, as suggested by the dilatation of the renal pelvis (arrows), the patient progressed to anuria and irreversible failure. **B,** After sonographic examination, lateral abdominal radiographs were obtained 5 days after excretory urography. The left kidney (K) had persisted in a nephrogram phase. The abscessed right kidney did not opacify. Prolonged elimination of contrast material is present in the urinary bladder. From Daley CA, Finn-Bodner ST, Lenz SD: Contrast-induced renal failure documented by color Doppler imaging in a dog. J Anim Hosp Assoc *30:*33, 1994.

Pyelonephritis and Hydronephrosis

Hydronephrosis, pyelonephritis, or pyelectasis from diuresis can cause renal pelvic dilatation that appears as an anechoic lumen in the center of the echogenic renal sinus (Fig. 11–38).[24–26] The midtransverse image plane is most reliable in confirming dilatation of the renal pelvis. An oblique dorsal or sagittal image plane through the hypoechoic renal crest or medullary papilla surrounded by diverticular tissue can mimic pelvic dilatation. In the midtransverse image plane, pelvic dilatation appears as a black C, as the walls of the renal pelvis are separated by small amounts of fluid (see Fig. 11–9), or as a black triangle in the hilus, with the enlarged proximal ureter forming the apex of the triangle as distention progresses (Fig. 11–39).[9,12] Advanced hydronephrosis may create cyst-like expansion of the kidney, which appears as a global anechoic structure with a thin circumferential rim of renal tissue and, occasionally, remnant linear septa of diverticular tissue (Fig. 11–40).[9,12,24] Through transmission is usually present. Pyelonephritis is unlikely to cause this extreme amount of pelvic dilatation. Otherwise, differentiation of hydronephrosis and pyelonephritis may not be possible with sonography. Deformity and hyperechogenicity of pelvic diverticula may be seen with scarring in pyelonephrosis (Fig. 11–41). Diuresis can create only mild separation of the renal pelvis.[24,25] The hypoechoic form of feline lymphosarcoma that invades the renal sinus has been reported to mimic pyelonephritis or hydronephrosis.[3,33]

Ureters and urinary bladder should be inspected carefully for identification of a possible obstruction if renal pelvic dilatation is detected. Hydroureter appears as a thin-walled anechoic tube extending from the renal pelvis along the dorsal abdominal wall

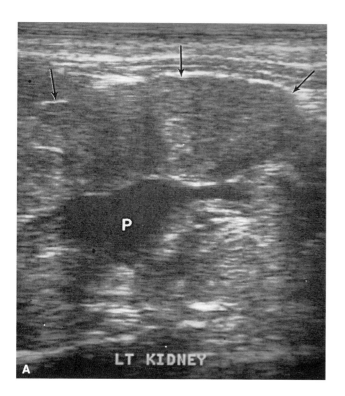

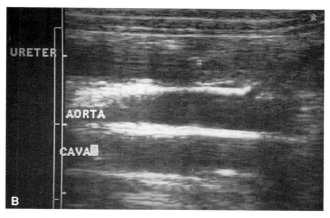

Figure 11–38

A, Mid-dorsal sonogram of the left kidney (arrows) of a febrile young dog with pyuria, hematuria, and leukocytosis. The dog had been incontinent since birth. The anechoic triangular area (P) is the dilated renal pelvis. Poor corticomedullary distinction with the kidney appears as a mottled echogenic structure. **B,** The dilated left ureter was followed caudal to the kidney paralleling the descending aorta and caudal vena cava. The ureter continued caudal to the bladder trigone, indicating ectopia. **C,** Urinary bladder wall (+) is thickened and echogenic with loss of the normal architecture. The mucosal layer (arrowheads) is hyperechoic and irregular. Low level echoes of cellular sediment are present in the lumen. The final diagnosis was unilateral ureteral ectopia and a secondary cystitis, ureteritis, and E. coli pyelonephritis.

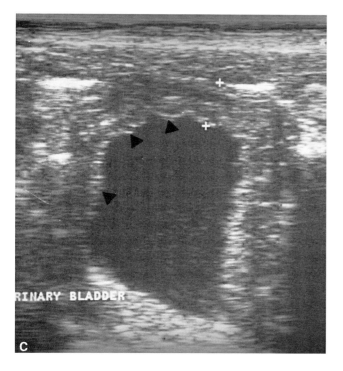

Figure 11–39

Midtransverse sonogram of a kidney (arrows) in a dog with hydronephrosis shows the dilated triangular, anechoic (fluid-filled) renal pelvis (P). The dilated proximal ureter (U) is seen as a parallel-walled anechoic tube extending from the renal pelvis. Absence of a color Doppler flow signal within the Doppler region of interest (ROI), even when angled more steeply, further distinguishes the ureter from a hilar blood vessel. High velocity flow is seen in an adjacent interlobar artery (arrowhead). The large red color signal (A) is a motion artifact caused by adjacent bowel peristalsis.

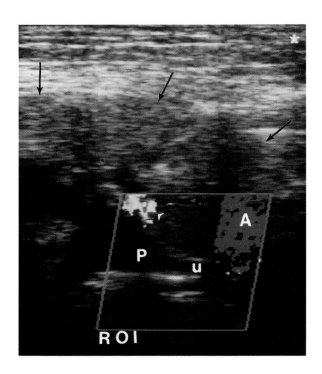

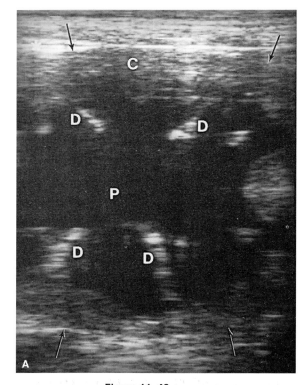

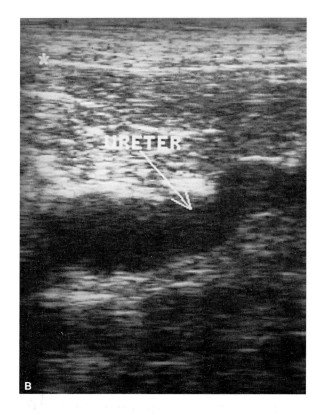

Figure 11–40

A, Midsagittal sonogram of a kidney (arrows) in a dog with a transitional cell carcinoma in the urinary bladder trigone. Advanced hydronephrosis is indicated by the anechoic cyst-like renal pelvis (P) replacing most normal renal tissue with only a thin rind of cortex (C) remaining. The hyperechoic septa (D) are distorted remnants of pelvic diverticula. **B,** The distended, tortuous, fluid-filled ureter (hydroureter) could be followed to the area of the obstructing trigonal mass.

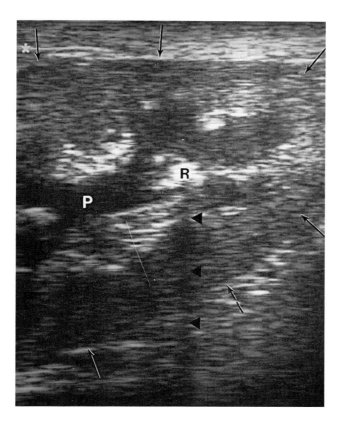

Figure 11–41

Midsagittal sonogram of a kidney (arrows) of a dog with chronic pyelonephritis. The renal pelvis (P) is dilated and deformed. Hyperechoic change around the pelvis represents peripelvic fibrosis and scarring. A focus of mineralization or small renolith (R) is present in a diverticulum and has a distal acoustic shadow (arrowheads). The overall echogenicity of the kidney is increased.

toward the bladder (see Fig. 11–38). If significant hydroureter is present, it is possible to follow the ureter to the bladder trigone. The walls of a dilated ureter may appear more tortuous and less uniformly parallel than blood vessels (see Fig. 11–40**B**). Additionally, Doppler evaluation can help differentiate a dilated ureter from blood vessel by looking for blood flow (see Fig. 11–39). An obstructive ureteral calculus appears as an echogenic focus with or without acoustic shadowing in the lumen of a dilated ureter (Fig. 11–42). A stenotic ureter is more difficult to diagnose and, if seen, may be a persistent abrupt termination of a dilated ureter. If the ureter cannot be followed distal to the kidney, the bladder trigone should be evaluated for causes of obstruction, such as a mass or ureterocele.

Diffuse Renal Disease

Diffuse renal disease can be the most difficult to evaluate sonographically and includes infiltrative renal disease and congenital renal disease. Diffuse infiltrative pathology of the kidney often creates a diffuse increase in echogenicity. Diseases that create hyperechoic change in the kidneys of cats include glomerulonephritis (see Fig. 11–31), chronic interstitial nephritis (see Fig. 11–9), pyogranulomatous change (feline infectious peritonitis) (Fig. 11–43), diffuse infiltrative lymphosarcoma, and microcystic polycystic disease.[1,3,9,12,22,24,33] Diseases that reportedly create a diffuse increase in echogenicity of the dog kidney include glomerulonephritis (Fig. 11–44), chronic interstitial nephritis (Fig. 11–45), nephrocalcinosis, amyloidosis, nephrosclerosis, lymphosarcoma, and end-stage renal disease.[1,3,9,12,22,24,31] Tubular necrosis is reported by some investigators to appear diffusely hypoechoic,[3,4,38] whereas in other studies, tubular necrosis did not alter the sonographic appearance of the kidney.[42,44]

Congenital disease of the kidney can be indistinguishable sonographically from chronic infiltrative renal disease, and may be suggested more by the age of the animal than by any distinct sonographic finding. Renal dysplasia, disorganized development of renal parenchyma because of anomalous differentiation, may be familial (beagle,

Figure 11–42

Oblique sonogram of the abdomen of a dog with acute abdominal pain and hydronephrosis of the right kidney. The dilated tortuous fluid-filled right ureter (U) was followed to an area caudal to the kidney and a 1-cm hyperechoic curvilinear structure (C) with distal acoustic shadowing (arrows) within the lumen of the ureter. The ureter could not be located caudal to this area. The presence of an obstructing ureteral calculus was confirmed at surgery.

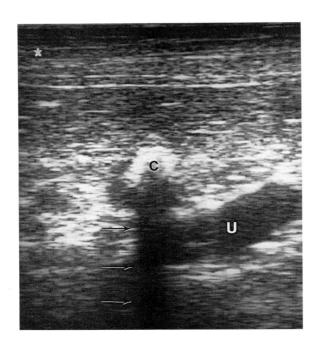

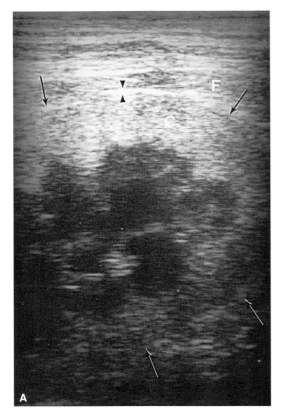

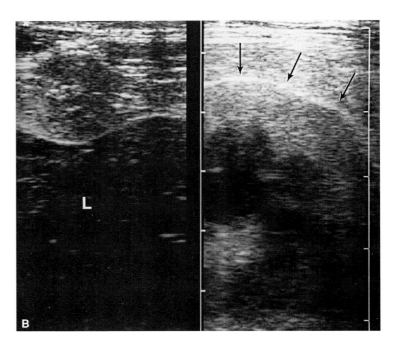

Figure 11–43

A, Lateral parasagittal sonogram of the left kidney of a cat with feline infectious peritonitis. The cortex (C) is isoechoic with perirenal fat (F) and the near field renal capsule is prominent (arrowheads). **B,** Split format sonogram of the caudal pole of the left kidney (arrows) and liver (L) allows side-by-side comparison of the relative echogenicity. Gain, depth, and focus is the same for each side of the image. Note that decreasing the gain to make the kidney appear less echogenic results in a nearly anechoic liver.

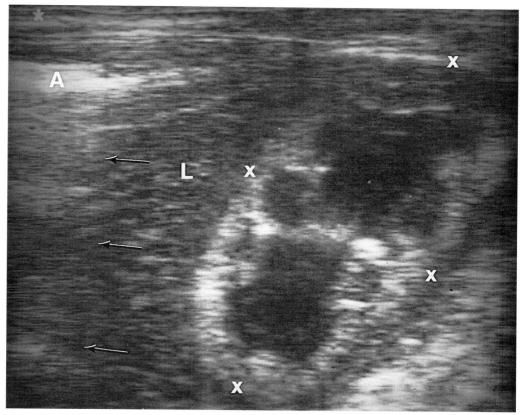

Figure 11–44

Midsagittal sonogram of the right kidney (X) of an older dog with glomerulonephritis. Note the diffuse increase in renal echogenicity relative to the hepatic parenchyma of the caudate liver lobe (L). Air within the lungs (A) causes a hyperechoic interface with distal acoustic shadowing filled with reverberation (arrows) cranial and ventral to the caudate lobe.

Figure 11–45

Lateral parasagittal sonogram of the left kidney (arrowheads) of an older dog with chronic interstitial nephritis. The diffuse increase in renal echogenicity makes it difficult to distinguish the hyperechoic kidney from surrounding echogenic fat. The kidney is small and irregularly shaped, and has a thickened cortex (C), reduced medulla (M), and acquired cortical cyst (arrow). The irregular hypoechoic focus in the caudal pole is an acute infarct (I).

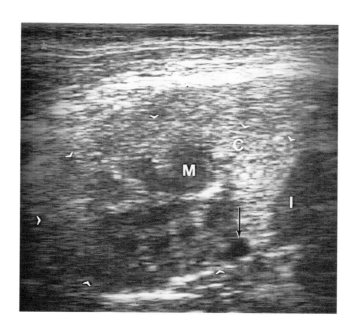

Bedlington terrier, cocker spaniel, dachshund, Doberman pinscher, German shepherd, Lhasa apso, malamute, Norwegian elkhound, shih tzu, Samoyed, and cats) or may be caused by fetal or neonatal infection or teratogenesis. Dysplastic kidneys are usually small (Fig. 11–46), but they may be normal in size. They are usually misshapen and hyperechoic because of large amounts of fibrous tissue infiltration. Internal architecture is abnormal with poor differentiation between the renal cortex, medulla, and pelvis. Frequently, cysts of varying sizes are present in the cortex or medulla and the ureters may be dilated (Fig. 11–47). Renal agenesis (beagles, cats) may be an incidental sonographic finding after a prolonged search for the missing kidney. The opposite kidney is often normal in appearance but enlarged because of compensatory hypertrophy. True renal hypoplasia is rare and may manifest sonographically as a small but normal appearing kidney in a young animal.

In general, diffuse infiltrative disease of the kidney is not reliably diagnosed using sonography alone. Such disease in its early stages may not result in sonographic changes. For reasons described previously, diffuse echogenic change in the kidney is nonspecific and subjective, and can be difficult to detect. Nonpathologic renal change, such as fatty infiltrate in the renal cortex of the cat, can create a hyperechoic appearance that is indistinguishable from pathologic change (Fig. 11–3).[19] If diffuse change in renal echogenicity is seen concurrent with clinical signs of renal disease, an ultrasound-guided renal biopsy may be necessary for confirmation and diagnosis. A more reliable sonographic indicator of pathology may be the lack of a well-defined medullary zone in patients undergoing diuresis (Fig. 11–48). This sign may indicate severe end-stage renal disease.[22] More research and controlled studies on this observation are required to confirm its value as a prognosticator.

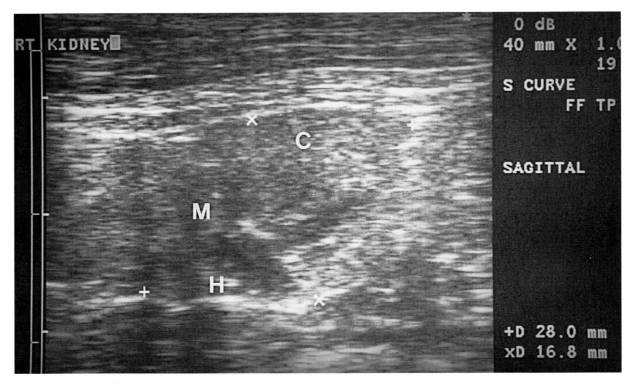

Figure 11–46

Mid-dorsal sonogram of an oblong echo complex structure (+, x) in the area of the right kidney in a 1-year-old Lhaso Apso with renal failure. The renal vein and artery had to be followed sonographically to this structure to confirm its identity as a small, abnormally shaped hyperechoic right kidney. The internal architecture of the kidney is abnormal, with a small deformed medulla (M) and a disorganized cortex (C) and renal hilus (H). Familial renal dysplasia was confirmed at necropsy.

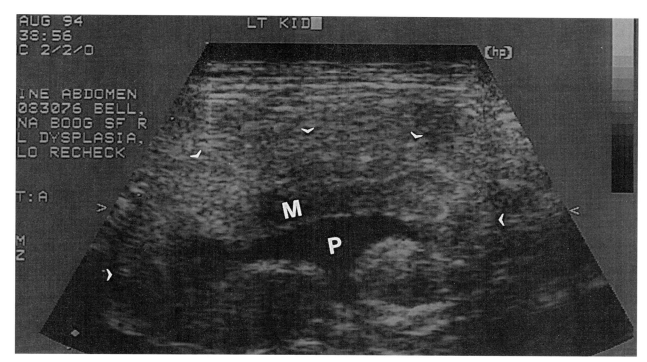

Figure 11–47

Mid-dorsal sonogram of the left kidney (arrowheads) of a 1-year-old azotemic dog. The kidney is small and diffusely hyperechoic. The internal architecture is abnormal, with a poorly defined medulla (M) and dilated renal pelvis (P). Cortical cysts were visible in other scan planes. Urine cultures were negative and renal dysplasia was diagnosed on the basis of biopsy results.

Figure 11–48

Midsagittal sonogram of the left kidney (arrowheads) in a 4-year-old dog with acute renal failure. The kidney was reliably identified by following the renal artery from the aorta to the hilus of the enlarged, mass-like, diffusely echogenic structure. The infiltrated medulla and cortex (+) could not be distinguished as separate areas. In spite of supraphysiologic diuresis, minimal urine accumulation was noted in the renal pelvis (arrows). Leptospirosis and acute nephritis were diagnosed on the basis of histopathologic findings.

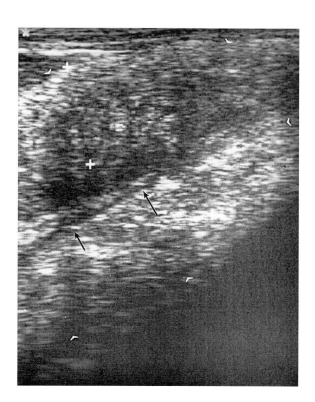

ULTRASOUND-GUIDED RENAL BIOPSY

Before biopsy, patients should undergo a complete historical and physical evaluation.[36] The extent of laboratory data required is variable, depending on the severity of the patient's condition. A baseline hematocrit and coagulation studies, such as prothrombin time, activated partial thromboplastin time, and platelet count, are recommended. Bleeding times or von Willebrand's factor analysis can be obtained if there is suspicion of a bleeding diathesis not identifiable by these parameters.[36,45]

Fine needle aspiration is recommended before obtaining a core biopsy, if patient cooperation allows, in case purulent material is present.[36] When possible, both aspiration and cutting biopsies are performed unless the small size of the mass or critical condition of the patient is prohibitive. For fine needle aspiration of the kidney, the animal can be sedated, but cutting core biopsies require the use of general anesthesia. In some types of biopsy needles, an aspirate can be obtained with a small-gauge spinal needle through the cannula of the cutting needle, eliminating the need for multiple punctures.

Once the site and transducer are prepared in sterile fashion, the sonographer takes the following steps. Scan the renal lesion and select a biopsy site. Place the target lesion near an edge of the transducer and maximize the size by adjusting depth. Note the depth of the target lesion on the monitor and select the appropriate needle length. Stabilize the transducer and insert the needle at a point immediately adjacent to the edge of the transducer. To be seen when inserted, the needle must be at the center of the transducer edge, parallel to the plane of the ultrasound beam, and at an angle varying from 20 to 45° from the long axis of the transducer, depending on the depth of the lesion (Fig. 11–49). Once the needle tip is visualized, guide it into the target lesion while continuously monitoring needle tip location and making small adjustments in needle trajectory. Fine positional changes can be made by withdrawing the needle several millimeters and redirecting its course. Hypoechoic or anechoic areas within the lesion are avoided as potentially necrotic, hemorrhagic, or abscessed, unless culture or drainage of the fluid is desired.

When the needle tip is in the target lesion, remove the stylet and apply continuous suction with a syringe. Syringe size varies from 5 to 30 ml. Smaller syringes create less vacuum for use in soft or semiliquid tissue, such as spleen or lymph nodes, and larger syringes are used in fibrous masses or when aspirating with an extension set. Although a vacuum is maintained, move the needle back and forth a few millimeters and slightly redirect it several times, without having the needle tip leave the mass. Negative pressure is released before removing the needle from the mass to prevent contamination from neighboring tissue or aspiration of the sample into the barrel of the syringe. The aspirated material is expelled onto a slide for cytologic analysis, and core samples are placed in an appropriate fixative. Performing multiple fine-needle aspirates (two to three) of a lesion increases the diagnostic yield and can usually be performed safely, even in a vascular organ such as the kidney. The procedure lasts 15 to 30 minutes.

An automated biopsy device[a] is helpful in obtaining a biopsy because of speed of sample acquisition.[46–48] During a manual Tru-Cut[b] biopsy, the kidney can be seen to move away from the biopsy needle. To prevent this movement, the kidney should be fixed in position before placing the tip of the needle within the capsule of the kidney.[47] A small skin incision may be made with a scalpel if a large-gauge cutting biopsy is to be performed. A small amount of sterile coupling gel on the stab incision prevents dissection of subcutaneous gas during introduction of the biopsy needle. Core biopsies of diffuse renal disease should be obtained from the cortical areas in the poles of the kidneys or in a sagittal plane along the lateral cortex, avoiding deep medullary tissue.[45] Color flow Doppler imaging can be used to avoid the larger interlobar vessels.[36] If Doppler is unavailable, however, the area of the pelvic diverticula, which is aligned with the interlobar vessels, is avoided during biopsy. The number of biopsy passes in the kidney is usually limited to two.[48]

[a] *Biopty, Bard Urological, C.R. Bard, Covington, GA*

[b] *Tru-Cut core biopsy needles, Travenol Laboratories, Deerfield, IL*

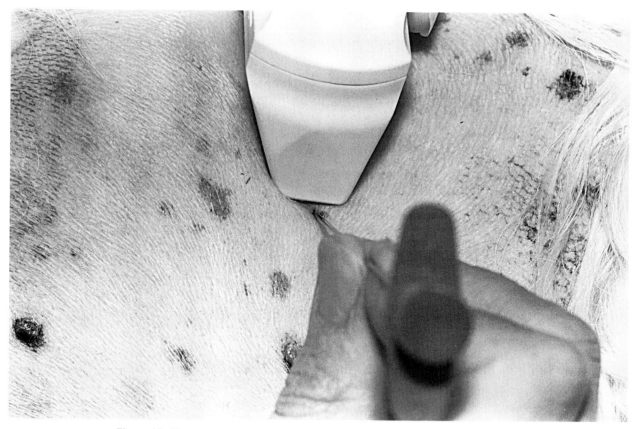

Figure 11–49

Correct placement of a biopsy needle for ultrasound-guided aspiration of the kidney using a phased linear array probe. An image of the kidney is obtained on the monitor showing the target tissue placed in the biopsy area. To remain within the sound beam throughout the biopsy, the needle is introduced just cranial to the cranial edge of the probe, in the center of the probe edge, at a 45° angle, and in the same geometric plane as the sound beam. The needle is visualized beginning at the entrance into superficial tissue until the needle tip enters the target tissue. During an actual biopsy, the needle, probe, and patient skin are aseptically prepared and surgical gloves are worn.

REFERENCES

1. Finn-Bodner ST: Nephrosonography and cystosonography. Ultrasound Symposium. Annual Meeting of the American College of Veterinary Radiology, Orlando, 1992.
2. Konde LJ, et al: Comparison of radiography and ultrasonography in the evaluation of renal lesions in the dog. J Am Vet Med Assoc *188:*1420, 1986.
3. Walter PA, Feeney DA: Renal ultrasonography in the dog and cat. Proceedings of the Annual Meeting of the American Veterinary Ultrasound Symposium Proceedings, 1988.
4. Walter PA et al: Ultrasonographic evaluation of renal parenchymal diseases in dogs: 32 cases (1981–1986). J Am Vet Med Assoc *191:*999, 1987.
5. Herrtage ME, Dennis R: Contrast media and their use in small animal radiology. J Small Anim Pract *28:*1105, 1987.
6. Walter PA, Feeney DA, Johnston GR: *Diagnosis and treatment of adverse reactions to radiopaque contrast agents.* In *Current Veterinary Therapy IX.* Edited by RW Kirk. Philadelphia: WB Saunders, 1986, pp. 47–52.
7. Feeney DA, Osborne CA, Jessen CR: Effects of radiographic contrast media on results of the urinalysis with emphasis on specific gravity. J Am Vet Med Assoc *176:*1378, 1980.
8. Daley CA, Finn-Bodner ST, Lenz SD: Contrast-induced renal failure documented by color Doppler imaging in a dog. J Am Anim Hosp Assoc *30:*33, 1994.
9. Ackerman N: Radiology and ultrasound of urogenital diseases in dogs and cats. Ames, IA, Iowa State University Press, 1991, pp. 1–25, 1991.

10. Walter PA, et al: Renal ultrasonography in healthy cats. Am J Vet Res *48:*600, 1987.

11. Wood AKW, McCarthy PH: Ultrasonographic-anatomic correlation and an imaging protocol of the normal canine kidney. Am J Vet Res *51:*103, 1990.

12. Feeney DA, Walter PA: Ultrasonography of the kidneys, adrenal glands and urinary bladder. American Institute of Ultrasound in Medicine Animal Ultrasound Course Proceedings, 1989.

13. Walter PA et al: Feline renal ultrasonography: Quantitative analyses of imaged anatomy. Am J Vet Res *48:*596, 1987.

14. Arkless R: The normal kidney reaction to intravenous pyelography. Am Radiol *107:*746, 1969.

15. Finco DR, et al: Radiologic estimation of the kidney size of the dog. J Am Vet Med Assoc *159:*995, 1971.

16. Nyland TG, et al: Ultrasonic determination of kidney volume in the dog. Vet Radiol *30:*174, 1989.

17. Barr FJ: Evaluation of ultrasound as a method of assessing renal size in the dog. J Small Anim Pract *31:*174, 1990.

18. Felkai CS, et al: Ultrasonographic determination of renal volume in the dog. Vet Radiol Ultrasound *33:*292, 1992.

19. Yeager AE, Anderson WI: Study of association between histologic features and echogenicity of architecturally normal cat kidneys. Am J Vet Res *50:*860, 1989.

20. Hartzband LE, Tidwell AS, Lamb CR: Relative echoity of the renal cortex and liver in normal dogs. Third Annual Ultrasound Symposium Proceedings, American College of Veterinary Radiology, 1989.

21. Boag BL, Atilola M, Pennock P: Renal sonographic measurements in the dog preceding and following unilateral nephrectomy. Vet Radiol Ultrasound *34:*112, 1993.

22. Konde LJ: Sonography of the kidney. Symposium on diagnostic ultrasound. Vet Clin North Am Small Anim Pract *15:*1149, 1985.

23. Konde LJ, et al: Ultrasonographic anatomy of the normal canine kidney. Vet Radiol *25:*173, 1984.

24. Lamb CR: A critical review of the role of ultrasonography in small animal renal disease. American Institute of Ultrasound in Medicine Advanced Small Animal Ultrasound Imaging Seminar, 1990.

25. Pugh CR, et al: Iatrogenic renal pyelectasia in the dog. Vet Radiol Ultrasound *35:*50, 1994.

26. Mann MJ: Hydronephrosis secondary to bladder distension. J Diagn Med Sonography *2:*87, 1990.

27. Biery DN: *Radiographic evaluation of the kidneys.* In *Canine Nephrology.* Edited by KC Bovee. Media, 1984, pp. 275–313.

28. Spaulding KA, Stone E: Color Doppler evaluation of ureteral flow dynamics in the dog as influenced by relative specific gravity. Proceedings of the Annual Scientific Meeting of the American College of Veterinary Radiology, Chicago, 1993.

29. Nyland TG, et al: Diagnosis of urinary tract obstruction in dogs using duplex Doppler ultrasonography. Vet Radiol Ultrasound *34:*348, 1993.

30. Platt JF, et al: Duplex Doppler ultrasound of the kidney: Differentiation of obstructive from nonobstructive dilatation. Radiology *171:*515, 1989.

31. Cartee RE, Selcer BA, Patton CS: Ultrasonographic diagnosis of renal disease in small animals. J Am Vet Med Assoc *176:*426, 1980.

32. Konde LJ, et al: Sonographic appearance of renal neoplasia in the dog. Vet Radiol *26:*74, 1985.

33. Walter PA, et al: Applications of ultrasonography in the diagnosis of parenchymal kidney disease in cats: 24 cases (1981–1986). J Am Vet Med Assoc *192:*92, 1988.

34. Osborne CA, et al: Renal lymphoma in the dog and cat. J Am Vet Med Assoc *158:*2058, 1971.

35. Ackerman N: Ultrasonographic appearance and early detection of VX2 carcinoma in rabbit kidneys. Vet Radiol *30:*88, 1989.

36. Finn-Bodner ST, Hathcock JT: Image-guided percutaneous needle biopsy: Ultrasound, computed tomography, and magnetic resonance imaging. Semin Vet Surg *8:*258, 1993.

37. Biller DS, Schenkman DI, Bortnowski H: Ultrasonographic appearance of renal infarcts in a dog. J Am Anim Hosp Assoc *27:*370, 1991.

38. Spies JB, et al: Sonographic evaluation of experimental acute renal arterial occlusion in dogs. AJR Am J Roentgenol *142:*341, 1984.

39. Tidwell AS, Ullman SL, Schelling SH: Urinoma (para-ureteral pseudocyst) in a dog. Vet Radiol *31:*203, 1989.

40. Miles KG, Jergens AE: Unilateral perinephric pseudocyst of undetermined origin in a dog. Vet Radiol Ultrasound *33:*277, 1992.

41. Barr FJ, et al: Hypercalcemic nephropathy in three dogs: Sonographic appearance. Vet Radiol *30:*169, 1989.

42. Biller DS, Bradley GA, Partington BP: Renal medullary rim sign: Ultrasonographic evidence of renal disease. Vet Radiol Ultrasound *33:*286, 1992.

43. Adams WH, et al: Early renal ultrasonographic findings in dogs with experimentally induced ethylene glycol nephrosis. Am J Vet Res *50:*1370, 1989.

44. Adams WH, Toal RL, Breider MA: Ultrasonographic findings in dogs and cats with oxalate nephrosis attributed to ethylene glycol intoxication: 15 cases (1984–1988). J Am Vet Med Assoc *4:*492, 1991.

45. Schelling CG: Ultrasound-guided interventional techniques. J Am Anim Hosp Assoc 1992.

46. Poster RB, Jones DB, Spirt BA: Percutaneous pediatric renal biopsy: Use of the biopsy gun. Radiology *176:*752, 1990.

47. Wiseman DA, et al: Percutaneous renal biopsy utilizing real time, ultrasonic guidance, and a semi-automated biopsy device. Kidney Int *38:*347, 1990.

48. Hager DA, Nyland TG, Fisher P: Ultrasound-guided biopsy of the canine liver, kidney, and prostate. Vet Radiol *26:*82, 1985.

12
CHAPTER

THE URINARY BLADDER
Susan T. Finn-Bodner

Lower urinary tract disease is a common and frequently recurrent problem in dogs and cats. Survey radiography followed by double contrast cystography are traditionally the recommended techniques to visualize the lower urinary tract. These examinations, however, are time consuming, expensive, invasive, and expose the patients and handlers to ionizing radiation. Additionally, contrast techniques require placement of a urinary catheter, patency of the urethra, and, frequently, sedation or anesthesia for a diagnostic examination.[1,2] Reported risks of cystography include air embolism, trauma to or rupture of the urethra or bladder, granulomatous contrast reactions, and iatrogenically introduced infection and inflammation.[3-9] In many instances, urinalysis and urine culture cannot be performed after cystography.

Sonography is rapid and painless, does not involve ionizing radiation, and can be performed without chemical restraint or bladder catheterization. The urinary bladder is ideally suited to this examination because of the superficial position and excellent acoustic properties of this fluid-filled organ. A recent study using excretory urography, double contrast cystography, and sonography to visualize the urinary bladder in dogs with transitional cell carcinoma found sonography was the only imaging technique with which lesions were detected in all patients.[2] The focus of this chapter is on the sonographic appearance of the normal anatomy and commonly encountered disease processes of the lower urinary system.

INDICATIONS FOR CYSTOSONOGRAPHY

Cystosonography can assess volume, size, and shape of the urinary bladder. Changes in wall outline (rupture, ureterocele, diverticulum, adjacent extramural mass), changes in wall thickness (inflammatory cystitis, infiltrative neoplasia, obstructive hypertrophy), identification of mural masses (neoplasia, polyp, inflammatory nodule, abscess, hematoma), and intraluminal defects (calculi, crystalline "sand," cellular debris, catheters, foreign bodies, blood clots) can be detected.[1,10,11] Indications for cystosonography include signs of lower urinary tract disease, difficulty in catheterization, suspected abnormalities of the trigone in patients with hydronephrosis or hydroureter, verification of catheter placement, quantification of postvoiding residual volume,[12,13] and as part of routine abdominal sonography.[1,14] Additionally, ultrasound-guided biopsy and aspiration of detected lesions can be performed simultaneously. Cystosonography should be considered the initial diagnostic step in the evaluation of the bladder, urethra, and associated lymph nodes and organs. Additional information or confirmation of pathology should be pursued if necessary with contrast cystography.

TECHNIQUES

It has been suggested that the bladder should be completely distended for its examination with ultrasound, ensuring such distention by scanning first thing in the morning, giving a diuretic, or filling the bladder with sterile saline.[2,10,11,14] Mild distention does facilitate in locating the bladder and differentiating it from other intrapelvic structures, but a completely distended bladder can be difficult to examine for several reasons. Superior sonographic resolution is obtained by using the highest frequency transducer that can penetrate to and image the bladder. The far wall of a large, fluid-filled bladder may be beyond the limits of inspection with a 7.5-mHz transducer in even a medium-sized dog (Fig. 12–1), whereas a mildly distended urinary bladder is still located easily and can be inspected systematically in most animals with a 7.5-mHz transducer. It is easier to miss a focal lesion in an overly distended bladder because of the total area that must be evaluated. Overdistention of the bladder can lead to compression or displacement of adjacent organs that should be inspected during the examination. Lastly, bladder wall morphology and thickness change with various levels of distention. In the completely distended bladder, the wall is stretched into a thin rim in which early mural change is difficult to detect (Fig. 12–2). It is easier to assess wall abnormalities if the bladder is only mildly to moderately distended. It is not ideal, however, to allow the patient to urinate immediately before the examination, creating a collapsed urinary bladder.

Placing the patient in dorsal recumbency is helpful but not absolutely necessary for sonographic examination of the urinary bladder. This position centers the bladder and avoids distortion of caudal abdominal anatomy that occurs when a full bladder falls to one side in response to gravity. Whichever position is most acceptable to the patient, reducing motion and struggling, is usually the best position to use. Whether the patient is in dorsal or lateral recumbency, the bladder should be inspected in longitudinal and transverse planes from both the caudoventral and caudolateral surface of the abdomen (Fig. 12–3) to prevent nonvisualization of a lesion in the bladder wall closest to the contact surface of the transducer.

Resolution in the near field is decreased by transducer-skin reverberation artifact, especially in animals with large amounts of subcutaneous fat, thick cornified skin, or der-

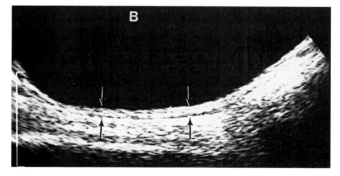

Figure 12–1

Sagittal sonogram of the overly distended bladder (B) of a normal dog. The degree of distention requires use of a lower frequency, lower resolution 5.0-mHz probe with its greater penetration. The far-field bladder wall (arrows) is difficult to evaluate. The near-field bladder wall is not visualized. The bladder wall is stretched into a thin, double-lined structure.

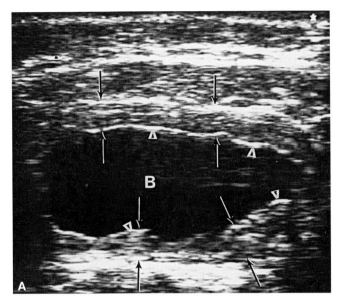

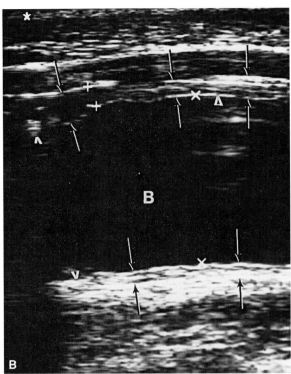

Figure 12–2

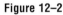

Sagittal sonograms of the urinary bladder (B) in a cat with cystitis. The bladder is mildly distended in **A** and completely distended in **B.** The sonographic changes suggestive of inflammatory disease, such as an irregularly thickened bladder wall (arrows) and hyperechoic mucosa (arrowheads), are easily appreciated in **A** but nearly masked by overdistention in **B**.

matitis. This artifact creates an amorphous haze in the near wall of the bladder that can easily be mistaken for a thickened bladder wall (Fig. 12–4). Decreasing zonal gain through this region on the ultrasound machine (Fig. 12- 5) or use of a standoff pad can help in severe cases of near-field reverberation (Fig. 12–6).[14] Massaging acoustic coupling gel into the animal's skin a few minutes before scanning enhances visualization in the near field by more closely coupling the ultrasound beam with superficial soft tissues. Side lobe artifact can also create "pseudo" thickening of the bladder wall. This artifact, caused by multireflector redirection of the sound beam by the highly reflective colon-air interface, results is an amorphous haze located anywhere in the bladder that can appear as an intraluminal mass or false thickening of an adjacent wall (Fig. 12–7).[15]

Urinary catheter placement has been recommended for cystosonography.[2] Such catheterization negates some of the noninvasive benefits of sonography relative to contrast radiography. If a catheter must be placed and sterile fluid is instilled, care is needed to avoid air bubbles, which will collect along the uppermost wall and create reverber-

Figure 12–3

Schematic of probe placement and the image planes used to perform a thorough sonographic examination of the urinary bladder.

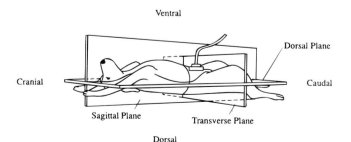

Figure 12–4

Sagittal sonogram of the urinary bladder in a cat with cystitis. The thickened ventral bladder wall (arrows) is less easy to assess than the dorsal bladder wall because of the amorphous haze and parallel linear echoes (arrowheads) caused by near-field reverberation artifact. This artifact can make assessment of the ventral bladder wall difficult and may result in overestimation of wall thickness. Electronic calipers measure wall and mucosal epithelium thickness.

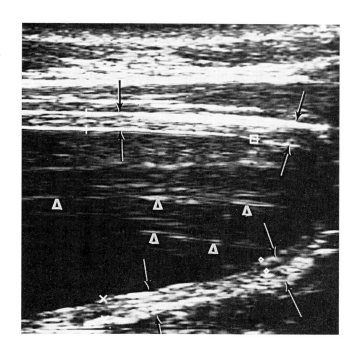

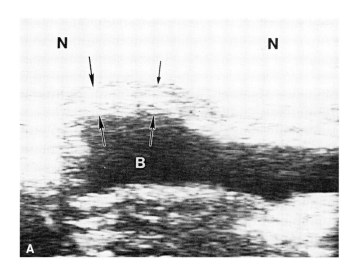

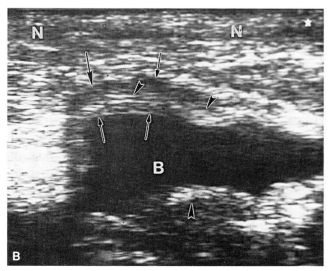

Figure 12–5

Sagittal sonogram of the urinary bladder (B) in a dog with Cushing's syndrome and chronic urinary tract infection. **A,** The gain has been set too high in the near-field (N), creating an artifactual hyperechoic appearance to the ventral body wall and bladder wall. Measurement of the ventral bladder wall (arrows) is difficult at this gain setting and the normally anechoic bladder lumen is filled with false echoes that could be misinterpreted as cellular sediment or crystals. **B,** The near-field gain has been decreased, allowing accurate assessment of the irregularly thickened wall (arrows), visualization of the hyperechoic change in the mucosal epithelium (arrowheads), and an anechoic lumen.

Figure 12–6

Sagittal sonogram of the urinary bladder (B) of the dog in Figure 12–5 after placement of a stand-off pad (P) on the ventral abdomen. The anechoic pad has increased the distance from the probe face to the area of interest, the ventral bladder wall (arrows). This change allows better resolution of the wall and decreases near-field artifact, which impedes visualization. The bladder wall is thickened and the mucosal epithelium (e) is hyperechoic in this cushingoid patient with chronic cystitis.

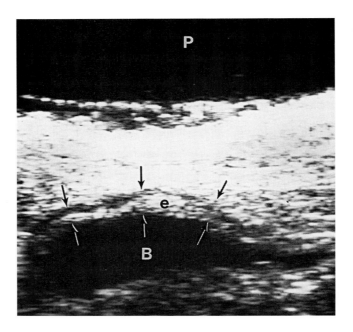

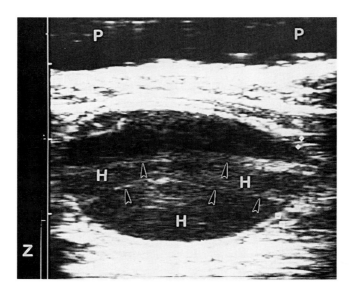

Figure 12–7

Sagittal sonogram of the urinary bladder in a normal cat. A stand-off pad (P) placed on the abdomen moves the area of interest out of the near-field. The acoustic power and gain are too high and the focal zone (Z) has not been moved into the region of the bladder. The amorphous "haze" (H) and parallel echogenic lines (arrowheads) create a "pseudomass" along the dependent bladder wall. This pseudomass is created by side-lobe artifact; an unfocused portion of the beam is strongly reflected from the nearby gas-filled colon and redirected, after multiple secondary reflectors, back to the transducer. The ultrasound system misinterprets the misdirected beam as a complex interface deep to the probe. This artifact, which can mimic wall thickening, a mass, or cellular sediment, can be decreased by minimizing acoustic power and overall gain and adjusting focus.

ation artifacts and potentially mask lesions (Fig. 12–8). Sterile saline that has been microwaved and then cooled is usually free of air bubbles. If a balloon-tipped catheter is used in the area of interest, the use of saline instead of air to distend the balloon is beneficial (Fig. 12–9). The walls of urinary catheters appear as parallel echogenic lines (Fig. 12–10).

Factors that may affect sonographic appearance of the urinary bladder are bladder distention, bladder location, patient position and conformation, pressure of adjacent intra-abdominal structures (feces-filled or gas-filled colon) (Fig. 12–11), and disease.[14] Transducer pressure on the body wall can also distort the normally round to pear-shaped appearance of the bladder (Fig. 12–12). Careful use of different probe angles and patient positions can often differentiate true pathologic wall distortion from artifact. The use of endocavity transducers, such as transvaginal, transurethral, and transrectal transducers, has been recommended for evaluation of human bladder disease[16–18] and may provide improved resolution with some increase in invasiveness.

Structures that effectively mimic the urinary bladder are periprostatic cysts and a fluid-filled uterus (Fig. 12–13). Locating the trigone area and urethra or passing a catheter into the bladder often allows differentiation of the bladder from a cyst. A fluid-filled uterus is often tortuous and can be followed cranially to a perirenal location.

NORMAL BLADDER ANATOMY

The regions of the bladder consist of a blunt vertex, rounded midportion, and neck or trigone. Female dogs, as well as cats of either gender, have an elongate bladder neck.[10] The entire bladder, except the neck, is covered by peritoneum. The median ligament connects the bladder to the ventral pelvic floor. On histologic examination of the completely collapsed bladder, the thickness of the transitional epithelium of the wall varies from 25 to 60 μm, whereas that of the entire bladder wall varies from 2 to 5 mm.[19,20]

Sonographically, the urinary bladder has been described as an anechoic structure surrounded by the smooth, regular outline of an echodense wall. The bladder wall appears as an acoustic interface of wall and serosal fat with no distinction between wall layers.[2] The impression of a nondefinable wall in early bladder imaging is probably related to the use of low frequency transducers (5.0 mHz or less), resultant inferior sono-

Figure 12–8

Sagittal sonogram of the urinary bladder of a cat that was catheterized to instill sterile saline solution. The linear hyperechoic focus (arrows) along the uppermost ventral bladder wall is an air bubble, introduced during catheterization. Note the reverberation artifact (arrowheads) and acoustic shadow (S) deep to the highly reflective air bubble.

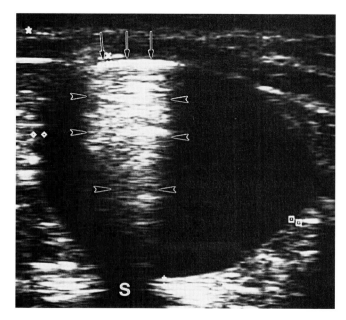

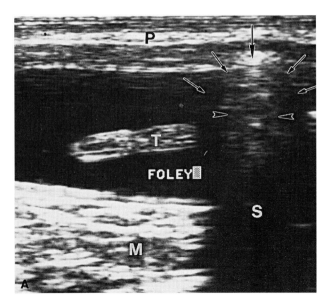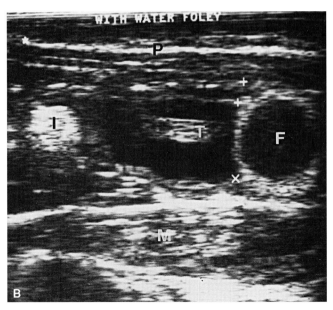

Figure 12–9

Sagittal sonogram of the urinary bladder of a dog with a balloon-tipped Foley catheter that was preplaced for contrast cystography. **A,** The air-filled balloon (small arrows) is seen as a near-field curvilinear hyperechoic focus (large arrow) with reverberation (arrowheads) and acoustic shadowing (S) deep to the initial interface. This artifact is impeding visualization of structures deep to the catheter balloon. **B,** Filling of the balloon with sterile saline allows clear visualization of the balloon and adjacent structures. Note the slight compression of the bladder wall around the balloon in the bladder neck compared to wall thickness (x–x, +–+) just cranial to the balloon. The hyperechoic circle just cranial to the bladder is gas-filled jejunum (I) in cross section. M, psoas muscles; P, peritoneum; T, catheter tip.

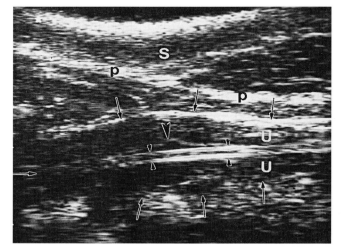

Figure 12–10

Sagittal sonogram of the caudal abdomen in a cat with cystitis and constant stranguria. The thick walls of the collapsed inflamed urinary bladder (arrows) are easier to detect after placement of a catheter (small arrowheads). Note the parallel-walled appearance of the catheter. A small amount of anechoic urine (large arrowhead) is in the bladder lumen surrounding the catheter. Even though empty, as is typical in animals with cystitis, the bladder can now be located and evaluated for calculi or crystalline "sand." S, subcutaneous fat and tissue; P, peritoneum; U, urethra.

Figure 12–11

Transverse sonogram of the urinary bladder (B) in a dog with a portosystemic shunt and a urate calculus (S). The bladder is poorly distended. A second curvilinear hyperechoic structure (C) with distal acoustic shadowing just lateral to the calculus could be misinterpreted as a second calculus. Close inspection shows that the bladder wall (arrows) curves over the extraluminal pseudocalculus, the colon (C), but passes under the true intraluminal calculus. This artifact occurs most commonly when the bladder is flaccid, allowing compression by the colon. If doubt still exists, the patient can be re-examined while standing. In this position, a true cystic calculus, free within the lumen, would fall to the now dependent ventral bladder wall.

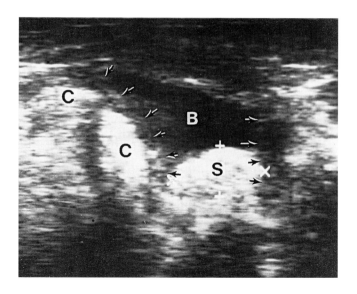

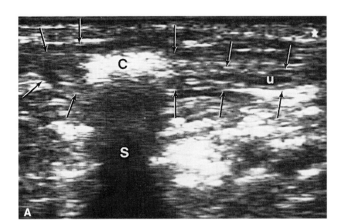

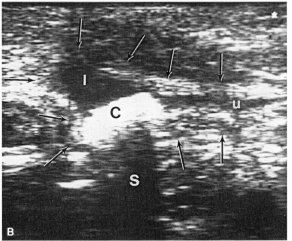

Figure 12–12

Sagittal sonogram of the urinary bladder in a dog with a cystic calculus and chronic cystitis. **A,** Excessive probe pressure causes collapse of the minimally filled urinary bladder (arrows) around the large solitary luminal calculus (C). The discrete curved hyperechoic surface of the calculus could be overlooked or misinterpreted as gas within the bowel in spite of strong acoustic shadowing (S). **B,** Release of probe pressure allows the bladder to "fill" with anechoic urine and the bladder and calculus can be identified.. Note the bladder wall curving around the calculus. Repositioning the patient or ballotment can demonstrate the mobility of the calculus, confirming its intraluminal nature. I, lumen; u, urethra.

Figure 12–13

Transverse sonogram of the urinary bladder in a cat in the first trimester of pregnancy. Both the bladder (B) and gestational sac are circular anechoic structures. The uterus can be followed from the uterine body into the uterine horns by turning the probe into a longitudinal plane and following the tubular uterus. Alternatively, a catheter can be placed within the bladder to identify this structure.

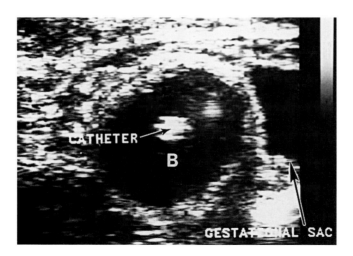

graphic resolution, or examination of the bladder in an overly distended state (Fig. 12–14). Technologically improved resolution and refined scanning techniques now allow sonographers to define the internal architecture of the heteroechoic wall.[10] In a more recent study,[19,20] the sonographic architecture of the bladder wall was described as having three to four subtly defined layers. The layers of the wall are (1) the brightly echogenic serosa/perivesicular fat interface, (2) the slightly heterogeneous, hypoechoic smooth muscle tunic, (3) the irregular, discontinuous circumferential echogenic line of the lamina propria submucosa that parallels the mucosal surface, and (4) the hypoechoic mucosal layer, the lamina epithelialis (Fig. 12–15). The mucosal and submucosal layers are well defined only when the bladder is nearly empty, with no tension deforming the wall. With increasing distention, the mucosal layer thins and becomes nonde-

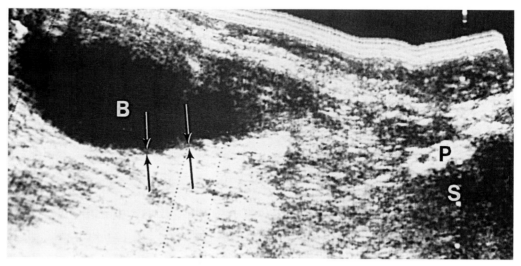

Figure 12–14

Sagittal static B-mode sonogram of the urinary bladder (B) of a normal dog. While performing an examination using this older technique, the probe was placed at the umbilicus, then swept caudal to the pubis (P). A short wait was necessary for the image to develop. Motion detection and fine tuning of probe placement was not possible without immediate image updating. The bladder wall (arrows) is visualized only as a boundary between the anechoic lumen and heteroechoic extraluminal structures. Note the acoustic shadow (S) deep to the pubic bone.

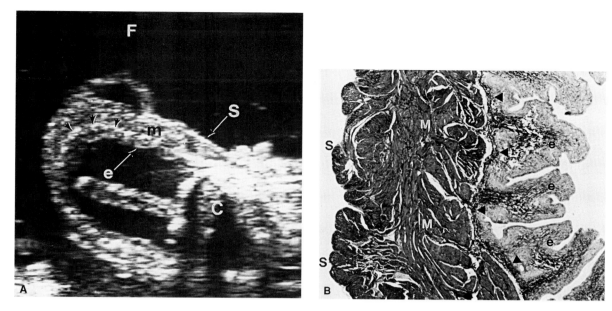

Figure 12–15

A, Sagittal sonogram in a normal cat shows the urinary bladder surrounded by anechoic fluid (F). A balloon-tipped Foley catheter (C) is inside the bladder. At minimal distention, the four-layer architecture of the bladder wall can be detected with high resolution ultrasound. **B,** Histology slide of the bladder in **A.** The increased amounts of collagen in the serosa and submucosa create their hyperechoic appearance. S, serosa; m, smooth muscle layer; e, epithelial mucosa; arrowheads, lamina propria submucosa.

tectable, blending with the echogenic submucosal layer and forming an echogenic boundary between the muscular layer and the bladder lumen. The wall then appears as two parallel echogenic lines with a hypoechoic center (Fig. 12–16). This appearance is noted best where the sound beam contacts the wall at a 90° angle.[20] The vertex is less well defined at all levels of distention, probably because of the off-incidence angle of the beam at this location (Fig. 12–17).[21]

Figure 12–16

Sagittal sonogram of the fully distended bladder (B) of a normal cat. A urinary catheter (c) was placed within the bladder for subsequent imaging studies. When compared to the bladder wall morphology in Figure 12–15, the mucosal layer has thinned and is imperceptible. The bladder wall (cursors) has become a three-layered structure with a thin, hyperechoic serosal covering (arrowhead), a thicker hypoechoic muscular wall (arrow), and a thin hyperechoic submucosal lining (arrowhead).

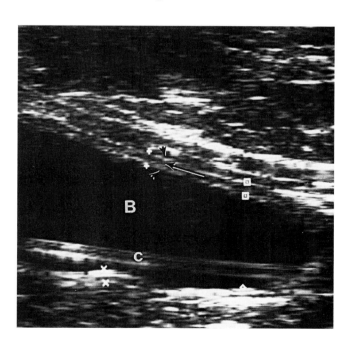

Figure 12–17

Sagittal sonogram of a cat with a fully distended urinary bladder (B) surrounded by anechoic fluid (F). The sound beam (S, line) exiting the probe placed on the ventral body wall is nearly parallel to the bladder wall at the vertex. This parallel course creates poor sound reflection, with little of the beam returning to the probe to register the presence of an interface. An artifactual defect created in the bladder wall at this point (arrows) could be misinterpreted as discontinuity or rupture of the bladder, particularly in animals with free abdominal fluid and a history of trauma. The vertex can be better evaluated by sliding the probe cranial (or caudal), angled back toward the vertical wall for more perpendicular reflection.

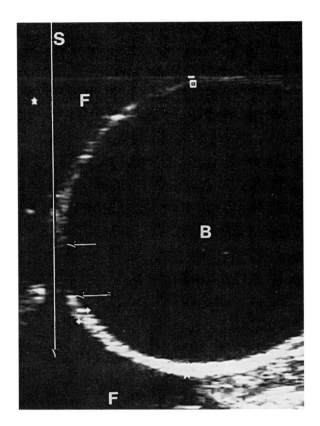

Urinary bladder wall thickness, as well as morphology, changes with the level of distention. In the normal cat, the mean and standard deviation of bladder wall thickness in millimeters across all levels of distention are as follows: vertex (1.7 ± 0.54), dorsal midwall (1.5 ± 0.56), ventral midwall (1.3 ± 0.57), dorsal trigone (1.7 ± 0.56), and ventral trigone (1.7 ± 0.48).[20] Predictably, all locations of bladder wall thin with increasing physiologic distention. The vertex as well as dorsal and ventral trigone are normally slightly thicker and less distensible than the dorsal and ventral midwalls. Normal bladder wall thickness in the dog has not been investigated, but it is probably less than or equal to 2 mm. Sonographically, the normal bladder wall, at all levels of distention, should be thin, smooth, and nearly uniform in thickness.[20]

The shape of the urinary bladder changes with distention. The nearly empty bladder has a smoothly undulant contour. As the bladder is distended, the shape becomes increasingly spheroid, elliptic, or pear-shaped (Fig. 12–18). The ellipsoid shape of the bladder enables accurate calculation of bladder volume, which can be used to evaluate postvoiding urine volume in the evaluation of micturition defects (Fig. 12–19).[12,13] The bladder lumen should be uniformly anechoic. An accumulation of perivesicular fat can be identified around the vertex of the bladder.[20] Similar accumulations of perivesicular fat are seen surrounding the bladder neck (Fig. 12–20).

The ureters enter the bladder obliquely at the ureterovesicular junction and are covered by a mucosal flap.[22] Sonographic inspection of the dorsal trigone in some animals will reveal a small, focal conical thickening at the ureteral papilla. Peristaltic bursts of urine emptying into the bladder in a 45° angle from the ureteral orifice, "ureteral jets," can be detected with color Doppler flow imaging (Fig. 12–21).[23,24] Ureteral peristalsis is controlled by one or more pacemakers, which are located in the recesses of the renal pelvis, and by the activity of the ureteropelvic junction, which determines whether a

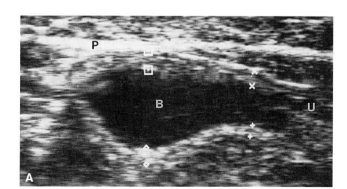

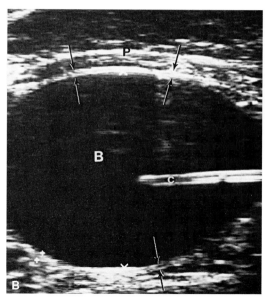

Figure 12–18

A, Sagittal sonogram of the nearly empty urinary bladder (B) of a normal cat. Size is indicated by the centimeter marks at left. The bladder wall (cursors) is collapsed, uniformly thickened, and smoothly undulant. P, peritoneum; U, urethra. **B,** Sagittal sonogram of the completed distended urinary bladder of the same cat as in **A.** A urinary catheter (c) was placed for subsequent imaging studies. The shape of the bladder becomes increasingly spheroid with distention. The normal bladder wall (arrows, cursors) has stretched into a thin, uniform, echogenic structure. P, peritoneum; U, urethra.

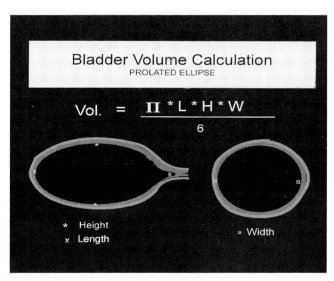

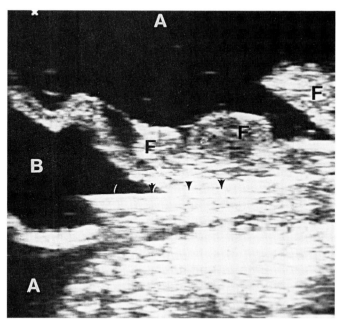

Figure 12–19

Sagittal and transverse images of the urinary bladder shows cursor placement and formula for calculation of bladder volume. The measurement cursors are placed at the lumen-mucosal boundary.

Figure 12–20

Sagittal sonogram of the urinary bladder (B) of a dog with free abdominal fluid (A). The anechoic fluid allows easy detection of the masslike accumulations of fat (F) present in many animals around the bladder neck. In extreme cases, this perivesicular fat could be misinterpreted as a mass or abnormal prostate in the male. A catheter is visible within the urethra and bladder neck (arrowheads).

Figure 12–21

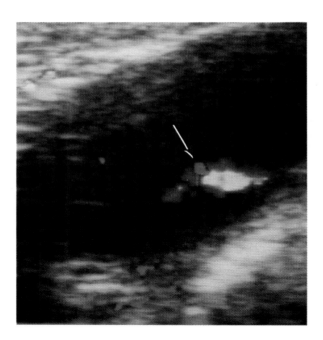

Transverse color Doppler sonogram of the bladder in a young female dog with urinary incontinence. A blue "jet" is seen as urine empties normally from the left ureteral orifice into the bladder. The probe has been angled slightly toward the right and the blue coloring identifies flow from left to right (as indicated by the color wheel). The right ureter also emptied normally. The absence of ectopia was confirmed with contrast radiography and at surgery to repair primary sphincter incontinence.

pacemaker stimulus initiates a peristaltic wave. During diuresis, every stimulus initiates a peristaltic wave.[22] Administration of furosemide before sonography changes the relative physical density between urine emptying from ureters and urine within the bladder, improving sonographic visualization of ureteral jets. The increased velocity, volume, and frequency of ureteral jets after diuretic administration also assists visualization.[24] In some animals, ureteral jets can be detected during gray scale imaging without Doppler evaluation because of protein, fat droplets, crystals, or cells within the urine or after diuretic administration has changed the physical density of the urine (see Fig. 12–40).

The walls of the urinary bladder can be followed caudally, to the level of the pubis, as the subtle parallel echogenic walls of the prostatic or membranous urethra (Fig. 12–22). At the pubis, acoustic shadowing by the soft tissue-bone interface obscures further visualization of the urethra (see Fig. 12–14). With patience and practice, the urethra can be visualized again, caudal to the pubis, and followed for variable distances in the male and female dog (Fig. 12–23). Placement of a urinary catheter allows quick confirmation of the urethra, but this step is not necessary for the experienced sonographer. The penile urethra can be examined by scanning from a lateral location around the prepuce, because the os penis does not completely encircle the urethra, allowing access to an acoustic window (Fig. 12–24). Sonography of the urethra can be sensitive and specific in identifying crystalline "sand" or small calculi. Intraoperative sonography can be used to assure removal of small calculi and "sand" during surgical lavage of the bladder.

DISEASE PROCESSES

Urinary bladder disease, as detected sonographically, can be classified as extramural, intraluminal, or mural. Extramural disease often is detected by its secondary affect on the bladder, such as compression by an enlarged prostate or periprostatic cyst. Only diseases of the bladder lumen or wall are discussed in this chapter. Associated urethral disease is mentioned only briefly.

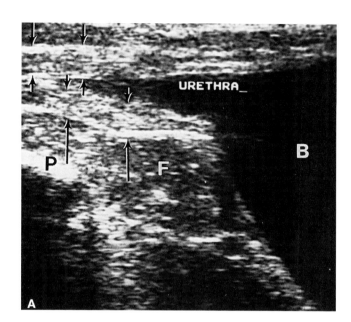
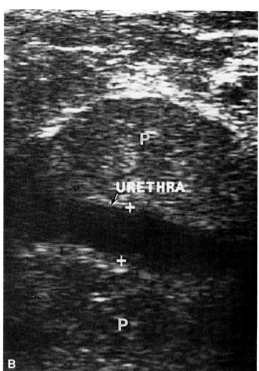

Figure 12-22

A, Sagittal transrectal sonogram of the urinary bladder neck (B) and proximal urethra in a normal dog. The probe was placed in the rectum, reversing the image with cranial to the right and caudal to the left. The anechoic neck of the bladder tapers into the parallel echogenic walls of the urethra (arrows). Heteroechoic perivesicular fat (F) is seen around the urethra and bladder neck. P, the hyperechoic surface of the pubic bone. **B,** Midsagittal sonogram of the prostatic urethra in a dog with urinary obstruction from an impacted calculus at the os penis. Notice the secondary dilatation of the urethra (+,+). The hypoechoic ellipses on both sides of the urethra are the lobes of the prostate (P).

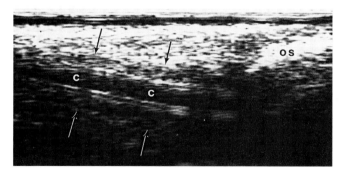

Figure 12-23

Sagittal sonogram of the caudal preputial area of a male dog. The urethra has been followed distally from the bladder, around the ischial arch, and to this level. Therefore, the image is reversed, with caudal to the left and cranial to the right. The hyperechoic curvilinear structure in the near field is the caudal aspect of the os penis. A urinary catheter (C) appears as a parallel-walled structure within the membranous urethra (arrows). The catheter is not well visualized in the penile urethra because of acoustic shadowing from the os penis.

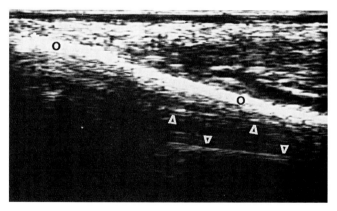

Figure 12-24

Parasagittal sonogram of the prepuce of a dog. The sound beam has been angled around the os penis (O), which appears as a long, hyperechoic linear structure. The area of the urethra and a catheter (arrows) in place within the urethra can be detected deep to the os penis. This technique can be used to evaluate the penile urethra for calculi in some animals.

Intraluminal Disease

Intraluminal disease of the urinary bladder includes: (1) crystals, crystalline "sand," and cellular debris; (2) calculi; (3) gas; (4) blood clots; and (5) foreign bodies. Most intraluminal disease is easily differentiated from mural disease sonographically by mobility. Repositioning the patient or digitally balloting the bladder should create motion and a change in location of intraluminal objects.[14] Occasionally, a polypoid mural mass in one cross-sectional image can be mistaken for an intraluminal structure, especially using static B-mode sonography.[11] Careful and complete ultrasound examination in at least two planes avoids confusion.

Crystals, Crystalline Sand, and Cellular Sediment

Sonographically, crystals, crystalline "sand" (feline urologic syndrome), fat droplets, and cellular sediment can all appear as mobile echogenic particles floating freely within the urinary bladder lumen (Fig. 12–25).[1] A technique to demonstrate mobility of these particles is to place the animal in lateral recumbency and to view the bladder with the transducer placed along the upper abdominal wall. The fingers of the other hand are placed under the bladder along the opposite abdominal wall. Wiggling the fingers in this position often resuspends heavier mobile material that has gravitated to the dependent wall. An alternate technique is to jiggle the caudal abdomen of the patient. The swirling of the echogenic particles resembles the liquid-filled Christmas globes that are turned upside down to make it snow (snow-globe sign) (Fig. 12–26).[1] Scanning while the animal is standing should show gravitation of heavier intraluminal material to the now dependent ventral bladder wall.

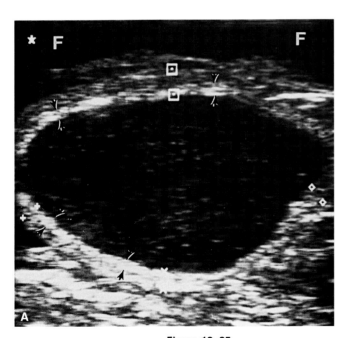
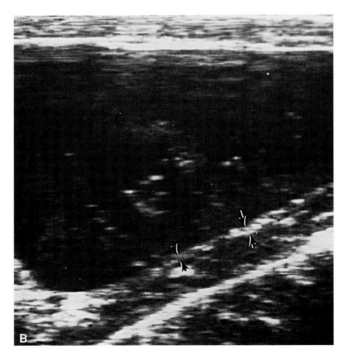

Figure 12–25

A, Sagittal sonogram of a cat with cystitis. The bladder wall (electronic calipers) is thickened and irregular, with a hyperechoic mucosal layer (arrowheads) surrounding the lumen. The low-level echoes floating within the lumen are caused by cellular debris and crystals. Free anechoic fluid (F) surrounds the bladder. **B,** Sagittal sonogram of a normal cat with numerous fat droplets in the urine. Note the "lacy" low-level echoes within the lumen. During real-time examination, the internal structure of the echoes were seen to move and shift. Change in bladder wall thickness (arrows) is not indicative of inflammation.

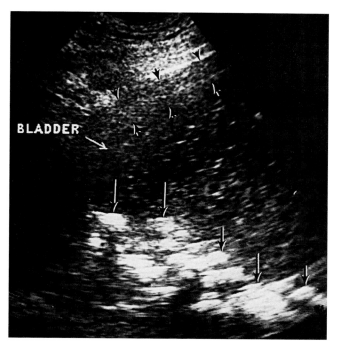

Figure 12–26

Sagittal sonogram of the caudal abdomen of a dog with severe bacterial cystitis and multiple cystic calculi. Initial evaluation of the bladder gives the impression of a complex mass rather than a fluid-filled bladder. Close inspection of the "mass" with real-time technique showed mobility of the internal echoes that correlated with patient movement (snow-globe sign). Note the thickened hypoechoic bladder wall and the multiple brightly hyperechoic curvilinear echoes of a stack of variably sized cystic calculi (arrows). Acoustic shadowing impedes evaluation of deeper calculi and the dorsal bladder wall.

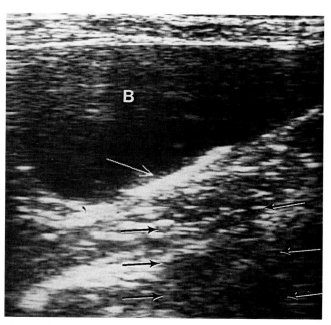

Figure 12–27

Sagittal sonogram of the urinary bladder (B) of a cat with crystalline "sand" within the bladder. The small hyperechoic particles have gravitated to the dependent wall as a hyperechoic layer (white arrow) with slight distal acoustic shadowing (black and white arrows). Patient repositioning or digital agitation of the bladder will resuspend the particles and differentiate the layer from a solid calculus.

Crystals and crystalline sand have been described as appearing more hyperechoic than cellular sediment,[10] but differentiation can be difficult. A large amount of crystals or sandy sludge, accumulating in the dependent portion of the bladder, may create an acoustic shadow because of their combined ability to block the sound beam (Fig. 12–27). Cellular sediment is more likely to "blend in" with and become imperceptible from the dependent bladder wall, creating artifactual thickening of the wall (Fig. 12–28). In cases of severe purulent cystitis, an exudate-urine interface may be detected, as heavier echogenic exudate settles to the dependent bladder wall, forming a horizontal line.[14]

Calculi

Diseases caused by uroliths are among the most common urinary tract problems of domesticated animals.[22] In dogs, several breeds are predisposed to formation of calculi, namely dachshunds, Dalmatians, cocker spaniels, Pekingese, basset hounds, poodles, schnauzers, and small terriers.[22] The presence of calculi may indicate primary bladder disease, such as infection (typically, struvite calculi), or systemic disease, such as primary hyperparathyroidism, hypercalcemic nephropathy (oxalate calculi), and portosystemic shunts (urate calculi) (see Fig. 12–11). Sonography is reported to have 100% accuracy in detecting calculi in human patients.[14] This technique can be used repeatedly to monitor dissolution of cystic calculi because of its noninvasive nature.

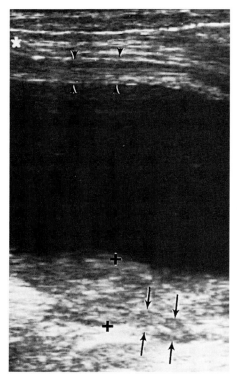

Figure 12–28

Sagittal sonogram of the urinary bladder in a dog with hematuria. Mild thickening, irregularity, and hyperechoic mucosal epithelium are seen in the ventral bladder wall (arrowheads). Note also the apparent asymmetric thickening of the dorsal bladder wall (+,+). Agitation of the bladder by repositioning the patient, however, resuspended the cellular material that had accumulated along the dependent wall and allowed measurement of a mildly thickened dorsal wall (arrows). The pseudothickening was created by an accumulation of hemorrhage.

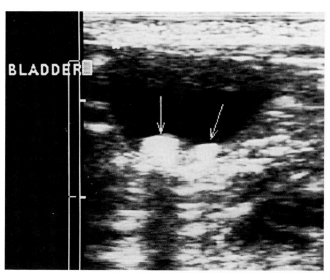

Figure 12–29

Transverse sonogram of the urinary bladder of a dog with cystitis and two cystic calculi (arrows). Note the hyperechoic discrete curvilinear surface of both calculi and the lack of acoustic shadowing beneath the smaller calculus. The ability to create an acoustic shadow is determined by calculus size, degree of mineralization, and location relative to the focal zone, but not by chemical composition.

Cystic calculi appear as curvilinear hyperechoic interfaces blocking much of the sound beam at the first fluid-calculus interface and creating a distal acoustic shadow (Fig. 12–29).[1] If several calculi have accumulated together, their combined interfaces create a hyperechoic undulant line (Fig. 12–30). The chemical composition of calculi does not correlate with the degree of acoustic shadowing or the echogenicity.[10,11] Calculi without calcium are equally hyperechoic; therefore, it is possible to use sonography to detect radiolucent as well as radiopaque calculi. The ratio of mineral to organic matrix within a calculus may affect the echogenicity and ability to block the sound beam. The mineral composition of a calculus cannot be determined on the basis of its sonographic appearance.

Cystic calculi are typically mobile within the bladder lumen; however, because of increased size, they are unlikely to float with agitation. Instead, calculi appear to roll away, marble-like, from an area of bladder being lifted by a finger beneath the dependent bladder wall. If the mobility of a suspect calculus is not easy to demonstrate while the patient is recumbent, standing the patient up will cause gravitation of an intraluminal calculus to the ventral bladder wall (Fig. 12–31).[14] Some calculi, such as the jagged-edged silicates, may adhere to the bladder wall and are then difficult to differentiate from a focus of dystrophic mineralization within the wall (Fig. 12–32).

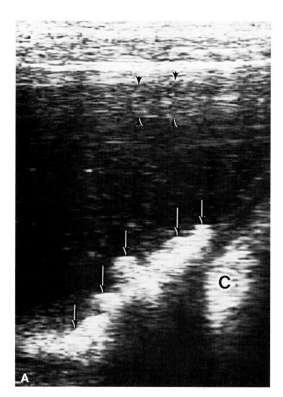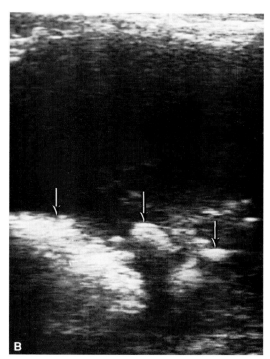

Figure 12–30

A, Sagittal sonogram of the urinary bladder of a dog with bacterial cystitis and multiple struvite calculi. The undulant hyperechoic line formed by the combined reflective surfaces (arrows) of the calculi could be confused with hyperechoic gas and feces in the adjacent colon (C). The ventral bladder wall is thickened and hypoechoic (arrowheads). The dorsal wall cannot be evaluated because of acoustic shadowing. **B,** Digital ballotment causes motion and momentary resuspension of the calculi (arrows), confirming their location within the lumen of the bladder.

Figure 12–31

Transverse sonogram of the urinary bladder (B) of the dog in Figure 12–12 with a chronic bacterial cystitis and a large solitary calculus (C). The dog was examined while standing and the calculus gravitated to the dependent ventral bladder wall, confirming its intraluminal nature. The bladder wall (arrows) is thickened and the mucosal epithelium is hyperechoic and irregular. The acoustic shadow creates an anechoic artifact in the dorsal bladder wall (arrowheads).

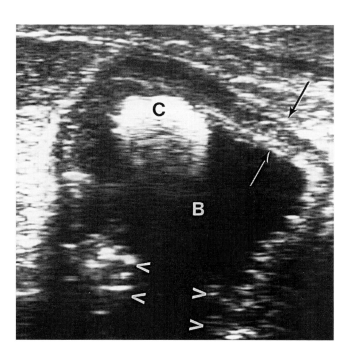

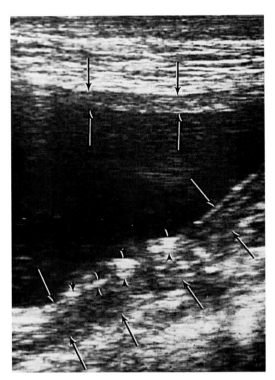

Figure 12–32

Sagittal sonogram of the urinary bladder in a dog with a chronic urinary tract infection. The bladder wall (arrows) is thickened and irregular. Multiple discrete hyperechoic foci are seen along the dependent dorsal bladder wall (arrowheads). Differential diagnoses for these foci include small calculi, crystalline accumulations, and mineralization or gas within the bladder wall. Digital ballotment of the bladder and repositioning of the patient did not result in a change in these foci. Therefore, adherent calculi (silicates) or intramural mineralization or gas was more likely than intraluminal disease. Biopsy revealed chronic transmural cystitis and dystrophic mineralization.

Cystic calculi may not cast an acoustic shadow if they are smaller than the active element diameter of the transducer, if thick or heterogeneous intervening tissue scatters the sound beam, or if the calculus is not in the focal zone of the transducer, especially if it is in the far field.[14] Large, highly reflective calculi have been reported to cause reverberation from its surface, much like a tissue-air interface, which can fill in an acoustic shadow.[10,11]

The appearance of urethral calculi is the same as that of cystic calculi, except they are not freely mobile. The urethra should be followed as far distally as possible during sonographic examination to detect additional calculi, because the most common sites of urethral impaction are the proximal end of the os penis in dogs and anywhere along the urethra in male cats.[22] The urethral walls can be seen to separate and appear displaced around impacted calculi (Fig. 12–33). Distention of the urethra with urine proximal to the calculus, multiple calculi in a row (steinstrasse, "stone street"), displacement of the urethral walls, or change in the sonographic appearance of the urethral walls may indicate obstruction. Sonographic re-examination after urination may indicate whether a urethral calculus is lodged. If urethral impaction is suspected, the ureters, renal pelvis, and kidneys should be examined to assess the extent of the obstructive nephropathy. Ultrasound has been used to identify calculi within the prostatic urethra and penile urethra of dogs that were not detected on radiographs because of their small size, radiolu-

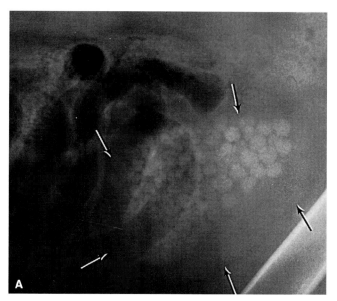
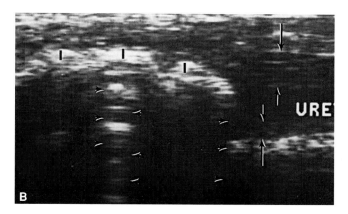

Figure 12–33

A, Lateral radiograph of the caudal abdomen of a male dog with chronic hematuria and acute dysuria (same dog in Fig. 12-30) reveals multiple, variably sized radiopaque calculi within the urinary bladder (arrows). **B,** Sagittal sonogram of the membranous urethra just proximal to the os penis of this dog reveals multiple urethral calculi. Notice the multiple hyperechoic curvilinear interfaces (I) and acoustic shadowing (arrowheads) of the calculi lined up within the urethra. Impaction of the urethra is suggested by separation of the urethral walls (arrows) and dilatation of the lumen with anechoic urine.

cent nature, or superimposition of radiographic shadows (Fig. 12–34). Sonography can be used to assure removal of urethral stones or "sand" after catheterization and retrograde lavage or during cystotomy.

Gas
Intraluminal gas bubbles introduced by urinary catheterization or produced by a gas-forming infection can also appear as small, floating hyperechoic foci in the bladder lumen. These foci rapidly gravitate to the uppermost bladder wall, however, and accumulate under the mucosal surface as a reverberating curvilinear hyperechoic interface (see Fig. 12–8).

Blood Clots
The sonographic appearance of clotted blood within the urinary bladder depends on the size and the chronicity of the clot. The fibrin mesh of blood clots appears mildly hyperechoic but do not cast acoustic shadows. Blood clots are frequently mobile within the bladder lumen (Fig. 12–35) and large clots often have complex, "lacy" internal patterns that give it a tissue-like appearance (Fig. 12–36).[10,11] Adherent blood clots may not differ in appearance from mural polyps or neoplasia. Blood clots associated with cystocentesis can adhere to the trauma site along the ventral or dorsal bladder wall. Occasionally, the entire lumen of the bladder is filled with a lacy, cobweb-like material that moves as a unit like gelatin. This appearance can be seen when a large, acute blood clot fills the bladder lumen, when urine protein content is high, or when fat droplets are present (see Fig. 12–25**B**).

Foreign Bodies
Foreign bodies that may be observed within the urinary bladder are catheters, metal ballistic foreign bodies (BBs), suture material, and grass awn. Catheters appear as parallel

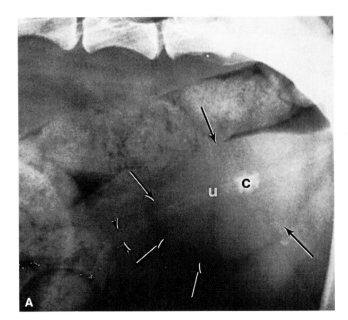 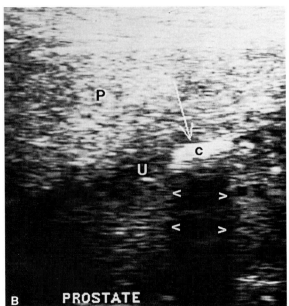

Figure 12–34

A, Lateral radiograph of the abdomen of a male dog with acute stranguria after surgery to remove multiple cystic calculi reveals a linear radiopaque urinary catheter (u) and a large, irregular radiopaque calculus (c) within a bladder-shaped soft tissue opacity (arrows). Close inspection reveals the catheter extends cranial to the apex of the "bladder," which was actually an enlarged prostate. **B,** Sagittal sonogram of the prostate (P) revealed a hyperechoic calculus (c, arrow) within the prostatic urethra (U). Note the distal acoustic shadow (arrowheads). The urinary catheter was seen in an adjacent scan plane passing around the calculus.

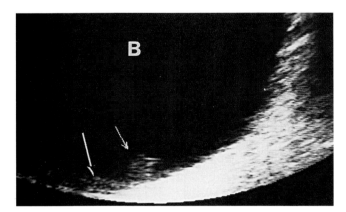

Figure 12–35

Transverse sonogram of the urinary bladder (B) of a dog with pelvic fractures and hematuria. The fullness of the bladder and the size of the dog required use of a 5-mHz probe, and compromised close evaluation of the bladder wall. No rupture or defects were seen within the wall, but blood clots (arrows) appeared as irregularly bordered, complex tissue-echogenicity masses, freely mobile within the lumen. Mural masses and polyps may have the same sonographic appearance but are not freely mobile. Adherent blood clots cannot be easily differentiated from mural masses.

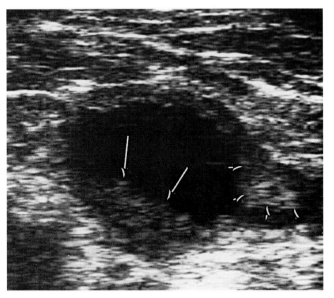

Figure 12–36

Sagittal sonogram of the bladder of a male cat with urinary obstruction that resulted in bladder rupture. The small rupture of the ventral trigone wall had sealed and was covered by an adherent, complex echogenic mass (arrowheads). A second freely mobile, "lacy," hypoechoic mass (arrows) was subsequently voided as a large blood clot. The adherent mass resolved over time and was presumed to be a hematoma.

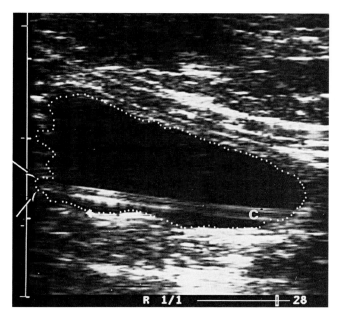

Figure 12–37

Sagittal sonogram of the urinary bladder of a cat. A urinary catheter (C) placed for imaging studies was passed too far into the urethra and is displacing or "tenting" the vertex (arrows). Before catheter placement, the vertex wall was smooth and semicircular. Catheter trauma has resulted in wall spasm and the rippled appearance of the vertex wall. The dotted line is electronically placed points to measure the bladder perimeter for volume calculation.

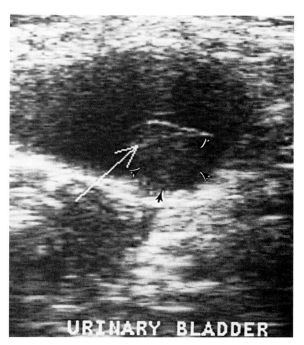

Figure 12–38

Transverse sonogram of the urinary bladder of a female dog with chronic cystitis and hematuria. At cystotomy, the branched linear, echogenic structure (white arrow) with an adherent hypoechoic mass (arrowheads) within the lumen proved to be a grass awn with adherent blood clot and fibrin.

hyperechoic lines that may form a loop within the bladder, depending on catheter length. An overly long catheter will cranially displace or "tent" the vertex of the bladder (Fig. 12–37). Sonography can be used to assist in correct catheter placement before an indwelling catheter is fixed in position, thereby avoiding iatrogenic damage. The sonographic appearance of a metallic foreign body (BB) is similar to that of a calculus other than it is circular, smooth, and extremely hyperechoic at the urine-foreign body interface. Sound reverberation can be seen distal to the metal foreign body within the acoustic shadow because of the highly reflective nature of metal. A grass awn can appear as mildly echogenic, small branching structure within the lumen (Fig. 12–38).

Mural Disease

Mural disease of the urinary bladder includes (1) congenital defects, such as ureteroceles, ectopic ureters, and patent urachus or urachal diverticula; (2) traumatic defects, such as partial or complete bladder rupture, mural hematomas, and herniation; (3) inflammatory defects, such as cystitis, inflammatory polyps, chronic bladder obstruction and muscular hypertrophy, mural abscess, and emphysematous cystitis; and (4) neoplasia.

Congenital Defects

Ureteroceles, which are intramural dilatations of the distal ureters in the bladder trigone, have been visualized in man and animals with sonography.[1,14] They appear as anechoic circular structures in the trigone with a thin, smooth echogenic wall (Fig.

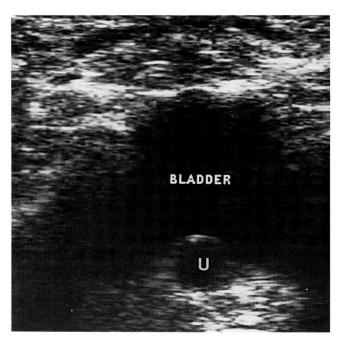

Figure 12-39

Oblique parasagittal sonogram of the urinary bladder of a young female dog shows intramural expansion of the left ureter, a ureterocele (U), in the bladder trigone.

12–39). A "small bladder within the larger bladder" at the trigone is a good visual analogy. They may be bilateral or unilateral. Although ureteroceles are truly mural abnormalities, projection into the lumen can make them appear intraluminal. Thinning of the adjacent bladder wall is difficult to detect. An associated hydroureter often can be followed from the bladder to the kidney, and an obstructive nephropathy and hydronephrosis may be present.

Ectopic ureter is the most common ureteral anomaly. The affected ureter may empty into the vas deferens, vesicular gland, or urethra of the male or the bladder neck, urethra, or vagina of the female.[22] Certain dog breeds have a high risk for the defect, including the Siberian husky, Newfoundland, Labrador retriever, West Highland white terrier, fox terrier, and miniature and toy poodle; the defect is familial in Siberian huskies and Labrador retrievers.[22]

Ectopic ureters usually do not affect the sonographic appearance of the bladder. They can be identified, however, as an anechoic tube or tubes with no evidence of Doppler-detected blood flow extending to an area other than the bladder trigone. Entry into the vagina is difficult to identify sonographically. Dilated ureters can be followed to the urethra in special cases. The actual opening into the urethra is difficult to isolate. Doppler-detected bilateral or unilateral absence of the normal "ureteral jets" after diuretic administration (Fig. 12–40; see also Fig. 12–21) suggests ectopia.[23,24] Contrast radiography remains a more valuable technique for detecting ectopic ureters. Ureteral anomalies may predispose a patient to hydronephrosis and urinary tract infection that may culminate in pyelonephritis,[22] making sonographic evaluation of the upper urinary tract important.

A patent urachus can appear in foals as an anechoic tubular structure that can be followed completely or partially from the umbilical area to the bladder lumen.[25] The sonographic appearance of a patent urachus has not yet been reported in dogs and cats, but it is most likely similar to the appearance in the foal. The fibrotic remnant of the urachus has been described as a heteroechoic structure extending from the ventral abdominal wall to the apex of the bladder.[10]

Diverticula of the urinary bladder may be congenital urachal remnants or they may be acquired defects owing to partial obstruction to urine outflow or to mural trauma. Urachal or traumatic diverticula of the bladder can be seen sonographically in both dogs

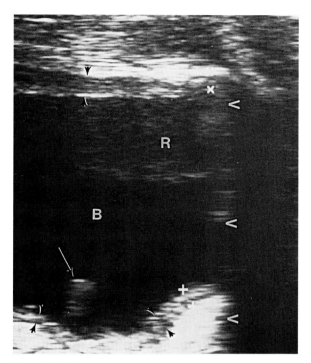

Figure 12–40

Transverse sonogram of the urinary bladder (B) of the young female dog in Figure 12–21 after furosemide administration. The change in physical density in the urine emptying from the right ureter relative to the urine in the bladder allows detection of the ureteral "jet" without color Doppler imaging. The bladder wall (black arrowheads) is slightly thickened from cystitis. Reverberation artifact (R) creates an amorphous haze along the ventral bladder wall. Adjacent colon creates a distal acoustic shadow (white arrowheads).

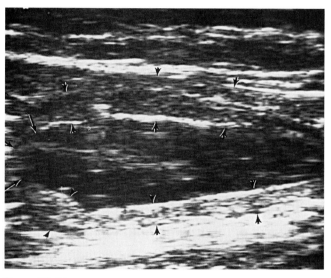

Figure 12–41

Sagittal sonogram of the urinary bladder in a 2-year-old cat with recurrent bacterial urinary tract infections. The bladder wall (arrowheads) is thickened and irregular with a hyperechoic mucosal epithelium. The bladder lumen appears stiff and angular and the lumen contains the numerous mobile low-level echoes of cellular sediment. The vertex of the bladder elongates abruptly into a thin-walled, conical structure (arrows). A urachal diverticulum was found on laparotomy.

and cats. Urachal diverticula are located at the vertex, where they represent incomplete closure of the urachus with an area of discontinuity in the muscle.[22] The ability of ultrasound to detect diverticula is reduced by the location of the defect at the vertex where the sound beam parallels the bladder wall and reflection back to the transducer is poor. Urachal diverticula have been described as anechoic, irregular intramural lesions,[10,11] although in my experience, they appear as persistent, conical thinning of the bladder wall at the vertex of the bladder (Fig. 12–41).[26,27] Traumatic diverticula can be seen at various locations in the bladder. Diverticula associated with concurrent cystitis from urinary stasis may have irregularity along the mucosal surface. Calculi may be present in the diverticulum. Diverticula are most difficult to recognize in the nearly empty bladder. They are best visualized with moderate bladder distention and usually persist as the bladder is progressively filled. A diverticula may acquire a balloon-like exaggerated appearance with progressive distention.[26,27]

Trauma

Rupture of the urinary bladder can occur after urethral obstruction, pelvic trauma, or iatrogenic overdistention. Sonographic differentiation of rupture of the bladder with release of urine into the abdomen from free abdominal fluid surrounding the bladder can be difficult unless the bladder wall is completely disrupted. A focal thickening or defect may be noted in the wall associated with the previous rupture (Fig. 12–42). Omentum, mesentery, or bowel may adhere to the rupture site. Discontinuity of the wall

Figure 12–42

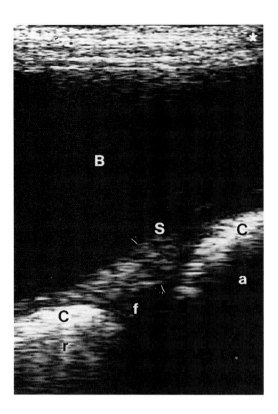

Sagittal sonogram of the urinary bladder (B) in a dog that had sustained pelvic trauma and bladder rupture. Free fluid was present elsewhere within the abdomen. At the rupture site (S, arrowheads), the bladder wall appeared intact, but thickened and irregularly hypoechoic. The gas-filled colon (C) was "fixed" to the rupture site and could not be displaced with probe pressure. A focal accumulation of fluid (f) was seen between colon and bladder wall. Acoustic shadowing (a) and reverberation (r) are seen distal to the gas-tissue interface of the colon. At laparotomy, the colon and omentum adhered to the rupture site.

is not a reliable sonographic sign of rupture because "echo drop-out" or loss of reflected echoes from a surface parallel to the sound beam and sound beam refraction can create an artifactual defect in the bladder wall when free fluid is present in the abdomen (see Fig. 12–17).[21] Partial rupture of the urinary bladder wall with subserosal accumulation of urine can be easier to detect as a focal anechoic halo associated with a portion of the wall.[26,27] Partial bladder ruptures in the trigone area may be visualized sonographically as temporarily nondiffusing accumulations of fluid around the bladder neck (Fig. 12–43).[26,27] Sonographic re-examination within 48 hours can assess persistent leakage or reabsorption of the urine.

Hematomas in the wall of the urinary bladder appear as a nonmobile, focal thickening that cannot be differentiated reliably from neoplasia or focal cystitis. The sonographic appearance of hematomas is age related. The "life span" of a hematoma begins as an anechoic focus in the acute stage. With formation of the fibrin clot in the subacute stage, the hematoma becomes hyperechoic (Fig. 12–44; see also Fig. 12–36). Within days, hematomas may acquire a complex appearance, with the formation of anechoic areas that reflect the beginning of hemolysis. In the chronic hematoma, reorganization and calcification recreates an echogenic appearance with possible acoustic shadowing.

Herniation of the urinary bladder into an inguinal or perineal hernia is identified sonographically as the absence of a bladder in the normal location and the presence of an anechoic, usually smooth-walled bladder-like structure inside the hernial sac. Identifying the urethra and following it into the hernial sac is difficult and the presence of a urinary catheter can be a useful guide if the urethra is patent. Centesis of urine from the anechoic structure in the hernial sac can be performed if confirmation is needed.

Inflammation

Inflammation of the lower urinary tract, usually involving inflammation of the bladder, is a common clinical problem in animals.[22] Predisposition to urinary tract infection occurs when there is stagnation of urine because of obstruction, incomplete voiding, glucosuria, or urothelial trauma. Other factors include catheterization, vaginoscopy, urinary

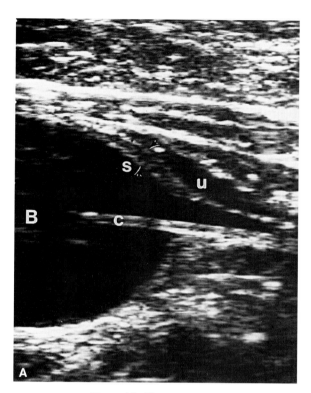
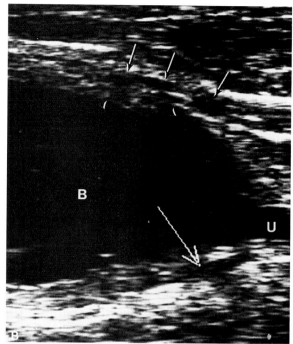

Figure 12–43

A, Sagittal sonogram of a cat with a urinary bladder (B) that had partially ruptured from overdistention during cystography. Note the catheter (C) in the urethra and bladder neck. Low-level echoes in the urine allowed visualization, with real-time ultrasound, of urine (u) diffusing through the injury site (S, arrowheads) and accumulating under the serosa. The actual defect in the wall was not detectable, but the wall appeared hypoechoic at the site. **B,** Re-examination of the rupture site 24 and 48 hours later showed gradual resorption of the anechoic fluid (arrow) and a persistent hypoechoic defect in the bladder wall. B, bladder; U, urethra.

incontinence, vaginitis, and administration of antibiotics or corticosteroids within the last 60 days.[22] The higher incidence in females may be associated with the short urethra. Etiologic agents involved in bladder infection include E. coli, Proteus, streptococci, staphylococci, mycoplasma, and blastomyces. A sterile hemorrhagic cystitis may occur in animals treated for neoplastic or immunologic diseases with cyclophosphamide.[22] Cystitis may be differentiated into acute and chronic forms.

Cystitis can create diffuse or focal irregular thickening of the urinary bladder wall.[2,14,26,27] Wall measurements must be correlated with bladder volume because wall thickness varies with distention.[19,20] In a study of induced cystitis in cats,[26,27] the sonographic changes detected in the bladder were (1) a circumferentially thickened, strongly defined, hypoechoic bladder wall with nonuniform wall thickness and loss of the parallel appearance of the mucosal and serosal surfaces; (2) increasing heteroechogenicity beginning at 15 days; (3) a stiffer, more angular bladder shape; (4) increased echogenicity and irregularity of the mucosal layer with chronicity; and (5) increased presence of cellular debris in the lumen (Fig. 12–45). Similarly, other investigators found the echogenicity of the bladder wall decreased with cystitis,[2,28] and described a hypoechoic zone below the mucosa.[10] These changes may be related to leukocyte infiltration and hemorrhage in all layers.[22] In chronic or severe cystitis, "heaping up" of the mucosal epithelium and fibrous thickening of the wall can create a hyperechoic, irregular appearance of the mucosal epithelium (Fig. 12–46).[14] This appearance may be related to superficial fibrinous or deep diphtheritic change or to proliferation of submucosal connective

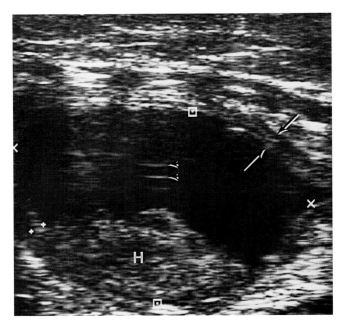

Figure 12–44

Sagittal sonogram of the urinary bladder of a cat with intermittent hematuria that had sustained bladder trauma 4 days previously. A large echogenic hematoma (H) associated with the dorsal bladder wall did not move with repositioning or ballotment, differentiating it from cellular material or a blood clot in the lumen. Resolution of the hematoma over a period of weeks differentiated it from mural neoplasia. Aspiration biopsy indicated old hemorrhage. Cursors indicate bladder dimensions and thickness of the mucosal epithelium; arrowheads denote reverberation artifact. The bladder wall (arrows) is mildly thickened.

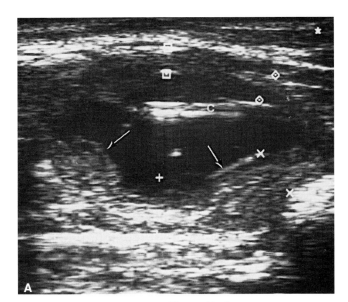
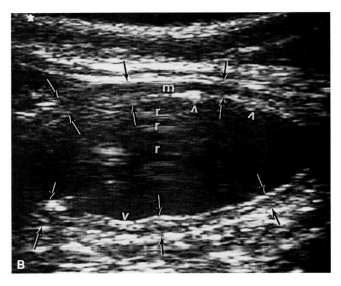

Figure 12–45

A, Sagittal sonogram of the urinary bladder of a male cat with acute cystitis. The bladder wall (cursors) is thickened, heteroechoic, and nonuniform in thickness. Masslike inflammatory nodules (arrows) are seen and the shape of the bladder is angular. A urinary catheter (c) was placed for other imaging studies. Escherichia coli was recovered from urine culture. **B,** Sagittal sonogram of the urinary bladder of the same cat 1 week later. The cat still had clinical signs of dysuria and urinalysis was abnormal, but urine culture was negative. The bladder wall (arrows) is still abnormal, with irregularity and increased echogenicity in the mucosal epithelium (arrowheads). The muscularis layer (m) is normoechoic. The lumen contains near-field reverberation artifact (r) and the low level echoes of cellular debris. The bladder shape is still slightly angular.

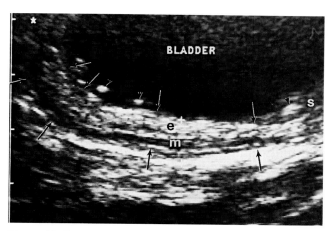

Figure 12–46

Sagittal sonogram of the urinary bladder of a dog with chronic severe cystitis and calculi (arrowheads). The bladder wall (arrows) is dramatically thickened (cursors). Fibrous thickening of the mucosal epithelium (e) has created a hyperechoic, irregular layer lining the bladder lumen. The muscularis (m) is the hypoechoic layer surrounding the thickened epithelium. Cellular sediment (s) is present in the dependent portion of the bladder, but much of the low-level near-field echoes is artifact.

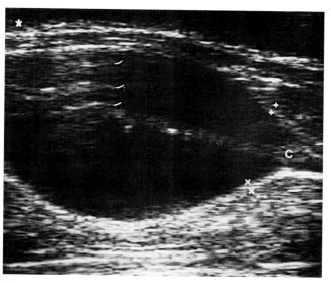

Figure 12–47

Sagittal sonogram of the urinary bladder of the cat with acute cystitis shown in Figure 12–45, 2 weeks later. The shape of the bladder and the thickness and appearance of the bladder wall (cursors) are normal. Note the parallel lines of reverberation artifact (arrowheads) in the near field of the bladder lumen. c, urinary catheter.

tissue.[22] Pathologic irregularity of the mucosa can be differentiated from the undulant, irregular appearance of the normal collapsed bladder wall by its persistent irregular appearance with increasing distention.

Selective inflammatory thickening of the urinary bladder wall has been seen on both double contrast cystograms and sonograms to affect the cranioventral wall.[10] I and other investigators have not detected a preferential location for wall thickening in cystitis, but rather have found diffuse circumferential involvement.[26,27] After resolution of inflammation, the sonographic appearance of the bladder wall may return to normal if the inflammation is not longstanding (Fig. 12–47).

Dystrophic mineralization of the urinary bladder wall can appear as a fixed hyperechoic focus with or without acoustic shadowing and without reverberation artifact (see Figure 12–32). Mass-like or nodular thickening of the bladder wall, which is indistinguishable from infiltrative neoplasia, can be seen with follicular or chronic polypoid cystitis and cyclophosphamide-induced hemorrhagic cystitis (Fig. 12–48). Occasionally, bladder wall thickening from muscular hypertrophy can be seen with chronic urinary outflow obstruction and inflammation, which can have a sonographic appearance similar to that of infiltrative neoplasia (Fig. 12–49). Mural wall abscesses can occur, particularly related to Corynebacterium infection, appearing as an anechoic cavity within a mass-like focal thickening of the bladder wall (Fig. 12–50). The wall around the cystic area can be complex and irregular.

Emphysematous cystitis develops in some dogs and cats, especially with diabetes mellitus, and is thought to be caused by fermentation of sugar by glucose-fermenting bacteria.[22] The sonographic appearance of this condition is multifocal, hyperechoic areas of intramural gas, with variable acoustic shadowing and reverberation, on multiple bladder walls (Fig. 12–51). Emphysematous cystitis can be differentiated from urinary catheter-introduced gas within the lumen by the involvement of bladder walls other than the

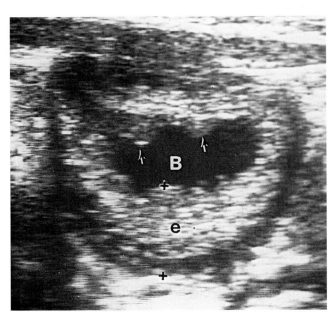

Figure 12–48

Transverse sonogram of the urinary bladder (B) of a dog being treated with cyclophosphamide for neoplasia. Note the severe thickening of the bladder wall (+) related to hemorrhagic cystitis. Mucosal epithelium (e) is diffusely thickened, irregular, and hyperechoic. The small hypoechoic masses (arrows) projecting into the lumen were inflammatory nodules.

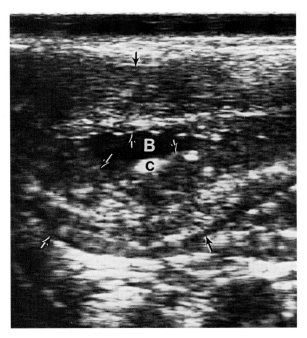

Figure 12–49

Sagittal sonogram of a severely thickened, echo-complex urinary bladder wall (arrows) in a dog with obstructive transitional cell carcinoma of the urethra. The lumen of the bladder (B) contains a small amount of anechoic urine and a single small calculus (c). Infiltrative neoplasia of the bladder was suspected. Biopsy of the bladder showed transmural cystitis and muscular hypertrophy, but no evidence of neoplasia.

Figure 12–50

Sagittal sonogram of the ventral wall (arrows) of the urinary bladder (B) of a male dog with severe necrotizing and emphysematous bacterial cystitis. The focal masslike thickening of the wall with an anechoic center (A) was found to be an abscess from which Corynebacterium sp. was cultured. The comet-tail reverberation resulting from the emphysematous change in the bladder wall (arrowheads) was also seen on survey radiography.

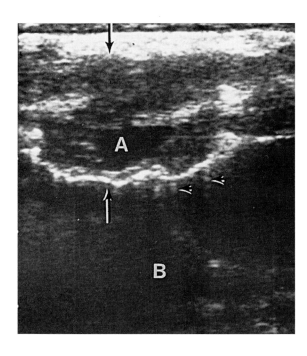

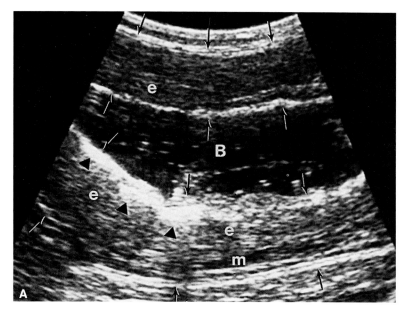

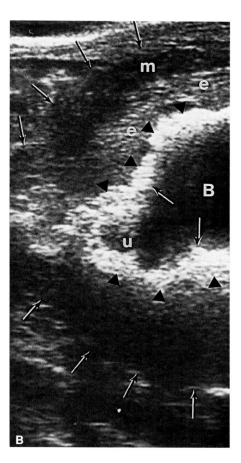

Figure 12–51

A, Transverse sonogram of the urinary bladder (B) in a nondiabetic dog with severe emphysematous bacterial cystitis. The thickened bladder wall (arrows) with extensive hyperechoic mucosal epithelium (e) was found to be necrotic and friable at laparotomy. The brightly hyperechoic foci bordering the lumen with distal reverberation are areas of emphysema (arrowheads). The bladder lumen contains multiple pinpoint hyperechoic foci that gravitate, during examination, to the upper wall and represent solubilized gas. **B,** Sagittal sonogram of the bladder vertex (B) showed the irregularly tapered outpouching of a urachal diverticulum (u). e, mucosal epithelium; arrowheads, mucosal emphysema; arrows, bladder wall; m, muscularis.

uppermost wall. The hyperechoic foci of emphysematous cystitis are also fixed in location, unlike intraluminal gas. Intraluminal gas may, however, be present in dogs with emphysematous cystitis.

Results of preliminary studies suggest sonography may be more sensitive and specific than double contrast cystography in detecting urinary bladder inflammation and resolution of bladder disease.[26,27] Sonography, therefore, is a valuable noninvasive technique for sequential imaging to assess response to antibiotic therapy.

Neoplasia

Tumors of the urinary bladder account for 0.5 to 1% of all canine tumors.[2,22] The Scottish terrier, Shetland sheepdog, beagle, and collie seem to be at greatest risk. Transitional cell carcinoma is the most common malignant tumor and may be papillary, polypoid, or sessile.[22] Adenocarcinoma, undifferentiated carcinoma, botryoid rhabdomyosarcoma,[2] squamous cell carcinoma, adenoma, papilloma, leiomyoma, leiomyosarcoma, fibroma, hemangiosarcoma, and fibrosarcoma also occur in the bladder.[22] These tumors usually affect older animals, with the exception of botryoid rhabdomyosarcoma, which tends to occur in the bladder of young, large breed dogs, especially St. Bernards.[22] Additionally, transitional cell carcinoma may develop in dogs in association with prolonged cyclophosphamide therapy.[22] Transitional cell carcinoma may occur in bladder diverticulum in man in association with stasis, chronic inflammation, and metaplasia.[29]

Three sonographic patterns of bladder tumors has been described in human patients.[14,30] One appearance is that of exophytic and echogenic or complex focal filling defects arising from the inner surface of the wall. The second type is that of a massive

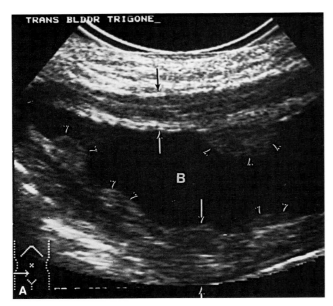

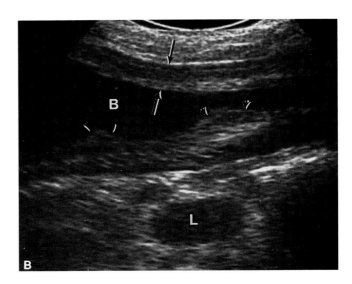

Figure 12–52

A, Transverse sonogram of the urinary bladder (B) in an older female dog with multifocal transitional cell carcinoma reveals multiple, variably sized hypoechoic masses with abrupt transition to the bladder wall (arrowheads). The circumferentially thickened bladder wall (arrows) and hyperechoic mucosal epithelium suggest chronic inflammation. Biopsy at the time of surgery showed diffuse nonresectable disease. **B,** Sagittal sonogram of the area dorsal to the bladder (B) of the dog in **A** revealed the elliptic hypoechoic mass of an enlarged sublumbar lymph node (L). Metastatic neoplasia was found during surgical exploratory and biopsy of the lymph node.

tumor obliterating the lumen of the bladder. Lastly, invasive tumors can appear as infiltrating wall lesions producing thickening of the wall, with unilateral loss of the concave inner borders of the bladder and little detectable intraluminal mass.[14,30]

The sonographic appearance of urothelial tumors in animals is complex and hypoechoic, with abrupt transition to normal wall (Fig. 12–52). In highly invasive or infiltrative tumors, this demarcation may not be appreciated and, especially, infiltrative muscular tumors may mimic cystitis.[2] Occasionally, neoplastic bladder masses are echogenic[14] or heteroechoic, especially if the disease process is advanced and if mineralization (Fig. 12–53), fibrous metaplasia, or necrotic areas are present in the tumor mass.[31] In one sonographic study of transitional cell carcinoma of the bladder in dogs, 66% had masses in the trigone, 70% in the dorsal wall, 10% in the ventral wall, and 30% in the proximal urethra.[2] Sixty percent of the animals had multifocal masses.

Botryoid rhabdomyosarcoma of the urinary bladder wall has been reported as a lobulated, heteroechoic mural mass located in the trigone and projecting into the bladder lumen as botryoid masses. Urinary obstruction is often a presenting sign.[10] Pedunculated mural masses can mimic intraluminal lesions; however, close sonographic inspection often discloses an attachment to the bladder wall with localized wall thickening.[10]

The diagnostic accuracy of sonography in detecting urinary bladder tumors depends on tumor size, tumor location, and to a degree, patient conformation. Masses ranging in size from 3 to 5 mm can be detected with adequate sensitivity.[2,14,32–34] Urothelial tumors are less echogenic than calculi, and unless they are polypoid, they may be overlooked or misinterpreted as inflammatory change or partially collapsed wall in a nondistended bladder.[30] When infiltrative tumors are suspected, full bladder distention may assist detection of the focal wall change. Masses in the neck and urethra may be harder to see when the pubic bone interferes with sound transmission.[6] This problem can be resolved

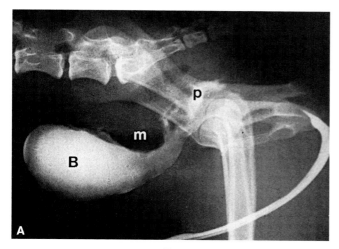

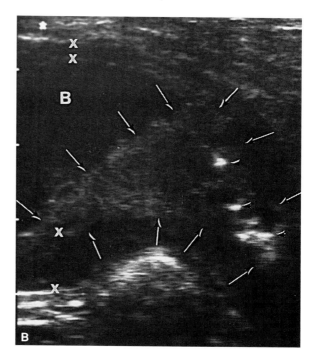

Figure 12–53

A, Lateral radiograph of a positive contrast cystogram/urethrogram in an older male dog with chronic hematuria and stranguria. A large, masslike filling defect (m) is seen in the dorsal bladder trigone. The prostatic urethra is poorly filled with contrast material, some of which has refluxed into the prostate (p). B, bladder. **B,** Sagittal sonogram of the bladder trigone (B) of the dog in **A.** A large hypoechoic mass (arrows) extends from the dorsal trigone wall and into the bladder neck and urethra. The hyperechoic foci (arrowheads) are areas of mineralization. The surrounding bladder wall (x) is thickened and hypoechoic. Hydronephrosis and hydroureter from urinary obstruction are evident bilaterally. Transitional cell carcinoma was diagnosed after biopsy.

with the use of transrectal sonography, but these transducers are not available commonly in veterinary practice. Detection of a mass in the vertex and near-field wall can require excellent technique to overcome the decreased sonographic resolution in these areas.[26,27] The prostate and urethra should be examined as completely as possible because tumors involving these structures can invade the bladder and appear to be a primary bladder mass (Fig. 12–54).

Sonographic differential diagnoses for urinary bladder neoplasia include polypoid or follicular cystitis, inflammatory nodules (see Figs. 12–45 and 12–48), blood clots (see Fig. 12–35), cellular sediment accumulated along the dependent wall (see Fig. 12–28), mural hematomas (see Figs. 12–36 and 12–44), and postsurgical reaction around suture material in the bladder wall (Fig. 12–55). Prominent ureteral papilla can mimic a small focal bladder mass in the dorsal trigone (see Fig. 12–21). Agitation of the bladder or repositioning the patient resuspends cellular sediment and changes the location of nonadherent blood clots, differentiating them from wall masses. All suspect bladder masses warrant biopsy (Fig. 12–56). Some bladder neoplasia, such as carcinomas, exfoliate tumor cells adequately to enable ultrasound-guided fine-needle aspiration biopsies to be of diagnostic utility. In one report, nonsurgical ultrasound-guided fine needle aspiration confirmed the presence of bladder neoplasia in six of six dogs.[2] More fibrous neoplasms, such as sarcomas, may require surgical biopsy. The sublumbar lymph nodes should be examined for enlargement, abnormal shape, or changes in homogeneous internal architecture, because approximately 50% of transitional cell carcinomas metastasize to

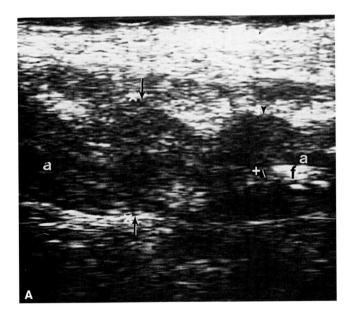

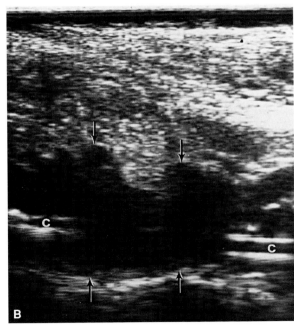

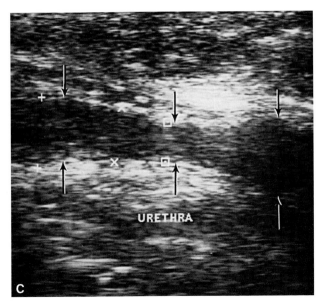

Figure 12–54

A, Sagittal sonogram of the urethra in a female dog with chronic stranguria and dysuria. (The urinary bladder of this dog is seen in Fig. 12–49.) Hydronephrosis and hydroureter were present bilaterally. The normally homogeneous, thin parallel walls of the urethra have been replaced by a thick, nodular heteroechoic tube (arrows, x–x). Urethral wall thickness (arrowheads, +–+) could be detected by small accumulations of anechoic fluid (a) in the lumen. The hyperechoic focus (f) is most likely mineralization or fibrosis. **B,** A urinary catheter (c) placed within the urethra allows confirmation of the tubular structure as urethra. Ultrasound-guided biopsy revealed the diagnosis of transitional cell carcinoma. **C,** Sagittal sonogram of the urethra (arrows) after treatment with an anti-inflammatory and antineoplastic agent (piroxicam, Feldene). Much of the masslike change in the urethra has resolved and the dog showed clinical improvement.

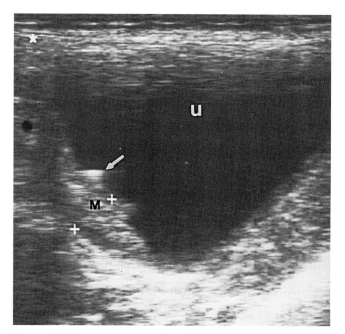

Figure 12–55

Sagittal sonogram of the urinary bladder (u) in a dog that had transitional cell carcinoma of the urethra demonstrated after biopsy during cystotomy and laparotomy. No lesions were seen within the bladder during surgery. Later re-examination with sonography showed a thickened nodular echogenic mass (m) near the bladder vertex (+,+). Ultrasound-guided biopsy (arrow shows the tip of the biopsy needle) was diagnostic of postsurgical change, organized hematoma, and fibroplasia, but no evidence of neoplasia. Subsequent sonographic examinations confirmed gradual resolution of the mass.

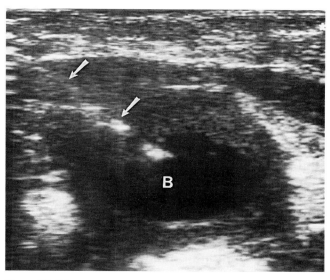

Figure 12–56

Sagittal sonogram of the urinary bladder (B) of a cat that had a fine-gauge needle (arrows) passed into the thickened bladder wall for aspiration and cytology. Once the needle has penetrated into the bladder lumen, it can be easily and accurately withdrawn into the thickened wall for aspiration. This technique may be more successful than aspiration during initial insertion when compression of the wall by the needle tip can mimic actual penetration.

Figure 12–57

Sagittal sonogram of the aortic bifurcation (Ao). The gain is set artificially high to evaluate internal architecture of the large (+,+), hypoechoic nodular mass (m) compressing and displacing (arrows) the terminal aorta. Ultrasound-guided biopsy was diagnostic of metastatic carcinoma in the external iliac lymph node.

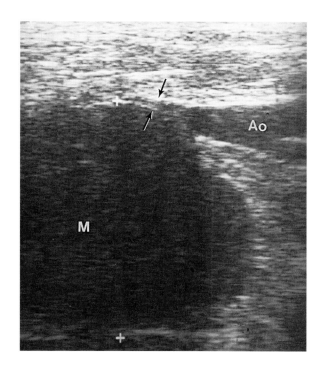

regional lymph nodes.[22] Enlargement or change in the appearance may be indicative of metastatic neoplastic disease. Ultrasound-guided fine needle aspiration of large sublumbar lymph nodes can be rewarding (Fig. 12–57).

REFERENCES

1. Finn-Bodner ST: Nephrosonography and cystosonography in Veterinary Medicine. Ultrasound Symposium. Proceedings of the Annual Meeting of the American College of Veterinary Radiology, Orlando, 1992.
2. Leveille R, et al: Sonographic investigation of transitional cell carcinoma of the urinary bladder in small animals. Vet Radiol Ultrasound *33:*103, 1992.
3. Barsanti JA, et al: Complications of bladder distention during retrograde urethrocystography. Am J Vet Res *42:*812, 1981.
4. Ackerman N, Wingfield WE, Corley EA: Fatal air embolism associated with pneumocystography in a dog. J Am Vet Med Assoc *160:*1616, 1972.
5. Park RD: The urinary bladder. In *Textbook of Veterinary Diagnostic Radiology.* Edited by DE Thrall. Philadelphia: W.B. Saunders, 1986, pp. 424–438.
6. Feeney DA, et al: Maximum distention retrograde urethrocystography in healthy male dogs. Am J Vet Res *45:*948, 1984.
7. Johnston GR, Feeney DA, Osborne CA: Urethrography and cystography in cats. Part 1. Techniques, normal radiographic anatomy, and artifact. Compend Cont Educ Pract Vet *4:*832, 1982.
8. Johnston GR, Feeney DA, Osborne CA: Urethrography and cystography in cats. Part II. Abnormal radiographic anatomy and complications. Compend Cont Educ Pract Vet *4:*931, 1982.
9. Thayer GW, Carrig CB, Evans AT: Fatal venous air embolism associated with pneumocystography in a cat. J Am Vet Med Assoc *176:*643, 1980.
10. Ackerman N: Radiology and ultrasound of urogenital diseases in dogs and cats. Ames, IA: Iowa State University Press, 1991, pp. 1–25.
11. Feeney DA, Walter PA: Ultrasonography of the kidneys, adrenal glands and urinary bladder. Proceedings of the American Institute of Ultrasound in Medicine Animal Ultrasound Course, 1989.
12. Orgaz RE, et al: Application of bladder ultrasonography. I. Bladder content and residue. J Urol *125:*174, 1981.
13. Griffiths CJ, Murray A, Ramsden PD: Accuracy and repeatability of bladder volume measurements using ultrasonic imaging. J Urol *136:*808, 1986.
14. Biller DS, et al: Diagnostic ultrasound of the urinary bladder. J Am Anim Hosp Assoc *26:*397, 1990.
15. Callen PW, Mahony BS: Ultrasound: Pelvis. In *Normal Variants and Pitfalls in Imaging.* Edited by JB Vogler, CA Helms, PW Callen. Philadelphia: WB Saunders, 1986, pp. 314–327.
16. Tsyb AF, Slesarev MD, Komarevtsev VN: Transvaginal longitudinal ultrasonograph in diagnosis of carcinoma of the urinary bladder. J Ultrasound Med *7:*179, 1988.
17. Gammelgaard J, Holm HH: Transurethral and transrectal ultrasonic scanning in urology. J Urol *124:*863, 1980.
18. Richmond DH, Sutherst JR, Brown MC: Screening of the bladder base and urethra using linear array transrectal ultrasound scanning. JCU *14:*647, 1986.
19. Finn-Bodner ST, et al: Sonographic architecture and morphometric evaluation of the normal feline urinary bladder wall. Proceedings of the Annual Meeting of the American College of Veterinary Radiology, Orlando, 1992.
20. Finn-Bodner ST, et al: Sonographic appearance and morphometric evaluation of the feline bladder. Vet Radiol Ultrasound, Submitted for publication, 1994.
21. Douglass JP, Kremkau FW: Ultrasound corner: The urinary bladder wall hypoechoic pseudolesion. Vet Radiol Ultrasound *34:*45, 1993.
22. Maxie MG: The urinary system. In *Pathology of Domestic Animals.* 4th Ed. Edited by KVF Jubb, PC Kennedy, N Palmer. San Diego: Academic Press, 1990.
23. Dubbins PA, et al: Ureteric jet effect: The echographic appearance of urine entering the bladder. A means of identifying the bladder trigone and assessing ureteral function. Radiology *140:*513, 1981.
24. Spaulding KA, Stone E: Color Doppler evaluation of ureteral flow dynamics in the dog as influenced by relative specific gravity. Proceedings of the Annual Scientific Meeting of the American College of Veterinary Radiology, Chicago, 1993.
25. Reef VB: Equine pediatric ultrasonography. Compend Cont Educ Pract Vet *13:*1277, 1991.
26. Finn-Bodner ST, et al: Transabdominal sonographic evaluation of experimentally induced cystitis of the feline urinary bladder. Proceeedings of the Annual Scientific Meeting of the American College of Veterinary Radiology, Chicago, 1993.
27. Finn-Bodner ST, et al: Transabdominal sonographic evaluation of experimentally induced cystitis of the feline urinary bladder. Vet Radiol Ultrasound, Submitted for publication, 1994.
28. Gooding GAW: Varied sonographic manifestations of cystitis. J Ultrasound Med *5:*61, 1986.

29. Williams, MJ, Gooding GAW: Sonographic diagnosis of a neoplasm in a bladder diverticulum. J Ultrasound Med *4:*203, 1985.

30. Cronan JJ, et al: Cystosonography in the detection of bladder tumors: A prospective and retrospective study. J Ultrasound Med *1:*237, 1982.

31. Love NE, Walshaw R: What's your diagnosis? J Am Vet Med Assoc *195:*1409, 1989.

32. Abu-Yousef MM, et al: Urinary bladder tumors studied by cystosonography. Radiology *153:*223, 1984.

33. Juul N, et al: Bladder tumour control by abdominal ultrasound and urine cytology. Scand J Urol Nephrol *20:*275, 1986.

34. Itzchak Y, Singer D, Fischelovitch Y: Ultrasonographic assessment of bladder tumors. I. Tumor detection. J Urol *126:*31, 1981.

THE REPRODUCTIVE SYSTEM

Mary B. Mahaffey, Barbara A. Selcer, and Robert E. Cartee

THE OVARIES—*Mary B. Mahaffey*

Normal Anatomy and Function

The ovary of the normal anestrus bitch is difficult to identify with ultrasound because it is small and its echogenicity is similar to that of surrounding structures.[1] The ovary is easier to visualize, however, during proestrus, estrus, and early metestrus. A 7.5-mHz transducer is necessary to obtain good quality images for evaluating parenchymal detail.[1–3] Some investigators have used 3.5-mHz[4] and 5.0-mHz[5] transducers to evaluate dog ovaries, but these transducers are unlikely to provide adequate image quality. (For all scans in this chapter, except as indicated, a 7.5-mHz transducer with a built-in standoff pad was used. Ventral is at the top and dorsal is at the bottom of all figures. For sagittal scans, cranial is to the left and caudal is to the right. The scale at right indicates centimeters.)

The ovaries can be scanned with the bitch in the standing position,[1] although I prefer to position the animal in dorsal recumbency. Tilting the sternum away from the side to be scanned facilitates finding the ovary.[2] The ovary is located caudal to the kidney by first finding the caudal pole of the kidney and then scanning the area of the pole from caudomedial to caudolateral in a sagittal plane. Once the ovary is identified, the transducer can be rotated 90° to obtain transverse images. The ovary may touch the kidney or be as much as 2 cm caudal to it, and may vary in position from directly caudal to caudomedial, caudolateral, or ventral to the caudal pole of the kidney.[2] The varied location of the ovary is probably caused by the pressure of transducer placement moving the ovary or kidney. Overlying bowel gas can interfere with visualization of the ovaries, but an adequate window can usually be found by repositioning the transducer. Image quality is better on scans of thin versus obese bitches,[2,3] on small versus large bitches, and on sagittal versus transverse views.[2]

At the beginning of proestrus, the ovaries are oval and have a fairly uniform echogenicity that is equal to or slightly greater than that of the renal cortex (Fig. 13–1).[2] Ovarian size increases during proestrus and estrus. The ovaries are easier to find if follicles are present.[2] Follicular development is first apparent from 2 to 7 (average 5) days after the onset of proestrus.[2] Follicles appear as small black dots that increase in size with time to an average maximum diameter of 0.6 cm (range of 0.3 to 1.1 cm) the day before ovulation.

The use of ultrasound to detect ovulation in the bitch has been reported by some authors,[2–5] but questioned by others.[1,6] In one study,[2] ovulation detected sonographically correlated with that predicted by progesterone and luteinizing hormone (LH) data in 9 of 10 bitches. Bitches were scanned daily. In another study, the accuracy of sonography in predicting ovulation in bitches was not as great, but the ability to detect ovulation improved dramatically the more experienced the sonographer and the better the equipment.[3] Ovulation is thought to take place when a decrease in the number of follicles is noted from one day to the next (Fig. 13–2).[2] If not already present, cystic (anechoic) structures, similar in appearance to follicles, develop and increase in size (up to 2.5 cm) after ovulation (Fig. 13–3). These structures gradually increase in echogenicity and fade away, and may represent follicles that did not ovulate, corpora hemorrhagica, fluid-filled

Figure 13–1

Sagittal abdominal sonogram of a bitch on the first day of proestrus. The ovary (black arrows) appears as an oval structure caudoventral to the kidney. Ovarian echogenicity is slightly greater than that of the renal cortex. (From Wallace SS, et al: Ultrasonographic appearance of the ovaries of dogs during the follicular and luteal phases of the estrous cycle. Am J Vet Res *53*:209, 1992.)

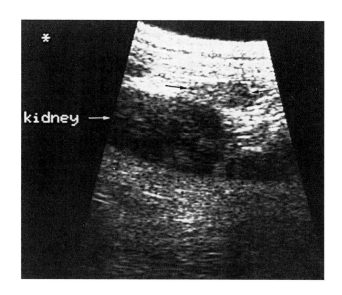

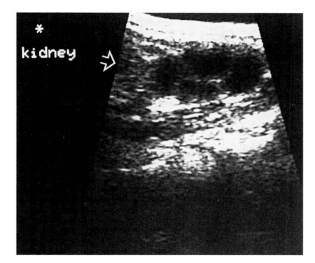
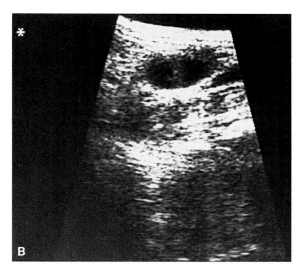

Figure 13–2

Sagittal sonograms of the left ovary of a bitch on days 11 **(A)** and 12 **(B)** after the onset of proestrus. Ovulation was thought to have occurred between the time sonography was performed on days 11 and 12. Note the decrease in number and size of follicles on day 12 compared to day 11. (From Wallace SS, et al: Ultrasonographic appearance of the ovaries of dogs during the follicular and luteal phases of the estrous cycle. Am J Vet Res *53*:209, 1992.)

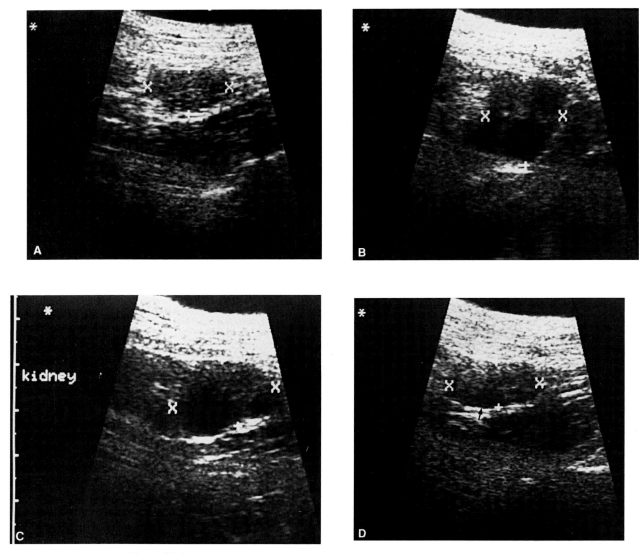

Figure 13–3

Sagittal sonograms of the right ovary of a bitch on days 14 **(A)**, 17 **(B)**, 19 **(C)**, and 25 **(D)** after onset of proestrus. Ovarian margins are identified by cursors. Ovulation was believed to have occurred between days 13 and 14. No follicles are seen on day 14. Three days later **(B)**, the ovary is larger and rounder and contains a large, cystic (anechoic) structure. On day 19, the ovary is slightly smaller and contains two cystic structures. By day 25, the ovary is smaller, more ovoid, and more uniform in echogenicity; however, a hypoechoic area is seen (arrow). Metestrus began on day 20. (From Wallace SS, et al: Ultrasonographic appearance of the ovaries of dogs during the follicular and luteal phases of the estrous cycle. Am J Vet Res *53:*209, 1992.)

corpora lutea, or cystic luteinized follicles.[2] The ovary increases in size and becomes more rounded after ovulation, but it gradually becomes smaller and oval during the later stages of metestrus (see Fig. 13–3). Although ultrasound can be used to evaluate the dog ovary during the heat cycle, it is not as convenient or as accurate as the progesterone assay as a means of detecting ovulation.[2,3]

Ovarian Abnormalities

The sonographic appearance of ovarian cysts has been reported.[7–9] Cysts are generally well-defined, thin-walled anechoic rounded structures with distant acoustic enhancement (Fig. 13–4). Because they resemble cystic structures normally seen after ovulation, sonographic findings should be correlated with clinical findings and history to determine if their presence is abnormal. The size of the cyst also may be helpful for differentiating between normal and abnormal, as the maximum size of normal cystic structures seen after ovulation is 2.5 cm^2 and abnormal cysts may be as large as 19 cm.[10] Functional follicular cysts may be associated with hydrometra and cystic endometrial hyperplasia, whereas cysts may make bitches susceptible to uterine infection.[11] Parovarian cysts (Fig. 13–5) arise from vestigial remnants of the embryonic Wolffian body.[12]

Ovarian neoplasms are uncommon in dogs. They may be bilateral, especially the adenomas and adenocarcinomas.[11] Granulosa cell tumors are usually unilateral and may be associated with cystic endometrial hyperplasia. In one report concerning the sonographic appearance of bilateral adenocarcinomas in a dog, the ovaries were enlarged (6 cm), irregularly marginated, and mostly solid, but they contained multiple small cysts.[13] An ovarian adenocarcinoma in a cat appeared similar to that described in the dog (Fig. 13–6). In another report,[7] functional ovarian tumors were described as having mixed echogenicity because of anechoic cysts, hypoechoic and hyperechoic tumor cells, and connective tissue. Specific cases or examples were not shown. Small cysts were also found in two bitches with granulosa cell tumors.[8,9] Sonography is useful for verifying the origin of ovarian masses and to check for abdominal metastasis, but not in differentiating tumor types[9] or between cystic ovaries and ovarian tumors containing small cysts.[14] Abdominal fluid may be found in some dogs with ovarian tumors.[13,14]

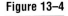

Figure 13–4

Sagittal sonogram of a 13-year-old bitch with a history of persistent estrus and vaginal discharge reveals multiple thin-walled anechoic cysts (closed arrows) within the left ovary just caudal to the kidney (open arrow).

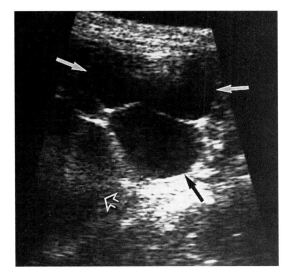

Figure 13–5

Sagittal sonogram of a 13-year-old bitch with a parovarian cyst caudal to the left kidney (not shown). The cyst, which is approximately 3 cm in diameter, is seen as a well-defined anechoic structure with distal acoustic enhancement.

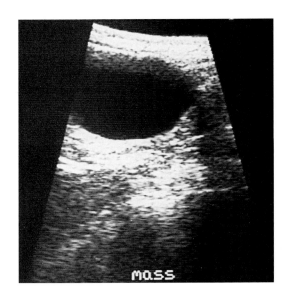

Figure 13–6

Sagittal sonogram of a 19-year-old cat with adeno-carcinoma of the left ovary. The ovary is seen as a large (7 cm), well-defined, mostly hypo-echoic mass (closed arrows) with anechoic foci caudoventral to the kidney (open arrow).

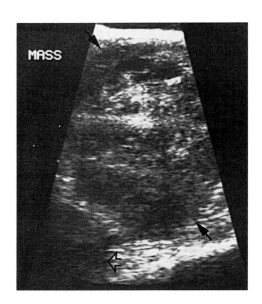

THE UTERUS

As for the ovary, the uterus of the dog and cat is best evaluated using a 7.5-mHz transducer with the patient in dorsal recumbency. The normal nongravid canine uterus is not readily identified with ultrasound. With practice, the cervix can be seen on transverse scans dorsal to the bladder and ventral or to the side of the colon, which usually contains gas (Fig. 13–7A). The cervix appears as a hypoechoic rounded structure that may have concentric rings. If it is followed cranially, the uterine body and bifurcation occasionally are seen (Figs. 13–7B and 13–8). It is difficult to follow each horn more than a few centimeters cranial to the bifurcation because it becomes obscured by surrounding bowel loops. When seen during anestrus, the uterus is homogeneously hypoechoic.[15]

The appearance of the canine uterus during proestrus, estrus, metestrus,[6] and postpartum[6,16,17] has been described. During proestrus, the uterus increases in diameter and appears as a hypoechoic tubular structure (see Figs. 13–7 and 13–8). Edema may be

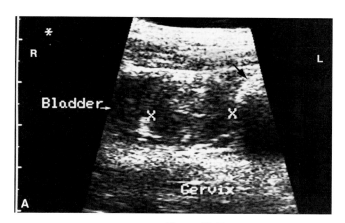 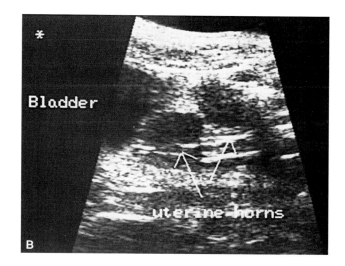

Figure 13–7

Transverse (cross-sectional) sonograms of the cervix **(A)** and uterine horns **(B)** of a 1-year-old bitch in proestrus. **A,** The cervix (between cursors) is a rounded, ill- defined, hypoechoic structure between the bladder on the right (R) and the colon (arrow) on the left (L). Although the colon normally lies dorsal to the cervix, which in turn lies dorsal to the bladder, the pressure of the transducer causes these structures to lie beside each other. **B,** The scan of the uterine horns was made by moving the transducer cranially from the cervix. The uterine horns are hypoechoic.

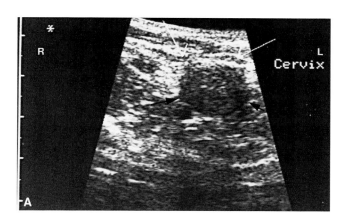 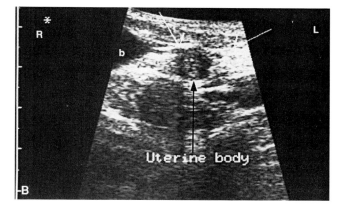

Figure 13–8

Transverse (cross-sectional) scans of the cervix **(A)** (arrows) and uterine body **(B)** (arrows) of a bitch in proestrus. The cervix is hypoechoic and is larger than the uterine body. b, urinary bladder; R, right; L, left.

responsible for this appearance.[6] During estrus, hyperechoic lines, possibly representing endometrial folds, radiate from the center of the uterus outward. In some bitches, fluid is found within the lumen (Fig. 13–9). The uterus becomes difficult to find during metestrus.

The postpartum uterus is easily identified.[6,16,17] The uterine wall initially has multiple alternating hyperechoic and hypoechoic layers, with the serosal and endometrial surfaces being hyperechoic (Fig. 13–10). The layered appearance is most prominent during the first week, after which the uterus gradually becomes more uniformly hypoechoic. Discrete, hypoechoic enlargements (1 to 4 cm in diameter in beagles) representing placental sites[17] become indistinguishable from the uterine wall by 4 to 5 weeks postpartum.

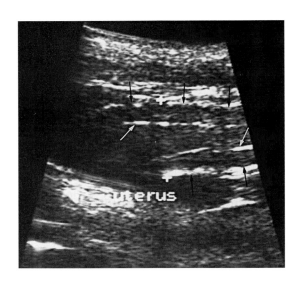

Sagittal (longitudinal) sonogram of the uterus of a bitch in estrus. Hypoechoic fluid is seen within the lumen. The mucosal surface (white arrows) is hyperechoic and the wall of the uterus is hypoechoic. Cursors and black arrows point to the serosal surface of the uterus.

Figure 13–10

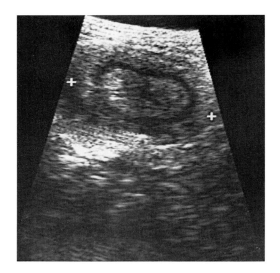

Transverse (cross-sectional) sonogram of the uterus (between cursors) of a bitch 4 days after whelping a litter. The uterine wall is thickened and consists of alternating hyperechoic and hypoechoic layers. The lumen (center) contains a small amount of hypoechoic fluid.

Uterine diameter is less between placental sites. Hypoechoic to anechoic fluid can be found in the lumen for at least 3 weeks.[16,18] Echogenic material within the lumen probably represents blood clots and residual fetal and maternal membranes.[16] Uterine diameter gradually decreases with time to approximately 0.5 cm (beagles) by 9 weeks postpartum. Uterine involution is complete by 15 weeks postpartum when the uterine horns are uniformly hypoechoic.[17]

Pregnancy

Sonography is useful for detecting pregnancy and evaluating fetal viability. Veterinary practitioners can become proficient at detecting pregnancy sonographically by scanning a few bitches on a weekly basis from 2 weeks after breeding until term. A 7.5- mHz transducer is necessary to identify fetal structures early in pregnancy and to evaluate anatomic detail in near-term fetuses. Because a fetus may become too large to fit entirely within a single 7.5-mHz image, a 5-mHz transducer is helpful in the later stages of gestation. Numerous articles have been written about sonographic detection of pregnancy in dogs.[5,15,19–29] Some discrepancy as to the gestational ages at which fetal structures can be identified is probably related to variations in the way gestational ages are determined, e.g., from breeding dates,[15,20,22] using vaginal cytologic data to estimate the date of ovulation retrospectively,[25] comparing to the day of parturition[23,29] of luteinizing hormone (LH) surge.[26,27] The most consistent results are obtained by estimating gestational age from the date of the LH surge[26,27] or retrospectively comparing to day of parturition.[29] When estimating from the LH surge, the gestational age at time of parturition ranges from 64 to 66 days.[30]

Pregnancy can be detected in dogs as early as 17 to 20 days after the LH surge (15 to 21 days after the first breeding) when the chorionic cavity (Fig. 13–11) is seen as a 1- to 2-mm anechoic spherical vesicle.[26] Specular reflections perpendicular to the sound beam may be seen. The term chorionic cavity may be used to designate either the gestational sac, yolk sac, or the allantoic cavity, depending on gestational age.[27] The embryonic mass does not appear until approximately 5 days later, when it is located at the periphery of the chorionic cavity and is 1 to 4 mm in length. The fetal heartbeat can be seen at the same time and the chorionic cavity becomes more ovoid (Fig. 13–12).[26] The uterus and placenta appear as a hypoechoic ring surrounding the chorionic cavity. The heart rate is about 120 to 140 beats per minute.[19] A few days later, the embryo moves away to the dependent portion of the chorionic cavity (see Fig. 13–12) and changes to a bipolar shape.[27] Fetal membranes become visible at about that time (see Fig. 13–12**B**). The only distinguishable fetal anatomic features seen before 30 days are the flickering heartbeat and an anechoic area in the head (Fig. 13–13) that may represent the developing fourth ventricle.[27] Fetal movement, skeletal development, and identification of internal organs occur between 30 and 50 days (Fig. 13–14). With time, the bladder, stomach, hypoechoic liver, chambers of the heart, hyperechoic lungs, and kidneys can be identified. After day 50, few new anatomic landmarks are detected.

Gestational age estimates based on the sonographic appearance of fetal and extrafetal structures of beagles[27] and cats[31] are presented in Tables 13–1 and 13–2, respectively. Besides the morphologic appearance, measurement of fetal and extrafetal structures has been used to estimate gestational age.[20,26,27,29] In beagles, the inner chorionic cavity diameter from 20 to 37 days and fetal head diameter from 38 to 60 days were the most accurate predictors of gestational age.[27] Gestational age estimates may be different for large and small breed dogs.[27] Fetal and body diameter measurements have been found to be accurate indicators of parturition date in cats.[32]

Sonography is sensitive for detecting pregnancy,[21,23,24,28,29,33] and is more accurate than palpation.[23,24] In a study of 121 bitches first scanned 20 to 30 days after the end of estrus, the authors reported 100% accuracy in determining whether or not bitches were pregnant.[33] Scans performed within the week prior to that time may be less accurate, with false negatives being the most likely error.[28] Therefore, to detect pregnancy, bitches should be scanned 3 to 4 weeks after the end of the estrus.

Accuracy in predicting litter size is poor (32 to 75%),[21,23,24,28,33] with underestimation of litter size being more common than overestimation. Possible explanations for inaccurate litter size estimation include that chorionic vesicles are too small, fetuses are obscured by overlying bowel gas or are otherwise overlooked, a fetus was counted more than once or mistaken for one already counted, or fetal death and resorption occurred.[34] Veterinarians disagree as to whether litter size estimates are more accurate in scans made during early pregnancy[23,28,33] or in those from middle to late pregnancy.[21,24] My experience has been that fetal counts are more accurate in scans made during early pregnancy. Most authorities agree, however, that litter size estimates are more accurate in small litters of about four or less than in large litters.[21,23,28,33]

Embryonic resorption is characterized by loss of the embryonic mass and heartbeat, collapse of the chorionic cavity with thickening and inward bulging of the uterine wall, increased echogenicity of the normally anechoic embryonic fluid, and reduced size of the chorionic cavity compared to adjacent ones (Fig. 13–15).[33] Resorption may occur in one embryo without adversely affecting others.

Sonography is also useful for evaluating fetal viability later in pregnancy. Slowing of fetal heart rate to less than twice the bitch's heart rate and decreased fetal movement

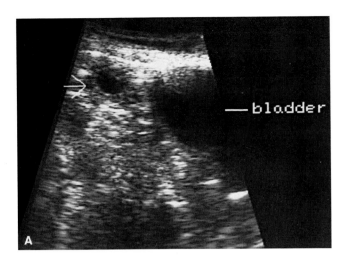
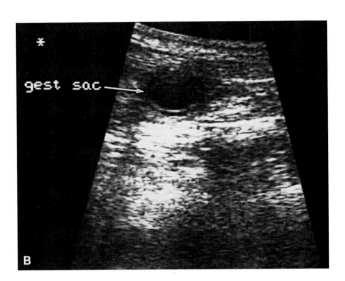

Figure 13–11

Sagittal sonograms of two different bitches approximately 15 days **(A)** and 19 days **(B)** after the first breeding dates. The chorionic cavity (gestational sac) (arrow) appears as a small spherical anechoic cavity. This finding is the earliest sonographic indication of pregnancy. The embryonic mass is not apparent at this stage.

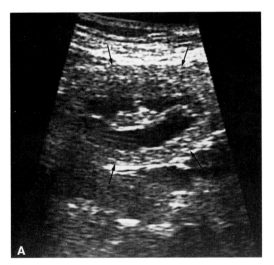
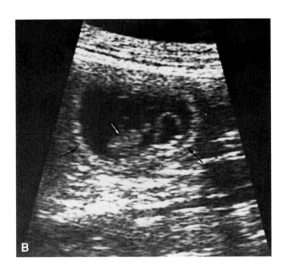

Figure 13–12

Sagittal abdominal sonograms of two different bitches approximately 3 weeks **(A)** and 4 weeks **(B)** after breeding. The uterus/placenta appears as a hypoechoic ring (arrows) around the chorionic cavity. The chorionic cavity is ovoid, a change from the spherical shape seen earlier in gestation. During real-time scanning, the flickering heart beat could be observed. **A,** The embryonic mass is in the center of the chorionic cavity. **B,** The embryo (white arrow) has moved to the periphery of the chorionic cavity and the fetal membranes are visible.

Figure 13–13

Sagittal abdominal sonogram of a bitch approximately 4 weeks pregnant. The uterus/placenta is the hypoechoic ring around the anechoic chorionic cavity. The fetal head (arrowhead) and a portion of the fetal body (arrow) are visible. The two anechoic foci within the head may represent the developing ventricular system.

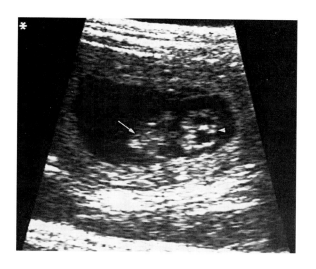

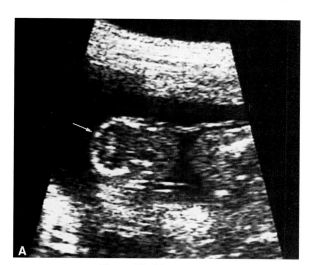

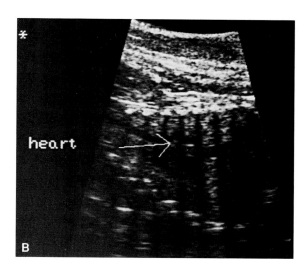

Figure 13–14

Long axis sonograms of near-term fetuses. Both fetuses are too large to fit entirely within the scan plane. **A,** The head (arrow) of a fetus can be identified. **B,** The thoracic cavity is seen in a dorsal plane. The hyperechoic ribs cast parallel acoustic shadows. The lungs are more echogenic than the heart. Individual cardiac chambers were seen during real-time scanning.

TABLE 13–1
Gestational Age Estimates Based on Sonographic Appearance of Fetal and Extrafetal Structures of Beagles

Pregnancy Feature	Days after LH Surge*	N*
Gestational sac	20	7
Uterine wall		
Echogenic at gestational sac	20 to 23	8
Placental layers	22 to 24	7
Zonary placenta	27 to 30	8
Embryo position		
Apposed to uterine wall	23 to 25	8
Dependent in chorionic cavity	29 to 33	8
Fetal membranes		
Yolk sac membrane	25 to 28	7
Allantoic membrane	27 to 31	7
Yolk sac tubular shape	27 to 31	8
Yolk sac folded cross section	31 to 35	6
Embryo and fetus		
Heart beat	23 to 25	8
Bipolar shape	25 to 28	8
Anechoic area in head	27 to 31	6
Choroid plexus	31 to 35	6
Limb buds	33 to 35	6
Fetal movement	34 to 36	5
Dorsal sagittal tube	30 to 39	6
Skeleton	33 to 39	4
Bladder	35 to 39	4
Stomach	36 to 39	4
Lung hyperechoic vs. liver	38 to 42	4
Liver hypoechoic vs. abdomen	39 to 47	4
Kidney	39 to 47	3
Eyes	39 to 47	4
Umbilical stalk	40 to 46	5
Intestine	57 to 63	4
Relative size relationships		
Body diameter 2 mm > head	38 to 42	4
Body diameter: chorionic cavity diameter > 1 : 2	38 to 42	4
Crown-rump length > placenta	49 to 42	4
Body diameter: outer uterine diameter > 1 : 2	46 to 48	5
Parturition	63 to 65	5

* LH, luteinizing hormone; N, number of pregnancies examined. (From Yeager AE, et al: Ultrasonographic appearance of the uterus, placenta, fetus, and fetal membranes throughout accurately timed pregnancy in beagles. Am J Vet Res 53:342, 1992)

indicate fetal distress.[8] Gas may be found within the uterus or fetus as early as 6 hours after fetal death,[35] and, if present, produces echogenic areas with shadowing. These areas should be differentiated from normal skeletal structures that also cause shadowing late in pregnancy. A macerated fetus may have few recognizable fetal structures,[31] appearing as an amorphous hypoechoic mass with echogenic debris (Fig. 13–16). Anechoic fluid in the thoracic cavity and subcutaneous tissues of a near-term fetus is compatible with hydrops fetalis (anasarca or lethal congenital edema).[36]

TABLE 13–2
Gestational Age Estimates Based on Sonographic Appearance of Fetal and Extrafetal Structures of Cats

Parameter	Days Post-Breeding	
	Earliest Day Identified	Range
Uterine enlargement	4	4–14
Gestational sac	11	11–14
Fetal pole	15	15–17
Cardiac activity	16	16–18
Fetal membranes	21	21–24
Fetal morphology	26	26–28
Fetal movements	28	28–30

From Davidson AP, Nyland TG, Tsutsui T: Pregnancy diagnosis with ultrasound in the domestic cat. Vet Radiol *27*:109, 1986.

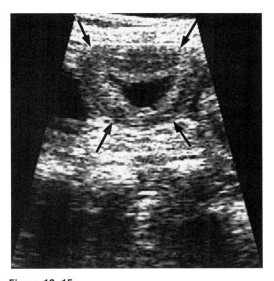

Figure 13–15

Sagittal abdominal sonogram of a bitch approximately 4 weeks pregnant shows five normal embryos and a chorionic cavity undergoing embryonic resorption (arrows). Embryonic resorption was characterized by an absence of fetal membranes and embryonic mass. The chorionic cavity was collapsed and smaller than the adjacent normal ones, which appeared similar to that seen in Figure 13–12**B**. The hypoechoic ring of the uterus/placenta bulged inwardly and was thicker than that of the normal embryos. On a scan performed 4 days previously, the chorionic cavity had normal shape, size, and fetal membranes, but no embryonic mass. Embryonic masses and heartbeats were found in the others, which appeared similar to those in Figure 13–12**A**.

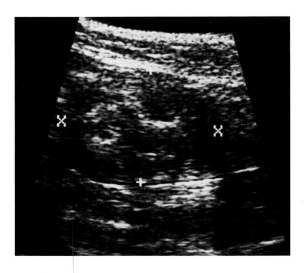

Figure 13–16

A sonogram of a macerated fetus in a cat with a bloody vaginal discharge and a palpable abdominal mass. The macerated fetus (cursors) appears as a mixed echogenic mass. No fetal structures are recognizable.

Uterine Abnormalities

Ultrasound is especially useful in the evaluation of the uterus of bitches with infertility and those suspected of having pyometra. In bitches with radiographic evidence of uterine enlargement, one can readily determine if enlargement is caused by pregnancy before fetal mineralization or by pyometra. In pyometra, the uterus appears as a well-defined tubular structure with distinct walls and a uniform hypoechoic to anechoic lumen (Fig. 13–17). Far enhancement implies that the luminal contents are fluid.[8] Occasionally, slight movement of cellular luminal contents caused by transducer placement can be seen. Echogenic debris may also be found (Fig. 13–18). If need be, the uterus can be differentiated from normal fluid-filled bowel by its lack of peristalsis and by following the horns caudally to the body. Serial sonograms are valuable to document evacuation of luminal contents and progressive decrease in uterine size in bitches treated medically for pyometra (Fig. 13–19). Because hydrometra and pyometra may appear similar sonographically, other diagnostic aids are needed to differentiate between the two conditions.

Ultrasound examination of the uterus and ovaries should be part of the routine evaluation of infertile bitches. In bitches failing to produce litters after breeding, sonographic evidence of implantation sites indicates conception and subsequent fetal resorption (Fig. 13–20A). Such bitches may appear healthy yet have pyometra and uterine wall cysts that protrude into the lumen (Fig. 13–20B).[37] In bitches with cystic endometrial hyperplasia/endometritis, anechoic cysts of varying sizes can be seen within an irregularly thickened uterine wall (Fig. 13–21).[34] A small amount of hypoechoic to anechoic fluid also may be present.

Sonography also may be helpful in confirming the location of uterine and vaginal masses. The number of reports describing such cases is low, so distinctive sonographic appearances for these masses have not been established. Uterine leiomyomas may be homogeneous and isoechoic to the uterine wall (Fig. 13–22).[8] Uterine leiomyosarcoma,[9] transmissible venereal tumor of the uterine stump,[9] and vaginal leiomyoma (Fig. 13–23) may appear as mixed echogenic masses, and uterine stump granulomas may be seen as poorly defined masses of mixed to increased echogenicity dorsal to the bladder (Fig. 13–24.[8]

Figure 13–17

A sonogram of the left uterine horn of a dog with pyometra. The uterus (arrows) contains hypo-echoic material with low-level echoes that moved in response to transducer pressure during real-time scanning. The curved white band overlying the dorsal part of the uterus is a transducer artifact (arrowhead).

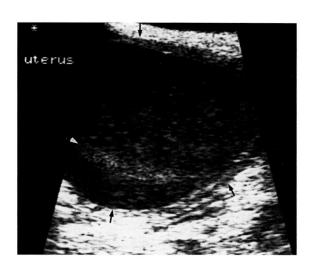

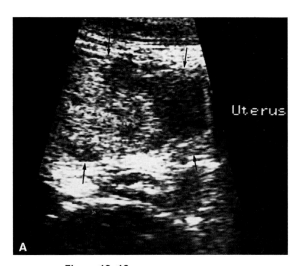 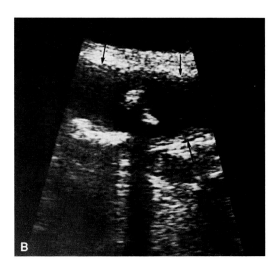

Figure 13–18

Sonograms of two bitches with pyometra. **A,** The uterus (arrows) contains hypoechoic fluid and echogenic debris that was thick and gelatinous when uterine contents were examined. **B,** The uterus (arrows) contains hypoechoic to anechoic fluid and echogenic foci with acoustic shadowing. The echogenic foci were bone remnants from a reabsorbed fetus.

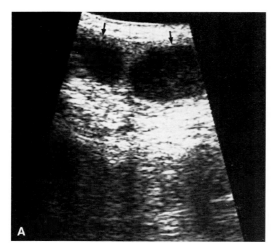
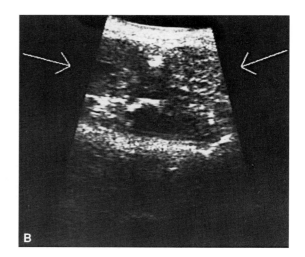

Figure 13–19

Transverse abdominal sonograms of a bitch treated for pyometra with uterine lavage, antibiotics, and prostaglandins. **A,** Before treatment. The uterine horns (arrows) are seen in cross-section and contain hypoechoic material. **B,** Transverse scan of the same area of the uterine horns 12 days later and after treatment. The uterine horns (arrows) are smaller and the luminal contents are more echogenic. The uterus continued to decrease in size with time. The dog was bred during the following estrus and whelped a normal litter.

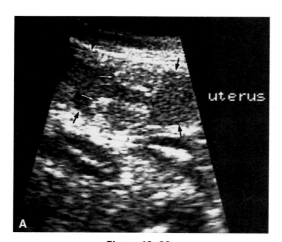
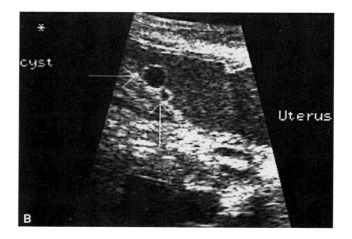

Figure 13–20

Sonograms of the uterus of a bitch presented for pregnancy evaluation 58 days after breeding. **A,** The uterus (black arrows) contains hypoechoic material. Echogenic foci (white arrows) represent an implantation site, indicating that conception and later fetal resorption occurred. **B,** Uterine wall cysts (arrows) containing anechoic fluid protrude into the lumen.

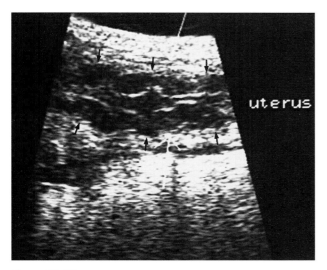

Figure 13–21

Long-axis sonogram of the uterus (black arrows) of a bitch with cystic endometrial hyperplasia/endometritis. The uterine wall is thickened and contains anechoic foci (endometrial cysts). The mucosal surface is echogenic and the lumen contains hypoechoic material.

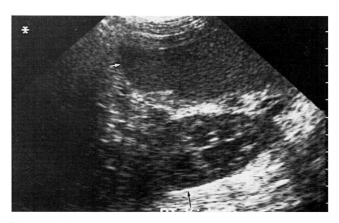

Figure 13–22

Sagittal abdominal sonogram (5.0-mHz transducer) of an 11-year-old female Rottweiler. A palpable abdominal mass was found on a routine physical examination. Sonographic examination revealed the mass (white arrow) was uniformly hypoechoic and occupied the caudal half of the abdomen. The black arrow points to the right kidney. The diagnosis was uterine leiomyoma.

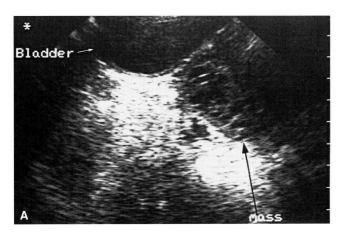
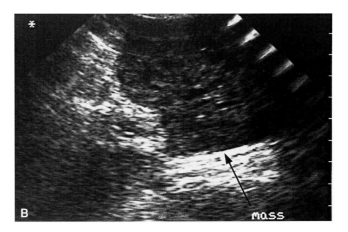

Figure 13–23

Sagittal abdominal sonograms (5.0-mHz transducer) of a 9-year-old female Chow with a history of anorexia. An abdominal mass was palpated during physical examination. **A,** A large, mixed echogenic mass with anechoic foci lies caudodorsal to the urinary bladder. **B,** Close-up of the mass. The diagnosis was vaginal leiomyoma.

Figure 13–24

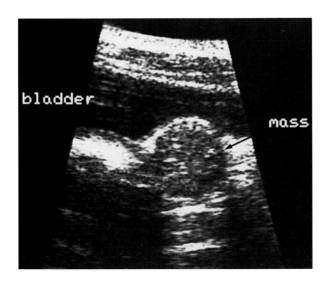

Sagittal abdominal sonogram of a 1-year-old spayed bitch with a vaginal discharge revealed a rounded, hypoechoic mass, approximately 2 cm in diameter, dorsal to the urinary bladder. The diagnosis was uterine stump pyometra.

THE PROSTATE—*Barbara A. Selcer*

Sonography can provide important diagnostic information in the evaluation of canine prostatic disease. Sonographic information alone is insufficient for accurate diagnosis or prognosis; these data should be used in combination with the history and findings from physical examination, radiographic data, and clinical laboratory test results. After all information is analyzed, a diagnosis or further diagnostic plans can be developed. Sonographic findings in prostatic disease are not pathognomonic. The principal value of the sonogram lies in tissue characterization, particularly in distinguishing solid from cystic disease. In addition, percutaneous biopsies or prostatic aspirations can be facilitated with sonographic guidance.

Anatomy

The prostate is the only accessory sex gland in the male dog. The size and weight of the prostate vary depending on the age, breed, and body weight of the patient. The prostate gland progressively enlarges with age. The three stages of development of the prostate gland are normal growth, hyperplasia, and senile involution.[38] The prostate is located within the pelvic cavity until the dog reaches sexual maturity, at which time with increased size, it extends into the abdominal cavity.[38] Because the prostate gland is androgen dependent, castration can alter prostatic size and location.

The prostate gland is bounded dorsally by the rectum and ventrally by the ventral abdominal wall and symphysis pubis. The ventral surface of the prostate is covered by a layer of fat and is retroperitoneal.[38] In mature dogs, the caudal one third of the dorsal surface of the prostate is attached to the rectum by a fibrous band.[38] Overall, the prostate is ovoid, with slight flattening of the dorsal surface. A median septum divides the gland into right and left halves. The urethra passes through the prostate slightly dorsal to the center portion of the gland. The prostate gland is composed of tubuloalveolar glands lined by columnar epithelium with multiple ducts entering the prostatic urethra. Two deferent ducts enter the cranial dorsal surface of the prostate and run caudoventrally, opening into the urethra at the colliculus seminalis.[38]

Sonographically, the normal prostate is spherical to ovoid with smooth, well-defined margins and uniform, coarse, medium to slightly hyperechoic echo texture (Fig. 13–25).[39–42] Canine prostatic glandular epithelium is described as hypoechoic compared to areas within the prostate with high collagen content that appear hyperechoic.[43] The

Figure 13–25

Sagittal sonogram of a normal canine prostate gland (outlined by cursor marks). The prostatic parenchyma has a mildly coarse, uniform, medium to slightly hyperechoic echo texture. *, cranial.

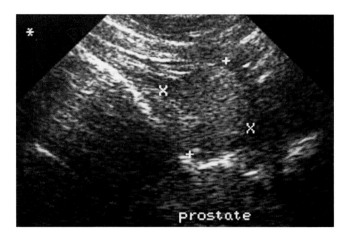

periurethral stromal regions, as well as the immature prostate gland in young dogs, appear more echogenic because of greater collagen content.[43] Unlike the prostate gland in man, in which several zones with different echogenic levels have been identified, the canine prostate gland does not appear to demonstrate this type of differentiation.[43–45] A hilar echo, presumably representing periurethral fibrous tissue and/or a confluence of echoes created by the prostatic urethra and prostatic ducts, has been reported. This hilar echo is described as a linear hyperechoic streak in the middle portion of the prostate gland.[39] In several prostatic diseases, the hilar echo is not visualized.[39–41]

Prostate size can be objectively evaluated sonographically, but it is more commonly measured on survey abdominal radiographs. The dorsoventral dimensions of the prostate should be less than 70% of the pubic sacral prominentory distance.[39,46] In man, sonographic volumetric measurements of the prostate have been made: 1 cm^3 of prostatic tissue is approximately equivalent to 1 g of prostatic weight.[44]

Indications

The value of diagnostic prostatic sonography lies in the evaluation of prostatic parenchyma, particularly in the classification of cavitary versus solid disease and diffuse versus focal or multifocal disease. It is useful to rule out certain processes based on changes in prostatic parenchyma, particularly to categorize disease as cavitary or noncavitary; to monitor prostatic size after therapy, to complement retrograde cystourethrography, and to facilitate percutaneous prostatic biopsy or aspiration.

Technique

Two prostatic scanning protocols have been developed: transrectal imaging and transabdominal imaging. Unlike prostatic scanning in man, for whom the transrectal approach is most common, transabdominal prepubic (suprapubic) scanning is most frequently used in veterinary medicine. Canine prostatomegaly usually results in caudal abdominal displacement of the prostate and provides easy access for transabdominal scanning.

Dogs are usually positioned in ventral or lateral recumbency. Hair adjacent to the prepuce is clipped and acoustic coupling gel is used to provide good transducer-skin contact. Scans should be performed in both transverse and sagittal sections. A full urinary bladder facilitates the examination by acting as a landmark for identification of the caudal urinary bladder and cranial prostate while also displacing intestinal viscera from the scan area. Frequently, a distended urinary bladder acts as a sonic window for enhanced prostatic visualization. A 7.5-mHz transducer is preferable to lower frequency transducers because the prostate, in most instances, is located superficially. In those cases in which greater depth penetration is required, use of a 5-mHz transducer may be appropriate. In general, sector scanners have smaller scan heads and are more convenient to use than linear array scanners, particularly if a portion of the prostate remains intrapelvic.

Using the distended urinary bladder as a landmark, scans are initiated in the caudal portion of the bladder, and the transducer is progressively moved caudally during the examination. Both the right and left lobes of the prostate should be evaluated in sagittal and transverse planes. When the prostate is not adequately visualized, a gloved finger may be inserted into the rectum and used to push the prostate forward.[2] A urethral catheter may also be of benefit in localization of the urethra and evaluation of prostatic lobe symmetry.[39] Colonic gas can create hyperechoic artifacts that might confuse prostatic evaluation. Water enemas before sonographic evaluation may decrease the possibility of this artifact.[47]

Prostatic Abnormalities

The following prostatic characteristics should be evaluated during sonographic examination:

1. Parenchymal echogenicity-isoechoic, hypoechoic, hyperechoic, anechoic
2. Parenchymal uniformity-uniform, focal, multifocal
3. Gland size and shape
4. Gland margination-smooth, irregular
5. Lesion margination-smooth, irregular
6. Prostatic lobe symmetry
7. Mineralization

These sonographic features can be used to categorize prostatic disease. The two major categories of prostatic disease include those in which the parenchyma is solid and noncavitary and those in which the lesions are cavitary or cystic. No sonographic features can reliably predict benign disease versus malignant disease versus infectious disease.[48] In most instances, prostatic biopsy, prostatic wash, prostatic aspiration, or a prostatic ejaculate is required for definitive diagnosis.

Prostatomegaly is a common finding in middle-aged to older intact male dogs. Dogs with prostatic disease often have hematuria, dysuria, tenesmus, or palpable prostatomegaly. The most commonly reported confirmed prostatic disease is bacterial prostatitis.[49] A frequent diagnosis in dogs is benign prostatic hypertrophy/hyperplasia (BPH), but its presence is uncommonly confirmed through biopsy.[49] The sonographic appearance of BPH, prostatic cysts, prostatic abscesses, paraprostatic cysts, bacterial prostatitis, and prostatic neoplasia have been reported.[39-41,44,47,50-52]

Benign prostatic hyperplasia/hypertrophy (BPH) is a common abnormality in aged, intact male dogs. Affected dogs are frequently asymptomatic. Mild prostatomegaly may be identified on rectal palpation. Sonographically, dogs with BPH demonstrate normal to slightly increased prostatic size. Sonograms frequently show symmetric enlargement of the lobes,[40,41,47] although asymmetry has been reported.[50] In canine BPH, the prostate uniformly appears slightly hyperechoic (Fig. 13-26),[39-41,47,50,51] although cystic lesions are also seen (Fig. 13-27). In man, BPH has a more varied appearance, with both hyper- or hypoechoic nodules reported.[44] In addition, small foci of prostatic calcification have been described in association with human BPH.[44] These changes are not reported with canine BPH.

Cavitary prostatic lesions are not pathognomonic and can be seen with prostatic cysts (see Fig. 13-27), prostatic abscesses (see Fig. 13-28), or paraprostatic cysts (see Fig. 13-29), prostatitis (see Fig. 13-30), prostatic neoplasia (see Fig. 13-31), or a combination of lesions (see Fig. 13-32). They can be focal or multifocal and range in size from a few millimeters to several centimeters in diameter. Cystic lesions are usually anechoic and demonstrate posterior enhancement; most have smooth to only slightly irregular mar-

Figure 13-26

Sagittal sonogram of the prostate of a dog with confirmed benign prostatic hyperplasia/hypertrophy. Overall prostatic echogenicity is increased. The cursor marks outline the prostate.

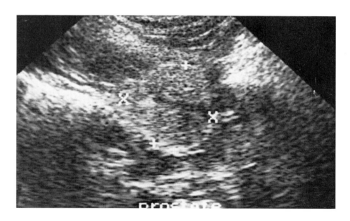

Figure 13-27

Sagittal sonogram of the prostate of a dog with confirmed benign cystic prostatic hyperplasia reveals small multifocal anechoic foci throughout the parenchyma (arrows). B, urinary bladder; *, caudal.

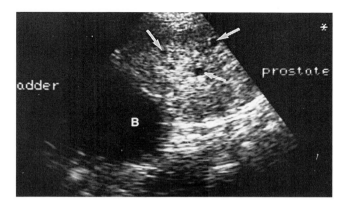

gins.[40,41,47] Some cystic lesions contain low-level internal echoes that may be the result of intracavitary hemorrhage or debris accumulation. Relatively large prostatic cysts are speculated to be prostatic retention cysts caused by obstruction of prostatic or ejaculatory ducts or hematocysts.[44,47]

Prostatic abscesses (Fig. 13–28) usually appear cavitary sonographically. Cavitary lesions can be solitary or multiple. In many instances, abscesses result in asymmetric enlargement of the prostate.[40,41,47,50] In contrast to prostatic cysts, the inner cavitary margins in prostatic abscesses are frequently irregular.[40,41,47,50] Cavitary prostatic abscesses range in echogenicity from hypo- to anechoic. If anechoic, posterior acoustic enhancement may be present.

Paraprostatic cysts (Fig. 13–29) are usually large cavitary structures adjacent to the prostate or the urinary bladder trigone region.[39–41,52] Paraprostatic cysts usually have a smooth margined and thin or thick walls.[39,52] Some cysts have internal septations.[39,52] They are frequently anechoic, demonstrating posterior acoustic enhancement, although low-level, internal echoes or a homogeneous hypoechogenicity may be present if they contain cellular material. Often, a stalk or attachment can be seen between the paraprostatic cyst and the prostate.[52] In many instances, only a broad attachment site is identified.[52] Paraprostatic cysts are speculated to form as a result of anomalous development of the Müellerian duct or as outpouchings of large prostatic retention cysts.[52]

Chronic prostatitis (Fig. 13–30) has a variable sonographic appearance. If abscessation is not present, prostatic scans can show diffuse or focal hyperechogenicity,[40,41,47] small (less than 1.5 cm in diameter) hypo- to anechoic foci,[47,50] or small, focal prominent hyperechoic foci.[40,44] Mixed echogenic patterns are also possible. Mineralization is infrequently identified. Chronic granulomatous prostatitis has been reported to have patchy

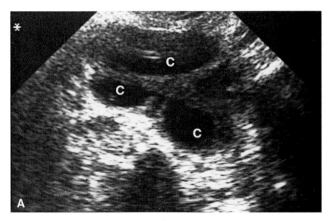
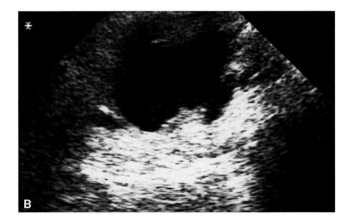

Figure 13–28

A, Transverse sonogram of a dog with a prostatic abscess demonstrates multiple large, thick-walled anechoic cavitary structures (C). Moderate posterior acoustic enhancement is seen deep to the cavitary lesions. *, left side of the dog. **B,** Transverse sonogram of the prostate of a dog with a prostatic abscess shows a large, irregularly marginated anechoic cavitary lesion. Posterior enhancement is seen deep to the abscess. *, left side of the dog).

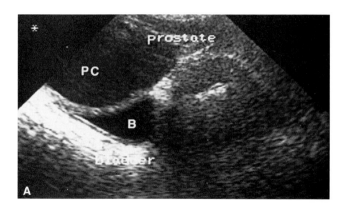

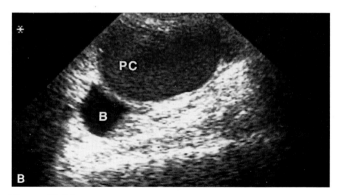

Figure 13–29

A, Sagittal sonogram of the prostate of a dog with a large paraprostatic cyst (PC). The cyst has compressed the cranial portion of the urinary bladder (B). Faint, low- level echoes are present within the cyst. *, cranial. **B,** Sagittal sonogram of the prostate of a dog with a paraprostatic cyst (PC) that contains internal, medium-level echoes relative to the anechoic urinary bladder (B). *, cranial. **C,** Sagittal sonogram of the prostate of a dog with a paraprostatic cyst (PC) reveals the cyst is largely cavitary, with thick internal septations. *, cranial; B, urinary bladder.

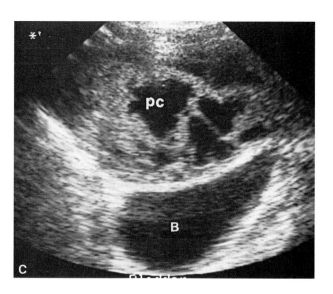

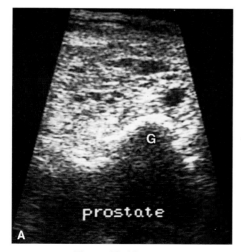
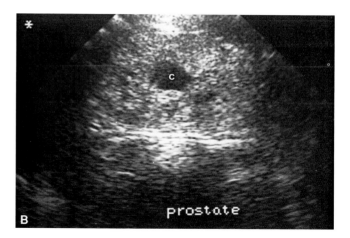

Figure 13–30

A, Transverse sonogram of the prostate of a dog with bacterial prostatitis. Small cavitary lesions are noted throughout the prostatic parenchyma. *, left side of the dog; G, colonic gas. **B,** Sagittal sonogram of the prostate of a dog with bacterial prostatitis reveals a solitary, irregularly marginated cavitary lesion (c) cranial to smaller hypoechoic areas. *, cranial.

echogenicity with focal, increased echogenic areas, possibly attributable to fibrosis.[39]

The two most frequently identified prostatic neoplastic diseases are prostatic adenocarcinoma (Figs. 13–31 to 13–33) and transitional cell carcinoma (Fig. 13–34). Sonographically, prostatic adenocarcinoma has been reported to produce symmetric and asymmetric prostatomegaly of mixed, nonuniform echogenicity.[39–41,47,50,51] Patchy echogenic areas with poor definition tend to coalesce, and cavitation, although infrequent, can be seen.[40] Multifocal, mineralized foci have been reported[39,40,47] and may demonstrate posterior acoustic shadowing. The shape of the prostate gland capsule is often irregular.[39,41] Doppler studies in human cases of prostatic carcinoma have demonstrated increased flow with low resistance.[44] Similar studies in dogs have not been performed.

Invasion of a transitional cell carcinoma of the bladder or urethra into the prostate may be identified during sonographic evaluation. As with prostatic adenocarcinoma, which involves parenchymal invasion, areas of mixed, nonuniform echogenicity can be seen with focal hyperechoic regions.[41] Mineralization may be present. Often, an irregular urethral margin is identified.

Ultrasound-Guided Prostatic Biopsy

Definitive diagnosis of prostatic disease usually requires, in addition to sonography, prostatic biopsy, prostatic aspiration, prostatic wash, ejaculation, or culture and sensitivity. The sonographic data can be useful in helping to determine whether core biopsy, needle aspiration, or noninvasive means should be pursued as further diagnostic tests. Ultrasound can also be of value in providing percutaneous guidance of needle placement in those cases in which prostatic biopsy or aspiration is warranted. Automated biopsy guns or manual biopsy instruments can be used. Obtaining a clotting profile before a biopsy is beneficial. In general, postbiopsy complication rates are low, although transient hematuria has been reported.[44,53,54]

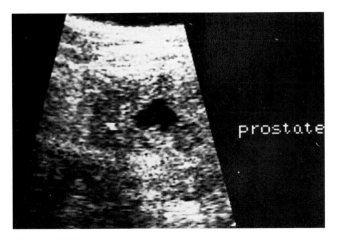

Figure 13–31

Transverse sonogram of the prostate of a dog with prostatic carcinoma shows an irregularly marginated cavitary lesion within the parenchyma. *, left side of the dog.

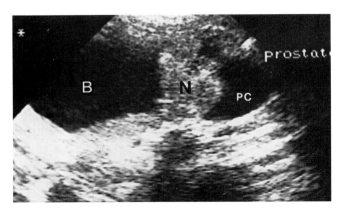

Figure 13–32

Sagittal sonogram of the prostate of a dog with prostatic carcinoma and a paraprostatic cyst (PC). The urinary bladder (B) is cranial to the mixed echogenic lesion. N, presumed neoplastic tissue.

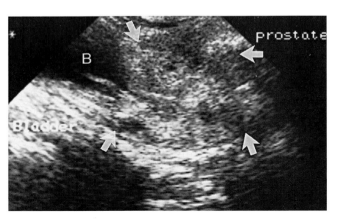

Figure 13–33

Sagittal sonogram of the prostate of a dog with prostatic carcinoma demonstrates a patchy, mixed echogenic pattern. Arrows delineate the margin of the prostate. *, cranial; B, urinary bladder.

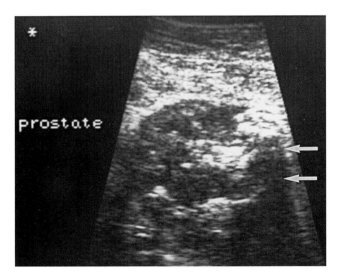

Figure 13–34

Sagittal sonogram of the prostate of a dog with prostatic parenchymal invasion from a transitional cell carcinoma. Note the mixed echogenic pattern within the prostate and numerous hyperechoic foci (some of which demonstrate posterior shadowing). *, cranial.

THE TESTICLES AND EPIDIDYMIS—*Robert E. Cartee*

B mode sonographic examination of the scrotum and testicle was reported as early as 1976, when Miskin and colleagues discussed the normal echo texture of both the testicle and epididymis in man.[1] These authors and others subsequently described the appearance and diagnosis of spermatoceles, hydroceles, epididymitis, and neoplastic diseases.[55-58] In 1981, Cunningham described the sonographic appearance of a sertoli cell tumor (fluid-filled spoke wheel appearance),[59] and the influence of epididymal cysts compressing the testicle and causing a false-positive diagnosis of a testicular lesion was presented in 1983.[60] The use of ultrasound in the diagnosis of testicular torsion was reported in 1975 and continues to be the subject of study.[61-65] Lymphoproliferative disease and choriocarcinomas of the scrotum and testicle have also been identified with B mode sonography.[66,67] Sonography may also be of value in the diagnosis of rupture or fracture of the testicle.[68]

The use of B mode sonography in the diagnosis of testicular disease in animals has also been investigated.[69-76] The normal sonographic appearance of boar and bull testicles showed them to be homogeneous hypoechoic structures with a hyperechoic mediastinum (Fig. 13–35).[69,70] Other than size, they resembled the human testicle, as did the epididymis (Fig. 13–36). The sonographic appearance of the testicle of the dog, reported in 1989, was similar to that reported in the boar and bull.[71] In another report of canine testicular and scrotal lesions diagnosed with the use of ultrasound, the sonographic appearance of neoplastic disorders, non-neoplastic noninfectious disorders, and non-neoplastic infection disorders were discussed.[72] In this study, seminomas and inter-

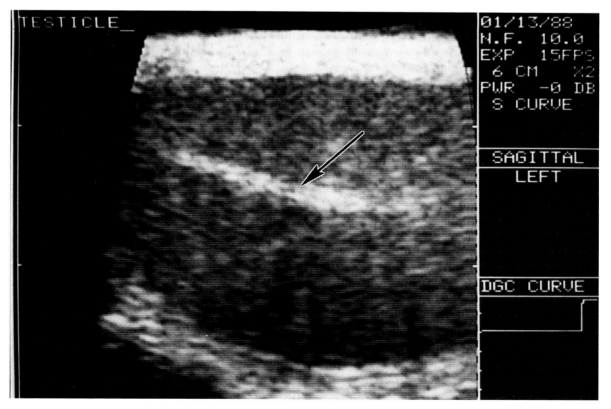

Figure 13–35

B mode sonogram of the normal echo texture of the testicle. Note the echogenic mediastinum testis (arrow).

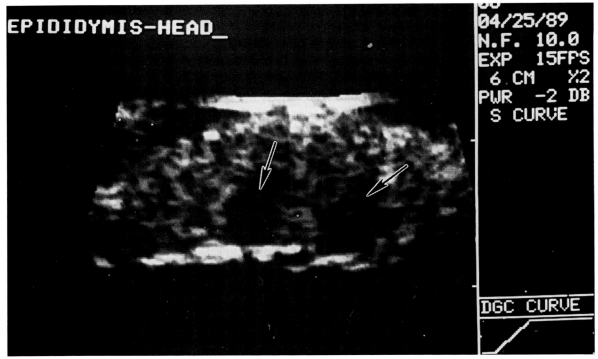

Figure 13–36

B mode sonogram of the head of the epididymis of the bull. Anechoic areas (arrows) indicate ductules.

stitial cell tumors yielded mixed echogenic patterns, whereas a hypoechoic appearance was characteristic of sertoli cell tumor. Typical anechoic areas were noted with hydroceles, whereas infectious processes resulted in both hypoechoic and hyperechoic patterns.[72] Testicular torsion in dogs was diagnosed using Doppler and B mode sonographic techniques.[73] Reduction in vascular flow in the testicular artery and a quickly occurring decrease in testicular echogenicity were reported in these animals. In an experimental study of ligation of the testicular artery in goats, a similar decrease in echogenicity of the testicle was noted.[74] A case report of the use of B mode sonography to examine a retained testicle in a horse also showed good measurement capability using ultrasound, but also showed a reduction in echogenicity from normal levels.[75]

The use of sonography to measure testicular size in bulls has proved to be reliable in the breeding soundness examination.[76] In one study, however, the sonographic appearance of testicular changes related to heat preceded the changes in semen evaluation values.[70] Examination of the testicle is done easily and quickly. The normal uniform echogenicity of all testicles in all species of animals allows early detection of changes (Fig. 13–37). Hypoechoic masses warrant biopsy or castration. Torsion is more likely present if the testicle shows echogenic changes. The mediastinum testes may be so reflective that a false hypoechoic area may appear (Fig. 13–38). Movement of the probe to the other side will quickly determine the true nature of the area. Inflammatory processes usually result in an initial increase in echogenicity followed by a decrease (Fig. 13–39). Anechoic fluid around the testicle suggests the presence of free blood or fluid attributable to hydrocele or testicular torsion (Fig. 13–40).

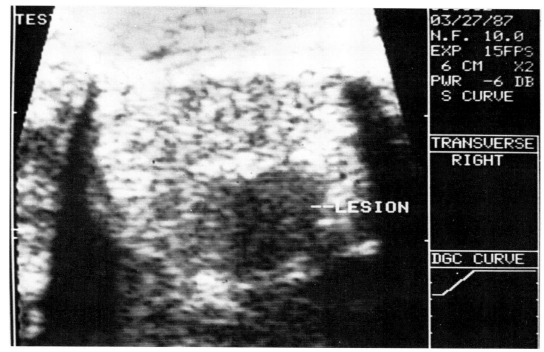

Figure 13–37

B mode sonogram of a canine testicle shows a hypoechoic lesion compatible with a sertoli cell tumor.

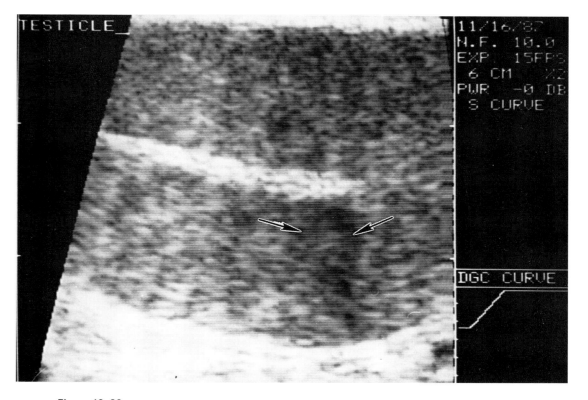

Figure 13–38

B mode sonogram of a testicle reveals a false hypoechoic area (arrows) that results from attenuation by the mediastinum testis.

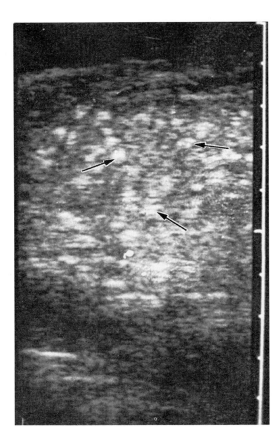

Figure 13–39

B mode sonogram of orchitis in a bull demonstrates a focal increase in echogenicity (arrows). This change may eventually be followed by a decrease reflecting degeneration of the parenchyma.

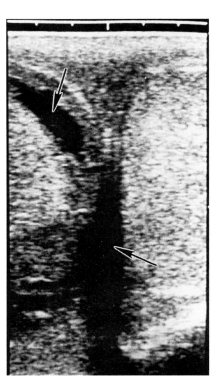

Figure 13–40

Sonogram of a hydrocele in a bull shows the anechoic fluid accumulations (arrows).

REFERENCES

1. England GCW, Allen WE: Ultrasonography and histological appearance of the canine ovary. Vet Rec *125:*555, 1989.
2. Wallace SS, et al: Ultrasonographic appearance of the ovaries of dogs during the follicular and luteal phases of the estrous cycle. Am J Vet Res *53:*209, 1992.
3. Renton JP, et al: Comparison of endocrine changes and ultrasound as means of identifying ovulation in the bitch. Res Vet Sci *53:*74, 1992.
4. Wilson J, Hayward JA: Real-time ultrasound scanning of bitches (letter to the editor). Vet Rec *116:*698, 1985.
5. Inaba T, et al: Use of echography in bitches for detection of ovulation and pregnancy. Vet Rec *115:*276, 1984.
6. England GCW, Allen WE: Real-time ultrasonic imaging of the ovary and uterus of the dog. J Reprod Fertil *39*(Suppl):91, 1989.
7. Wrigley RH, Finn ST: Ultrasonography of the canine uterus and ovary. In *Current Veterinary Therapy X.* Edited by RW Kirk. Philadelphia: WB Saunders, 1989.
8. Poffenbarger EM, Feeney DA: Use of gray-scale ultrasonography in the diagnosis of reproductive diseases in the bitch: 18 cases (1981–1984). J Am Vet Med Assoc *189:*90, 1986.
9. Rivers B, Johnston GR: Diagnostic imaging of the reproductive organs of the bitch. Vet Clin North Am Small Anim Pract *21:*437, 1991.
10. Rowley J: Cystic ovary in a dog: A case report. Vet Med Small Anim Clin *75:*1888, 1980.
11. Jubb KBF, Kennedy PC: The female genital system. In *Pathology of Domestic Animals,* 2nd Ed., New York: Academic Press, 1970.
12. Smith HA, Jones TC, Hunt RD: The genital system. In *Veterinary Pathology,* 4th Ed. Philadelphia: Lea & Febiger, 1972.
13. Goodwin JK, et al: Bilateral ovarian adenocarcinoma in a dog: Ultrasonographic-aided diagnosis. Vet Radiol *31:*265, 1990.
14. Barr F: Imaging of the reproductive tract: Uterus and ovary. In *Diagnostic Ultrasound of the Dog and Cat.* Boston: Blackwell Scientific, 1990.
15. Stowater JL, et al: Ultrasonic features of the dog uterus and fetus. Abstract. J Reprod Fertil Suppl *39:*329, 1989.
16. Pharr JW, Post K: Ultrasonography and radiography of the canine postpartum uterus. Vet Radiiol Ultrasound *33:*35, 1992.
17. Yeager AE, Concannon PW: Serial ultrasonographic appearance of postpartum uterine involution in Beagle dogs. Therio *34:*523, 1990.
18. England GCW, Allen WE: Diagnosis of pregnancy and pyometra in the bitch using real-time ultrasonography. Vet Annual *30:*217, 1990.
19. Johnston SD, et al: Prenatal indicators of puppy viability at term. Compend Cont Educ Pract Vet *5:*1013, 1983.
20. Cartee RE, Rowles T: Preliminary study of the ultrasonographic diagnosis of pregnancy and fetal development in the dog. Am J Vet Res *45:*1259, 1984.
21. Bondestam S, et al: Evaluating the accuracy of canine pregnancy diagnosis and litter size using real-time ultrasound. Acta Vet Scand *25:*327, 1984.
22. Taverne MAM, Okkens AC, van Oord R: Pregnancy diagnosis in the dog: A comparison between abdominal palpation and linear-array real-time echography. Vet Q *7:*249, 1985.
23. Shille VM, Gontarek J: The use of ultrasonography for pregnancy diagnosis in the bitch. J Am Vet Med Assoc *187:*1021, 1985.
24. Toal RL, Walker MA, Henry GA: A comparison of real-time ultrasound, palpation, and radiography in pregnancy detection and litter size determination in the bitch. Vet Radiol *27:*102, 1986.
25. Spaulding KA, Whitacre M, Van Camp S: Sonographic pregnancy diagnosis in the bitch. Proceedings of the 8th Meeting of the International Veterinary Radiology Association, Sydney, Australia, 1988.
26. Yeager AE, Concannon PW: Association between the pre-ovulatory luteinizing hormone surge and the early ultrasonographic detection of pregnancy and fetal heartbeats in Beagle dogs. Therio *34:*655, 1990.
27. Yeager AE, et al: Ultrasonographic appearance of the uterus, placenta, fetus, and fetal membranes throughout accurately timed pregnancy in Beagles. Am J Vet Res *53:*342, 1992.
28. England GCW, Allen WE: Studies on canine pregnancy using B-mode ultrasound: Diagnosis of early pregnancy and the number of conceptuses. J Small Anim Pract *31:*321, 1990.
29. England GCW, Allen WE, Porter DJ: Studies on canine pregnancy using B-mode ultrasound: Development of the conceptus and determination of gestational age. J Small Anim Pract *31:*324, 1990.
30. Concannon P, Rendano V: Radiographic diagnosis of canine pregnancy: The onset of fetal skeletal radiopacity in relation to times of breeding, preovulatory luteinizing hormone release, and parturition. Am J Vet Res *44:*1506, 1983.

31. Davidson AP, Nyland TG, Tsutsui T: Pregnancy diagnosis with ultrasound in the domestic cat. Vet Radiol *27:*109, 1986.

32. Beck KA, Baldwin CJ, Bosu WTK: Ultrasound prediction of parturition in queens. Vet Radiol *31:*32-35, 1990.

33. England CGW: Ultrasound evaluation of pregnancy and spontaneous embryonic resorption in the bitch. J Small Anim Pract *33:*430, 1992.

34. Konde LJ: Diagnostic ultrasound in canine pregnancy and uterine disease. Proceedings of the Annual Meeting of the Society of Theriogenology, 1988, pp. 247–249.

35. Farrow CS, Morgan JP, Story EC: Late-term fetal death in the dog: Early radiographic diagnosis. J Am Vet Radiol Soc *17:*11, 1976.

36. Allen WE, England GCW, White KB: Hydrops fetalis diagnosed by real-time ultrasonography in a bichon frise bitch. J Small Anim Pract *30:*365, 1989.

37. Fayrer-Hosken RA, et al: Early diagnosis of canine pyometra using ultrasonography. Vet Radiol *32:*287, 1991.

38. Evans HE, Christensen GC: *Miller's Anatomy of the Dog.* Philadelphia: WB Saunders, 1993, pp. 514–516.

39. Barr F: *Diagnostic Ultrasound in the Dog and Cat.* Oxford: Blackwell Scientific, 1990, pp. 65–77.

40. Feeney DA, Johnston GR: Two-dimensional, gray-scale ultrasonography-applications in canine prostatic disease. Vet Clin North Am *15:*1159, 1985.

41. Feeney DA, et al: Canine prostatic disease-comparison of ultrasonographic appearance with morphologic and microbiologic findings: 30 cases (1981–1985). J Am Vet Med Assoc *190:*1027, 1987.

42. Cartee RE, Rowles T: Transabdominal sonographic evaluation of the canine prostate. Vet Radiol *24:*156, 1983.

43. Cooney JC, et al: Ultrasonography of the canine prostate with histologic correlation. Theriogen *38:*877, 1992.

44. Bree RL: *Diagnostic Ultrasound.* St. Louis: Mosby Yearbook, 1991, pp. 261–388.

45. Hamper UM, Sheth S: Prostate ultrasonography. Semin Roentgenol *28:*57, 1993.

46. Feeney DA, et al: Canine prostatic disease-comparison of ultrasonographic appearance with morphologic and microbiologic findings: 30 cases (1981–1985). J Am Vet Med Assoc *190:*1018, 1987.

47. Feeney DA, et al: Canine prostatic ultrasonography - 1989. Semin Vet Med Surg *4:*44, 1989.

48. Burks DD, et al: Transrectal sonography of benign and malignant prostatic lesions. AJR Am J Roentgenol *146:*1187, 1986.

49. Krawiec DR, Heflin D: Study of prostatic disease in dogs: 177 cases (1981–1986). J Am Vet Med Assoc *200:*1119, 1992.

50. Foss RR, et al: A new frontier—veterinary ultrasound: The prostate part II. Med Ultrasound *8:*15, 1984.

51. Olson PN, et al: Disorders of the canine prostate gland: Pathogenesis, diagnosis, and medical therapy. Compend Cont Educ Pract Vet *9:*613, 1987.

52. Stowater JL, Lam CR: Ultrasonographic features of paraprostatic cysts in nine dogs. Vet Radiol *30:*232, 1989.

53. Rifkin MD, Resnick MI: *Ultrasonography of the Urinary Tract.* Baltimore: Williams & Wilkins, 1984, pp. 297–335.

54. Hager DA, Nyland TG, Fisher P: Ultrasound-guided biopsy of the canine liver, kidney and prostate. Vet Radiol *26:*82, 1985.

55. Miskin M, Bain J: B mode ultrasonic examination of the testes. JCU *2:*307, 1976.

56. Miskin M, Buckspan M, Bain J: Ultrasonographic examination of scrotal masses. J Urol *117:*185, 1976.

57. Sample WF, et al: Gray scale ultrasound of the scrotum. Radiology *127:*225, 1978.

58. Shawker TH: B mode ultrasonic evaluation of scrotal swellings. Radiology *118:*417, 1976.

59. Cunningham J: Echographic findings in sertoli cell tumor of the testis. JCU *9:*341, 1981.

60. Rifkin MD, Brownstein KP: Abnormal echogenicity of the testicle caused by epididymal cysts. J Ultrasound Med *2:*539, 1983.

61. Pedersen JF, Hold HH, Hald T: Torsion of the testis diagnosed by ultrasound. J Urol *113:*66, 1975.

62. Milleret R: Doppler ultrasound diagnosis of testicular and torsion. JCU *4:*425, 1976.

63. Perri AJ, et al: An evaluation of the role of the Doppler stethoscope and the testicular scan in the diagnosis of torsion of the spermatic cord. J Urol *15:*275, 1976.

64. Cohen HL, et al: Torsion of the testicular appendage. J Ultrasound Med *11:*81, 1992.

65. Grois BR, Cohen HL, Schlessel JS: Perinatal diagnosis of bilateral testicular torsion: Beware of torsions simulating hydroceles. J Ultrasound Med *12:*479, 1993.

66. Philips G, Kumai-Subaiya S, Sawitsky A: Ultrasonic evaluation of the scrotum in lymphoproliferative disease. J Ultrasound Med *6:*169, 1987.

67. Sequin DR, Longmaid III HE: Sonographic appearance of testicular choriocarcinomas. J Diagn Med Sonogr *3:*229, 1987.

68. Steinberg RH: Ultrasound of the fractured testis. J Diagn Med Sonogr *3:*239, 1987.

69. Cartee RE, et al: Ultrasonographic evaluation of normal boar testicles. Am J Vet Res *47:*2543, 1985.

70. Powe TA, et al: B mode ultrasonography of testicular pathology in the bull. Agri Pract *9:*43, 1988.

71. Pugh CR, Konde LJ, Park RD: Testicular ultrasound in the normal dog. Vet Radiol *31:*195, 1990.

72. Pugh CR, Konde LJ: Sonographic evaluation of canine testicular and scrotal abnormalities: A review of 26 case histories. Vet Radiol *32:*243, 1991.

73. Hricak H, et al: Experimental study of the sonographic diagnosis of testicular torsion. J Ultrasound Med *2:*349, 1983.

74. Eilts BE, et al: Ultrasonographic evaluation of induced testicular lesions in male goats. Am J Vet Res *50:*1361, 1989.

75. Jann HW, Rains JR: Diagnostic ultrasonography for evaluation of cryptorchidism in horses. J Am Vet Med Assoc *196:*297, 1990.

76. Eilts BE, Pechman RD: B mode ultrasound observations of bull testes during breeding soundness examinations. Theriogenology *30:*1169, 1988

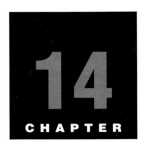

CHAPTER 14

THE INTEGUMENT, MUSCLES, TENDONS, JOINTS, AND BONES

Robert E. Cartee

THE INTEGUMENT

The use of sonography in the evaluation of the skin of animals has not been well reported. In man, studies with high frequency probes (20 to 50 mHz) have shown sonography is of value in the evaluation of skin and subcutaneous diseases.[1-4] Subepidermal edema, epidermoid cysts, and subcutaneous tumors have all been identified with ultrasound.[1-4] Wound healing characteristics have also been described.[1] Sonographic techniques have been used successfully to measure subcutaneous fat thickness in man and in sheep.[4-7] Measurements of dolphin skin and blubber have also been described. Frequencies of 7 and 10 mHz have been used to study some subcutaneous phenomena.[4] Skin and subcutaneous examination with ultrasound is best performed using a standoff pad or water bath. The epidermis is characteristically hyperechoic whereas the dermis and subcutaneous structures are variably hypoechoic (Fig. 14–1).

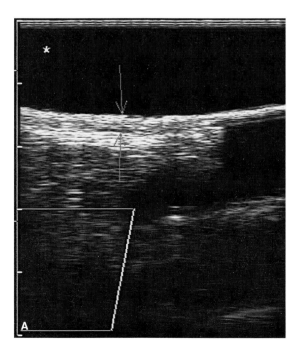

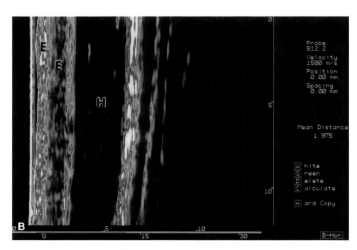

Figure 14–1

B mode sonograms of normal skin. **A,** Canine study, using 7.5 mHz. **B,** Equine study, using 20 mHz. E, epidermis/dermis; H, hypodermis.

MUSCLES

The use of sonography to evaluate muscle disease in animals has not been studied extensively, but the sonographic findings in man are well known. Normal muscle has been described as hypoechoic with hyperechoic lines indicative of fascia and fibrous connective tissue (Fig. 14–2**A**). Ruptures have been visualized as irregularities in the normal linear pattern. Hemorrhage in muscle may be anechoic at first, becoming hyperechoic coincident with thrombus formation.[4] Tumors of muscle have been diagnosed and characterized (Fig. 14–2**B**). Lipomas showed increased echogenicity and sarcomas were

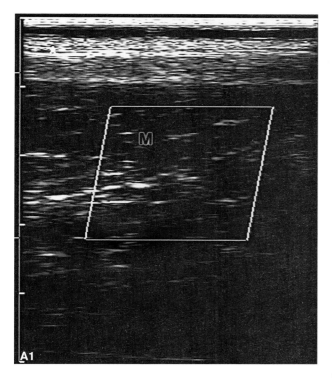

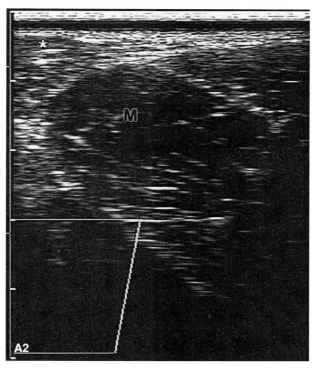

Figure 14–2

B mode sonograms of a normal canine quadriceps femoris muscle (M). **A1,** long axis. **A2,** short axis. **B,** Muscle mass (arrows).

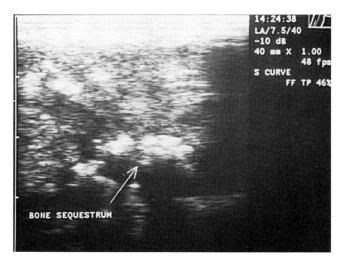

Figure 14–3

B mode sonogram of a foreign object (arrow) embedded in muscle. Note the acoustic shadow.

hypoechoic. Gas formation in certain muscle infections has been reported. Rhabdomyolysis was described as patchy areas of decreased echogenicity.[4]

Ultrasound has been used in studies of muscle hypertrophy and atrophy,[8] to measure animal subcutaneous fat, and to measure muscle thickness in beef carcasses.[9] Foreign objects embedded in muscles have been localized sonographically and bony sequestra have been described. A hyperechoic area with acoustic shadowing characterized these objects (Fig. 14–3).[10,11]

TENDONS

The use of diagnostic sonography in the evaluation of tendon disease has been studied in both man and animals. In man, trauma, inflammation, and postoperative patterns have been described.[4] Traumatic interruptions were hypoechoic, whereas calcifications and bony occlusions were hyperechoic with variable acoustic shadowing. Blurring of the contours and decreased echogenicity were reported in association with inflammatory conditions.[4]

In 1984, two groups of veterinary investigators described the B mode appearance of equine tendons in the metacarpal and metatarsal regions.[12,13] The normal superficial digital flexor tendon was hypoechoic, whereas the deep digital flexor tendon, the check ligament, and the suspensory ligament were all hyperechoic. This contrasting echogenicity was especially evident on transverse scanning. In 1986, Henry and colleagues reported the sonographic appearance of iatrogenic injuries of the check ligament and the superficial flexor tendon.[14] Early injury showed thickening of the tendon or ligament with discrete hypoechoic areas of hemorrhage, edema, and fiber disruption. Loss of the normal linear pattern was noted. As healing progressed, the hypoechoic areas decreased in size and became more echogenic. Dissection showed these areas contained more fibrous tissue. Rantanen and Genovese characterized the lesions in tendons in horses relative to their levels of black and white (anechogenicity and echogenicity).[15] "Blacker" lesions were described as most severe.

In 1987, a report in the human literature cautioned against the use of echogenicity for characterization unless the area was in the central axis of the beam.[16] In 1989, Spurlock and co-workers further described the appearance of tendinitis in the superficial digital flexor tendon of horses. They reported that the hypoechoic areas corresponded to areas of hemorrhage and necrosis. Hyperechogenicity was also seen as healing progressed.[17]

In 1991, Steyn and colleagues reviewed the sonographic appearance of and the scanning techniques for evaluation of the palmar metacarpal tendon and ligaments of the horse. They described the use of a centimeter tape attached to this region, distal to the accessory carpal bone, as a method of determining exact locations for future evaluation of the same area.[18] They included the palmar annular ligament in one measurement of the entire area from the palmar aspect of the superficial digital flexor to the skin surface. In another study of this area, thickening of the palmar annular ligament and distention of the digital sheath were identified using sonography.[19] Another author suggested the injection of saline in the digital sheath as one method of highlighting the structures in this area for sonographic evaluation.[20] In a review study of foals, distention of the tendon sheath with flocculent hypoechoic to echogenic fluid was reported to suggest septic tenosynovitis.[21]

In a detailed study of the pastern, both sonography and magnetic resonance imaging were used to evaluate normal and abnormal tendons and ligaments. The findings were compatible with those of previous reports of increased thickness and heterogeneous echogenicity after injury.[22] A study in which the sonographic appearance was compared with histopathologic findings in the superficial digital flexor tendons of horses showed that fibroplasia and granulation tissue were hypoechoic and chronic fibrosis was hyperechoic. The study showed that peritendinous lesions were readily apparent, intratendinous lesions were hyperechoic foci, and intertendinous lesions were difficult to assess.[23]

Sonographically, the typical palmar or plantar flexor tendon ligament complex (FTLC) consists of a hypoechoic superficial digital flexor and a more echogenic deep digital flexor. The interosseous is typically hyperechoic as is the check ligament (Fig. 14-4). Disruptions or tears in the flexor tendon typically appear as hypoechoic focal areas with increased thickness of the tendon (Fig. 14–5). In some cases, the tendon may be injured so severely that a part is displaced (Fig. 14–6). Tenosynovitis may be indicative of an increase in the anechoic fluid in the tendon sheath (Fig. 14–7). Healing tendons may show increased echogenicity because of fibrous tissue formation (Fig. 14–8).

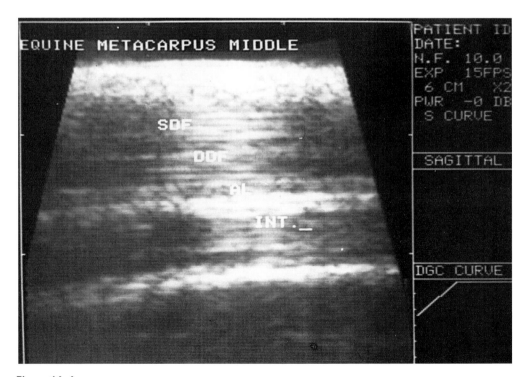

Figure 14–4

B mode sonogram of normal flexor tendons, check ligament, and suspensory ligament of the horse at the middle of the cannon bone. SDF, superficial digital flexor; DDF, deep digital flexor; AL, check ligament; INT, suspensory ligament (interosseous).

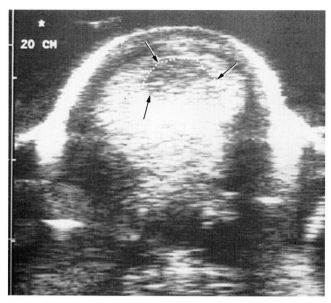

Figure 14–5

B mode sonogram reveals a hypoechoic area (arrows) in the superficial digital flexor tendon that represents a lesion.

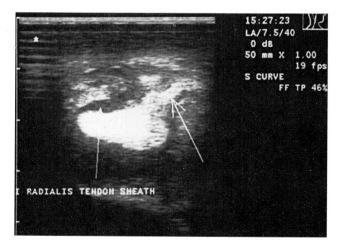

Figure 14–6

B mode sonogram shows severe displacement of the extensor carpi radialis tendon (arrow) in a horse.

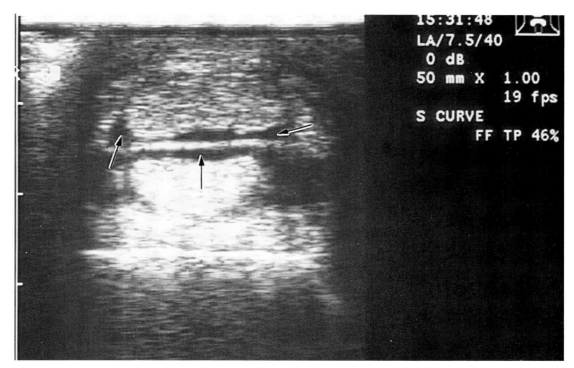

Figure 14–7

B mode sonogram of tenosynovitis with distention of the digital sheath. Arrows, anechoic area.

Figure 14–8

B mode transverse sonogram of a healing superficial digital flexor tendon (S). Note the increased level of echogenicity. D, deep digital flexor tendon.

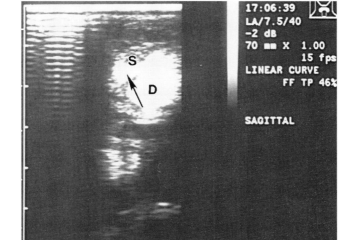

JOINTS AND BONES

In man, sonography has been used to examine the hip, the knee, and the shoulder.[24] Diagnosis of rotator cuff tears in the shoulder and congenital dislocation of the hip, as well as aspiration of hip joint fluid in pediatric patients, have all been performed using sonographic techniques.[25] Abnormal fluid accumulations adjacent to bone were assessed sonographically and were associated with osteomyelitis.[26]

The use of sonography in the examination of the interphalangeal joint, the navicular bursa, and the navicular bone of horses was first reported in 1982.[27] The bursa and joint space were described as sonolucent. In 1989, echogenic masses adjacent to the anechoic region in the dorsal pouch of the metacarpophalangeal joint were considered indicative of proliferative synovitis.[28] In a 1990 study of the equine stifle joint, ultrasound was used to identify the patellar ligaments, collateral ligaments, femoral trochlear ridges, and menisci.[29] These authors indicated that joint effusion, synovial thickening, articular cartilages, and subchondral defects were all detectable sonographically.[29] More studies of joint evaluation and bone sonography in animals are needed.

REFERENCES

1. Altmeyer P, El-Gamal S, Hoffman K: *Ultrasound in Dermatology.* Berlin: Springer, 1992.
2. Forster FK, et al: Ultrasonic assessment of skin and surgical wounds utilizing backscatter acoustic techniques to estimate attenuation. Ultrasound Med Biol *16:*43, 1990.
3. Olerud JE, et al: Correlation of tissue constituents with the acoustic properties of skin and wound. Ultrasound Med Biol *16:*55, 1990
4. Fornage BD: *Musculoskeletal evaluation.* In *General Ultrasound.* New York: Churchill Livingston, 1992, pp. 1–57.
5. Hayes PA, et al: Subcutaneous fat thickness measured by magnetic resonance imaging, ultrasound and calipers. Med Sci Sports Exerc *20:*303, 1987.
6. Heckmatt JZ, Pier N, Dubowitz V: Measurement of quadriceps muscle thickness and subcutaneous tissue thickness in normal children by real-time ultrasound imaging. JCU *16:*171, 1988.
7. Fukunaga T, et al: Study for measurement of muscle and subcutaneous fat thickness by means of ultrasonic B mode method. Jpn J Med Ultrasonics *16:*170, 1989.
8. Heckmatt JZ, Pier N, Dubowitz V: Assessment of quadriceps femoris muscle atrophy and hypertrophy in neuromuscular disease in children. JCU *16:*177, 1988.
9. Hanby PL, Stouffer JR, Smith SB: Muscle metabolism and real-time ultrasound measurement of muscle and subcutaneous adipose tissue growth in lambs fed diets containing a beta-agonist. J Anim Sci *63:*1410, 1986.
10. Cartee RE, Rumph PF: Ultrasonographic detection of fistulous tracts and foreign objects in muscles of horses. J Am Vet Med Assoc *184:*1127, 1984.
11. Shah ZR, et al: Ultrasonographic detection of foreign bodies in soft tissues using turkey muscle as a model. Vet Radiol Ultrasound *33:*94, 1992.
12. Pharr JW, Nyland TG: Sonography of the equine palmar metacarpal soft tissues. Vet Radiol *25:*265, 1984.
13. Spaulding KY: Ultrasonic anatomy of the tendons and ligaments in the distal - metacarpal - metatarsal region of the equine limb. Vet Radiol *25:*155, 1984.
14. Henry GA, Patton CS, Guble DO: Ultrasonographic evaluation of iatrogenic injuries of the equine accessory (carpal check) ligament and superficial digital flexor tendon. Vet Radiol *27:*132, 1986.
15. Genouese RL, et al: Clinical use of diagnostic ultrasound of the equine limb. Equine Lameness Symposium Proceedings, 1986, pp. 17–28.
16. Fornage BD: The hypoechoic normal tendon: A pitfall. J Ultrasound Med *6:*19, 1987.
17. Spurlock GH, Spurlock SL, Parker GA: Ultrasonographic gross and histologic evaluation of a tendinitis disease model in the horse. Vet Radiol *30:*184, 1989.
18. Steyn PF, McIlwraith CW, Rawcliff N: The ultrasonographic examination of the palmar metacarpal tendons and ligaments of the equine digit: A review - Part I. Equine Pract *13:*24, 1991.
19. Dik KJ, Van Den Belt AJM, Keg PR: Ultrasonographic evaluation of fetlock annular ligament constriction in the horse. Equine Vet J *23:*285, 1991.
20. Redding WR: Ultrasonographic imaging of the structures of the digital flexor tendon sheath. The Compendium *13:*1824, 1991.
21. Reef VB: Equine pediatric ultrasonography. The Compendium *13:*1277, 1991.
22. Denoix JM, Crevier N, Azevedo C: Ultrasound examination of the pastern in horses. Proceedings of the American Association of Equine Practitioners, 1991, pp. 363- 381.

23. Marr CM, et al: Ultrasonographic and histopathological findings in equine superficial digital flexor tendon injury. Equine Vet J 25:23, 1993.
24. Montana MA, Richardson ML: Ultrasonography of the musculoskeletal system. Radiol Clin North Am 26:1, 1988.
25. Okeefe D, Mamtora H: Ultrasound in clinical orthopaedics. J Bone Joint Surg [Am] 74:488, 1992.
26. Abiri MM, Kirpekar M, Ablow RC: Osteomyelitis: Detection with US. Radiology 169:795, 1988.
27. Hauser ML, Rantanen NW, Modransky PD: Ultrasound examination of distal interphalangeal joint, navicular bursa, navicular bone and deep digital tendon. Equine Vet Sci 2:95, 1982.
28. Steyn PF, et al: The sonographic diagnosis of chronic proliferative synovitis in the metacarpophalangeal joints of a horse. Vet Radiol 30:125, 1989.
29. Penninck DG, et al: Ultrasonography of the equine stifle. Vet Radiol 31:293, 1990.

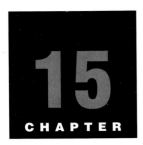

SONOGRAPHY OF EXOTIC ANIMALS

Robert E. Cartee and Pamela L. Johnson

GENERAL APPLICATIONS

The use of ultrasound in exotics dates back to 1975, when a 2-mHz transducer was used to perform cephalometry on 67 pregnant rhesus monkeys to determine normal versus suboptimal standards for intrauterine growth. Macaques and orangutans have been evaluated sonographically to determine pregnancy and embryonic loss, to predict fetal gestational age, and to assess normal fetal growth and development. Signs of pregnancy occur as early as 11 days, with positive identification on gestational days 16 to 18. Similarly, pregnant baboons have been monitored for studies in embryology as well as for normal changes in maternal blood pressure throughout gestation. Another form of prediction of gestational age was performed on baboons by measuring femur length and biparietal diameter. Previously, these studies necessitated the use of surgical procedures or blind injections, thereby increasing the risk of spontaneous abortion.

Obstetrically, real-time sonography is reliable for demonstrating placental implantation, cord insertion, fetal position, and viability. In one lowland gorilla, sonography proved the presence of fetal heart activity, ultimately preventing an inappropriate and potentially dangerous intervention. The value of this technology is no longer limited to obstetrics, however; sonography is also used in the assessment of urologic and abdominal disorders. Echocardiology is another application, for which ultrasound is used in the recognition of cardiac disorders and abnormalities. Sonography is also considered the best noninvasive technique for diagnosing soft tissue masses in the abdomen and pelvis, and is beneficial in the evaluation of lesions deep within solid organs.

Studies in primates designed to demonstrate the effects of ultrasound on the nervous system during and after a procedure showed that lower frequencies stimulate the central nervous system and higher frequencies tend to decrease central nervous system activity. Complete adaptation occurs within 3 minutes of continuous exposure, however, with no evidence that ultrasound promotes a risk to the integrity of neural tissue.[1-14]

Because of its increased availability, versatility, and invaluable assistance in diagnosis, sonography is now used to evaluate everything from deer to tapirs to reptiles, and most recently, marine mammals.

Deer

There have been several applications on red deer. With the use of an intrarectal linear array transducer during early pregnancy and a transabdominal sector scanner in late pregnancy, several observations have been made. Pregnancy was determined at day 30 with intrarectal scanning and at day 50 with transabdominal scanning. Sonographically derived fetal head diameter measurements predicted calving dates with a high degree of accuracy.[13] In a more detailed study, similar results were confirmed by recording measurements of uterine diameter, amniotic sac diameter, crown rump length, head length and diameter, nose length, chest depth and width, and placentoma base-apex length and width. The mean error of the calving date predictions for 132 deer was 0.97 days. Other species of deer have also been studied.[15–20]

Reptiles

In Indigo snakes, it is possible to detect heart movement and major blood vessels using a 5-mHz probe. Circulatory movements observed through exposed areas of shell membrane of Siamese crocodile eggs allowed documentation of in utero egg development without sacrificing the female or the eggs.[22] Ovary and egg imaging has been useful in several different species of turtles and tortoises, including the Kemp's Ridleys, Western Swamp tortoises, California desert tortoises, and Galapagos tortoises. Because many of these reptiles are endangered, these techniques have been and continue to be helpful in species preservation. In 1991, it was discovered that ultrasound could be used for monitoring ovarian function in reptiles. In one report, sonography was found to be of value in predicting litter size and embryo viability in the Cuban boa.[21–28]

Fish

Sonography provides an alternative method of determining gender in live fish. Previous methods involved radioimmunoassay of sex hormones, immunoagglutination techniques, or sacrificing the fish and examining them. These are all impractical because of time required, cost, or loss of specimens. Sonography does not allow positive identification of the ovary and testes in juvenile fish, but in mature salmon, it provides a rapid, noninvasive, accurate means of gender identification. This information is extremely valuable in fish industries. It has been suggested that these methods can also include other applications in fish, such as disease diagnosis (kidney inflammation), tissue bruise depth, and maturation and physiologic studies. Ultrasound has been helpful in detecting various parasites in fish tissue and has been used to monitor oocyte maturation.[29–31]

In studies at Auburn University, the abdominal organs of fish were studied and visualized. The ovary and testicle were difficult to distinguish, but the liver and gallbladder were easily seen (Fig. 15–1).

Other Animal Species

Laboratory species such as ferrets, rabbits, and rats have also been examined sonographically.[32–35] Other isolated instances of the use of sonography in zoo animals and wild animals have been reported, most related to pregnancy diagnosis but some involving the diagnosis of disease processes.[36–47]

Marine Mammals

The most recently reported benefit of the use of sonography has been in marine mammal diagnosis and research.[48–51] Although little has been done and even less has been published in this area, the use of ultrasound in these mammals has advantages.

Technique
Many aquatic animals require less preparation for the sonographic examination because of their lack of hair. Water, an excellent medium for transmittance, eliminates the need for some other coupling medium and, at the same time, allows the creature to stay in its environment. Because of their high intelligence level, with proper husbandry and train-

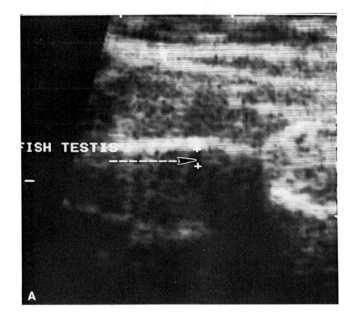

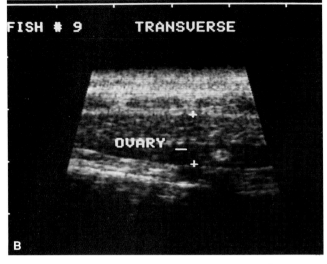

Figure 15–1

Sonograms of a spoonbill catfish. **A,** A 10-mHz scan of the testicle (arrow). **B,** A 10-mHz scan of the ovary (cursors). **C,** A sagittal 10-mHz scan of the abdomen. L, liver.

ing, most of these animals require no physical or chemical restraint for the examination. One of the minor negative aspects of this application occurred in one study performed outdoors. Without proper shading of the monitor, the clinician tended to increase the gain setting, causing distortion of the image of the structure being examined.[48]

As with other animals, a variety of transducers must be available. The type of transducer used depends on the variety and size of the species and, more particularly, the selection of organs to be examined. A 3.5-mHz probe is a good standard when evaluating the pleural surface of a dolphin (10 cm depth), whereas a 7.5-mHz (3 to 5 cm) probe provides high resolution with a shorter depth of field for studying the dolphin eye. Linear array imaging, normally used for transrectal imaging, is not feasible in marine mammals, but it can be used for structures in the abdominal cavity and to detect fluid in the thoracic or abdominal cavity.[48]

With trained animals, the examination procedure is relatively easy and usually of short duration. With dolphins, two trainers maintain stabilization in the water; one keeps eye and vocal contact while supporting and adjusting position by moving the head and pectoral fin and the other supports the peduncle. For longer procedures, the animal is manually restrained on foam pads, without the need for anesthesia. Pinnipeds can be trained for lateral and ventral recumbency as well as a vertical position on a stand. This kind of nonrestrained access prevents undo stress to the animal.[48]

As mentioned previously, no skin preparation is necessary with cetaceans. If the procedure is done out of the water, however, a coupling gel is used over the area to be scanned. Pinnipeds, with their extremely dense coat, often required sedation to be shaved. With generous amounts of coupling gel, however, sedation can be avoided. In some species, a blubber layer limits transduction of ultrasound. In these cases, for the best penetration, the use of lower frequency capacities, such as 2.0 to 3.5 mHz, are beneficial.[48,49]

Respiratory System

For evaluation of pulmonary parenchyma, radiography is considered more reliable than sonography, although some investigators have shown an advantage in using sonography for detecting pleural effusion.[48] In these cases, 3.5- to 5.0-mHz scanners were recommended for adult Tursiops. A 2.0- to 3.5-mHz probe was used for killer whales and pilot whales. For immature dolphins, otters, and smaller pinnipeds, a 5.0-mHz transducer was preferred. Clinically normal dolphins often show a slight irregularity or roughening of the ventral pleural surface, and this finding is not necessarily cause for concern. Follow-up scans ruled out possible inflammation.

When the lung is air filled, it is difficult to find a suitable cardiac window. The best probe position for viewing the heart seems to be on the ventral surface under the pectoral fin.[48]

The greatest cause of death in captive dolphins is bacterial pneumonia. In the evaluation of abnormalities resulting from such a condition, sector scanners were able to image in several planes with minimal acoustic shadowing and gave better results than linear array scanners.[48] Interruptions in the brightly echogenic line on the lung surface led to the diagnosis of pulmonary abscess. Biopsies are also possible with the aid of an ultrasound-guided needle. Other conditions recognized sonographically include chronic bronchopneumonia and pleural effusion. Echocardiology is performed on marine mammals, although no existing normal values are available.

Genitourinary Tract

Ultrasound has played an important role in managing reproduction in marine mammals. To reduce stress and obtain the best acoustic window, the recommendation is to examine pregnant dolphins in the water. The best window for visualization of the fetus is low on the lateral abdomen. Ovaries in T. truncatus are small and are acoustically similar to the surrounding tissue. Even when using the kidney as a landmark, ovaries are difficult to identify.[48,50,51]

In the male delphinid, the testicles are similar in appearance to human testicles and are located in the ventral abdominal wall. The acoustic window is low on the lateral abdominal wall near the genital slit. In juvenile Tursiops, the cigar-shaped testicles are 2 to 3 cm in diameter.[48]

As expected, the distended bladder is easily identified, and sonography is an excellent tool for detecting any abnormalities. The kidneys in delphinids are multilobar, lack an echogenic capsule, and often are difficult to recognize. Sea lion kidneys are more easily distinguished than those of the dolphin. In males, the testicles are landmarks to assist in the location of the kidney. To obtain an image of the complete kidney, a short axis sweep in two or more planes is preferred. Kidney diseases in marine mammals include renal calculi, cysts, neoplasms, and abscesses, but glomerular disease is rare in marine mammals.[48]

Gastrointestinal Tract

The sonographic appearance of the liver is similar to that of other species with one notable difference. In seals and sea lions, the hepatic venous sinus appears large. Clinicians theorize that this anatomic variation allows for heat conservation. For a complete examination, the liver should be viewed from both sides in longitudinal and transverse planes. Hepatomegaly can be detected by scanning the caudal border of the liver in a longitudinal plane. An increase in echogenicity is thought to be an indication of generalized liver disease. Hepatic abscessation or neoplasia appears as focal hypoechoic regions. Accuracy in the sonographic diagnosis of liver disease is continually improving and is limited only by the number of biopsies and necropsies performed to date.[48]

The spleen in T. truncatus is deep to the left lobe of the liver; small (8 cm), round, and smooth; and slightly more echogenic than the liver. It should be noted that the spleen is loosely attached and its position varies slightly. The pinniped spleen appears similar to that of the dog. Documentation in splenic abnormalities is limited at present, but it is increasing as more marine mammals are examined.[48]

Neoplasia

Neoplasia in marine mammals is becoming more and more prevalent. Some authors suggest that this increase is related to environmental chemical pollution. Sonography is currently used in the evaluation of thoracic and abdominal neoplasia in other species and will no doubt become standard practice in such cases involving marine mammals.[48]

Other Applications

Other possible uses for sonography in marine mammals include examination of eyes, muscle, blubber, and subcutaneous tissues.[48] For example, total blubber weight was estimated in southern elephant seals and this value was used to measure losses at different stages of lactation. Recent work at the navy research and development (NRaD) division in San Diego produced new images of the dolphin eye, skin, liver, kidney, and testicle and of fetal viability (Fig. 15–2). The dolphin eye, liver, and testicle were similar in appearance to those of other species. The dolphin kidney lacked cortical medullary regions and continued multiple hyperechoic focal regions. The skin was thick, but layers of epidermis and hyperdermis were visible. Advanced fetal development was detected easily in dolphins and fetal activity was apparent.

Two unique studies at Auburn involved imaging of the hepatopancreatic gland of the prawn (Fig. 15–3) and the fetuses of the brown bat (Fig. 15–4). In studies of the ostrich, sonograms showed in utero eggs, the liver, and the pectin of the eye (Fig. 15–5). In a study in snakes, abdominal sonograms showed developing reptile eggs and an obstructed lower digestive tract (Fig. 15–6). In examinations of exotic large cats, the kidneys of the tiger and jaguar were found to be identical to those of the common house cat (Fig. 15–7).

Because of the safety, simplicity, versatility, economic availability, and accuracy of sonography, its potential use in exotics is almost endless. As it is true in human clinical practice, the use of this technique is becoming more and more routine and indispensable in the diagnosis of many diseases in these species.

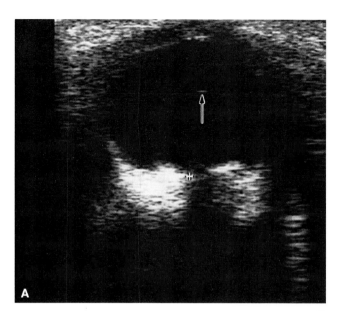

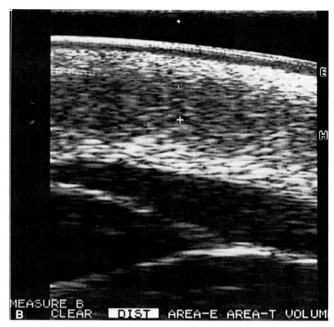

Figure 15–2

Sonograms of a dolphin. **A**, A 5-mHz scan of the eye. Arrow indicates the posterior lens capsule. **B**, A 7.5-mHz scan of the skin. E, epidermis/dermis; H, hypodermis. **C**, A 5-mHz scan of the liver (L). **D**, A 5-mHz scan of the kidney. Arrows indicate the hyperechoic regions not usually seen in other domestic species. **E**, A 5-mHz scan of the testicles (T). **F**, A 5-mHz scan of a viable fetus (arrow) in utero. Cursors indicate the width of the cranial vault.

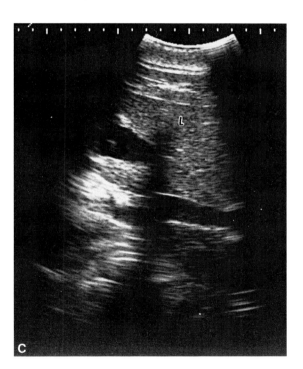

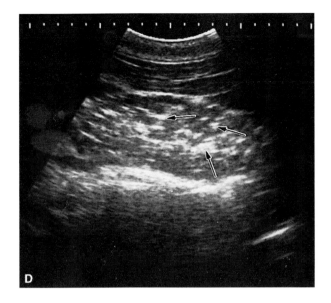

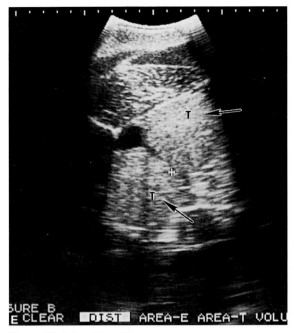

Figure 15–2 *(continued)*

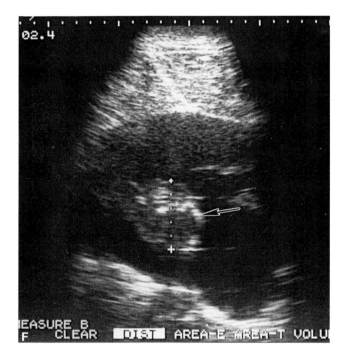

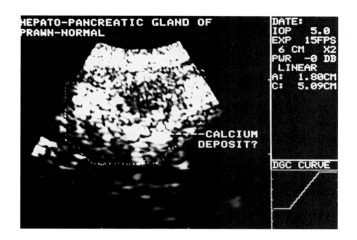

Figure 15–3

A 10-mHz scan of the hepatopancreatic gland of a prawn. Cuticle removal was necessary to scan this organ. A hyperechoic area may have been a calcium deposit.

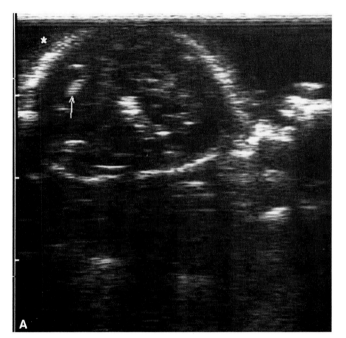

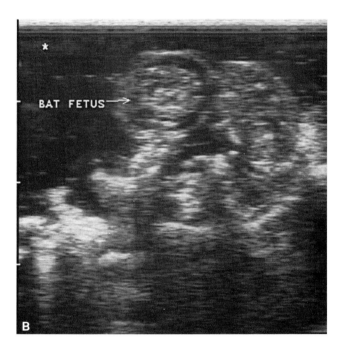

Figure 15–4

Sonograms of a brown bat. **A,** A 7.5-mHz scan of the abdomen. Arrow indicates the rib cage of one of the developing embryos. **B,** Surgically exposed uterus scanned with a 7.5-mHz probe in a water bath.

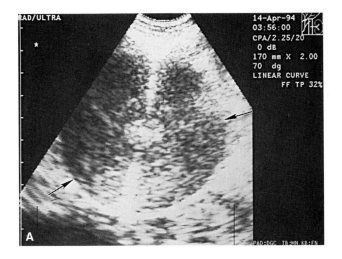

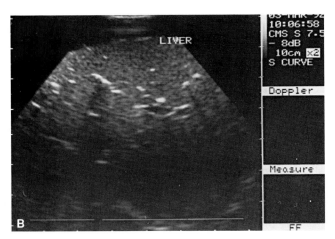

Figure 15–5

Sonograms of an ostrich. **A,** A 2.25-mHz scan of the caudal abdomen shows the spherical developing egg (arrow). Note the hyperechoic central structure. **B,** A 7.5-mHz scan of the liver. **C,** A 7.5-mHz scan of the eye shows the large pectin (arrow) in the vitreous (V). A, anterior chamber; L, lens.

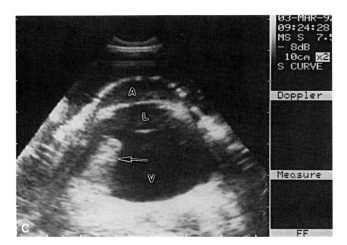

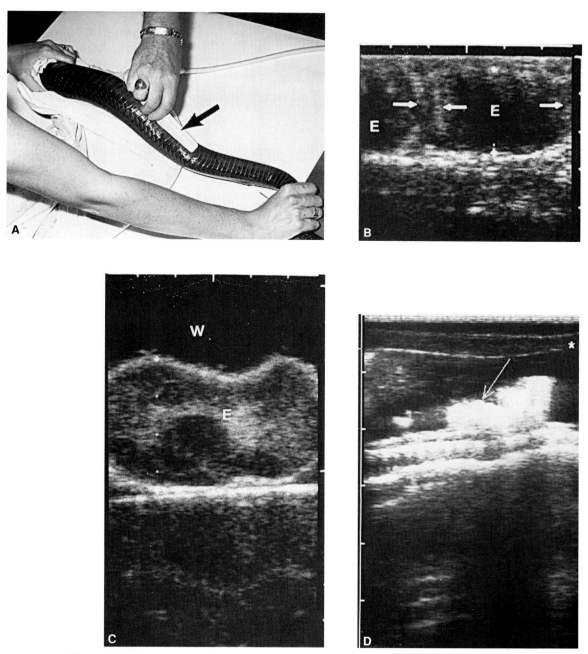

Figure 15–6

A, Placement of a 5-mHz probe on the ventral abdomen of the Eastern Indigo snake for diagnosis of pregnancy. **B,** In utero appearance of the eggs (E) (5 mHz). **C,** Water bath scan (5 mHz) of the snake egg. W, water. **D,** Arrow indicates large hyperechoic fecolith in the lower bowel of a small boa constrictor.

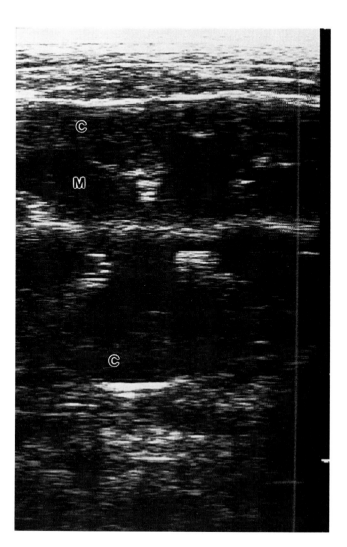

Figure 15–7

A 5-mHz scan of the left kidney of a tiger. C, cortex; M, medulla.

REFERENCES

1. Sabbagha RE, Turner H, Chez DA: Sonar biparietal diameter growth standards in the rhesus monkey. Am J Obstet Gynecol 1:371, 1975.
2. Tarantal AF, Hendricks AG: Use of ultrasound for early pregnancy detection in the rhesus and cynomolgus macaque. J Med Primatol 17:105, 1988.
3. Tarantal AF, Hendricks AG: Characterization of prenatal growth and development in the crab-eating macaque by ultrasound. Anat Rec 222:177, 1988.
4. Conrad SH, Sackett GP, Burbacher TM: Diagnosis of early pregnancy in *Macaca fascicularis.* J Med Primatol 18:143, 1989.
5. Cho F, et al: Early pregnancy diagnosis by the ultrasonographical device and observation of fetal growth in cynomolgus monkeys. Jikken Dobutsu 36:223, 1987.
6. Tarantal AF: International ultrasound in pregnant macaques; embryonic fetal application. J Med Primatol 19:47, 1990.
7. Hu JH, Ulrich WD: Effects of low-intensity ultrasound on the central nervous system of primates. Aviat Space Environ Med June, 1976, p. 640.
8. James Jr AE, et al: The use of diagnostic ultrasound in evaluation of the abdomen in primates with emphasis on the rhesus monkey. J Med Primatol 5:160, 1976.
9. Stoskopf MK, Sanders RC: Application of diagnostic ultrasound in nonhuman primates. Annual Proceedings of the American Association of Zoo Veterinarians, 1980, pp. 110–113.
10. James Jr PE, et al: Radiologic imaging of human diseases in exotic animals. JAMA 235:184, 1976.

11. Karesh WB: The use of ultrasonography in zoo medicine. Annual Proceedings of the American Association of Zoo Veterinarians, 1983.

12. O'Grady JP, et al: Practical applications of real time ultrasound scanning to problems of zoo veterinary medicine. J Zoo Ann Med *9:*52, 1978.

13. Adler J, et al: Graviditatsuberwachung mittels ostriol bestimmung und ultra schalluntersuch ung bei einem sumatra-orang-utan (Pongo Pygmaevs Abeli). Erkrankungen Zootiere *28:*203, 1986.

14. Brans Y, et al: Maternal blood pressure and fetal ultrasonography in normal baboon pregnancies. J Med Primatol *19:*641, 1990.

15. White IR, et al: Diagnosis of pregnancy and prediction of fetal age in red deer by real-time ultrasonic scanning. Vet Rec *124:*395, 1989.

16. Wilson PR, Bingham CM: Accuracy of pregnancy diagnosis and prediction of calving date in red deer using real-time ultrasound scanning. Vet Rec *126:*133, 1990.

17. Jabbour HN, Veldhuizen FA, Green G, Asher GW: Endocrine responses and conception rates in fallow deer (Dama Dama) following oestrous synchronization and cervical insemination with fresh or frozen-thawed spermatozoa. Jrnl of Reprod and Fertility *89*: 2, 495–502, 1993.

18. Sempere AJ, Renand G, Baritoan F: Embryonic development measured by ultrasonography and plasma progesterone concentrations in Roe deer. Anim Reprod Sci *20:*155, 1989.

19. Bingham CM, Wilson PR, Davies AS: Red time ultrasonography for pregnancy diagnosis and estimation of fetal age in farmed red deer. Vet Rec *126:*102, 1990.

20. Mulley RC, et al: Pregnancy diagnosis of fallow deer by ultrasonography. Aust Vet J *64:*257, 1987.

21. Smith CR, et al: Radiographic and ultrasonographic scanning of gravid eastern indigo snakes. J Herpatol *23:*426, 1989.

22. Schildger BJ, et al: The use of diagnostic imaging methods in reptiles. Berl Munch Tierarztl Wochenschr *104:*20, 1991.

23. Sainsbury AW, Gili C: Ultrasonographic anatomy and scanning techniques of the coelonic organs of the bosc monitor. J Zoo Wildl Med *22:*421, 1991.

24. Kuchling G, Bradshaw SD: Ovarian cycle and egg production of the Western swamp tortoise Pseudemydura-umbrina testudines chelidae in the wild and in captivity. J Exp Zool *229:*405, 1993.

25. Penninck DG, et al: Ultrasonography of the California desert tortoise (Xerobates Agassizi): Anatomy and application. Vet Radiol *32:*112, 1991.

26. Rostal DC, et al: Ultrasound imaging of ovaries and eggs in Kemp's Ridley sea turtles. J Zoo Wildl Med *21:*27, 1990.

27. Robeck TR, et al: Ultrasound imaging of reproductive organs and eggs in galapagos tortoises Geochelose-elephantopus. Zoo Biol *9:*349, 1990.

28. Tolson PJ, et al: Determination of litter size and embryo viability in the cuban boa, *Epicrates angulifer,* by use of imaging ultrasonography. Proceedings of the American Reptile Symposium, 1983, pp. 118–123.

29. Hafsteinsson H, et al: Application of ultrasound waves to detect sealworms in fish tissue. J Food Sci *54:*244, 1991.

30. Boyce NP: Ultrasound imaging used to detect cysts of Henneguya-Salminccola Protozoa Myxozoa in the flesh of whole Pacific Salmon. Can J Fish Aquatic Sci *42:*1312, 1985.

31. Shields RJ, et al: Oocyte maturation and ovulation in the Atlantic halibut. Aquaculture Fish Management *24:*181, 1993.

32. Peter AT, et al: Real-time ultrasonographic determination of pregnancy and gestational age in ferrets. Lab Anim Sci *40:*91, 1990.

33. Inaba T, Mori J, Torii R: Use of echography in rabbits for pregnancy diagnosis. Nippon Juigaku Zasshi *47:*523, 1985.

34. Inaba T, Inoue A: Use of echography in rats for pregnancy diagnosis. Nippon Juigaku Zasshi *47:*525, 1985.

35. Tello de Meneses R, Mesa MD, Gonyaley V: Echocardiographic assessment of cardiac function in a rabbit: A preliminary study. Ann Rech Vet *20:*175, 1989.

36. Adams GP, et al: Feasibility of characterizing reproductive events in lare non domestic species by transrectal ultrasonic imaging. Zoo Biol *10:*247, 1991.

37. Tachibana M: Observation of images of pregnancy by real-time ultrasonography in dairy cattle, pigs, sheep and brown bears. Jpn J Vet Res *34:*160, 1986.

38. Durrant BS, Hoge ML: Ultrasonography in a Przewalski's Horse Mare, Eques pizewalski. Theriogenology *29:*240, 1988.

39. Bourke DA, Adam CL, Kyle CE: Ultrasonography as an aid to controlled breeding in the llama (Lama glama). Vet Rec *130:*424, 1992.

40. Gizejewski Z, Skowron M, Snochowski M: Ultrasonographic control of ovulatory time in female hybrids of European bison and domestic cattle after oestrus synchronization. Proc Int Symp Ungulates *129:*569, 1991.

41. Fialoc L, Hojovcova M, Chvatal O: Pregnancy diagnosis in domestic and exotic animals using ultrasonics. Veterinarstri *3:*116, 1986.

42. Gorman NT: Oncology. Contemp Issues Small Anim Pract *9:*1, 1986.

43. Scientific Report, 1984–1987. UK Zoological Society of London. Regents Park, London, 1988.

44. Stoskopf MK: Clinical imaging in zoological medicine: A review. J Zoo Wildl Med *20:*396, 1989.

45. Fiola L, Hogovcova M, Chvatal O: Pregnancy diagnosis in exotic animals by means of ultrasound. Verhandlungsbericht-des-Internationalen-Symposiums-uber-die- Erkrankungen-der Zootiere *26:*69, 1984.

46. Bonlay GH, Wilson OL, DuBoulay GH: Diagnosis of pregnancy and disease by ultrasound in exotic species. Symposium of the Zoological Society of London *60:*135, 1988.
47. Chaduc F, Franck M, Mercier-Parisot P: Feasibility and development of sectional echography for monitoring reproduction and clinical investigations in zoo animals. Internationalem Symposiums uber die Erkrankwogen der Zoo und Wildtiere *23:*277, 1990.
48. Dierauf LA, ed: *CRC Handbook of Marine Mammal Medicine*, Boca Raton, FL, CRC Press, 1992, pp. 235–263.
49. Gales NJ, Burton HR: Ultrasonic measurement of blubber thickness in southern elephant seal. Aust J Zool *35:*207, 1987.
50. Locave G, Boudroeijnpark A: A survey of management practices for dolphin pregnancy with two examples of birth complications. Aquatic Mammol *17:*37, 1991.
51. Williamson P, Gales NJ, Lister S: Use of real time B-mode ultrasound for pregnancy diagnosis and measurement of fetal growth rate in captive bottlenose dolphins. J Reprod Fertil *88:*543, 1990.

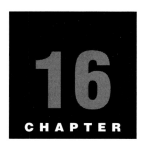

THE MARKET STATUS
AND FUTURE APPLICATIONS
OF SONOGRAPHY

Ken W. Marich

Diagnostic ultrasound has become a permanent part of imaging technology in veterinary medicine. From its birth in the 1940s as a nonimaging Doppler technique used for military purposes, i.e., sonar, medical sonography has evolved over the last five decades into a highly sophisticated science that now enjoys the role of most cost-effective diagnostic imaging tool. The science of diagnostic ultrasound has progressed in its development through the experimental era (1940s and 1950s), the imaging era (1960s and 1970s), and the Doppler era (1980s and 1990s). From the earliest two-dimensional compound images obtained with whole body immersion,[1] image quality has steadily improved with direct contact scanning, gray-scale tissue differentiation, digital scan conversion, real-time sector scanning, and electronic array technology. Echo Doppler techniques have also improved, evolving from simple audio output of frequency shifts to spectral displays from continuous wave (CW) Doppler, quantitative spectral analysis of range-gated pulsed wave (PW) Doppler, color Doppler imaging, and ultrasound angiography.[2,3]

The application of ultrasound in veterinary medicine began in the late 1970s and experienced rapid growth in the 1980s. During this period, many ultrasound systems were installed at veterinary teaching institutions as diagnostic instruments for both small and large animals, for reproductive examinations, for use in the food production industry, and for basic animal research to further the understanding of disease processes. With the increased exposure of veterinary students to diagnostic ultrasound and the introduction of lower priced ultrasound systems, the technology gained wider attention in the veterinary marketplace. Now in the 1990s, all teaching institutions have ultrasound systems, with many owning several high performance, multifunctional units incorporating multiple probe types and various Doppler capabilities, including color Doppler imaging. The future looks bright for diagnostic ultrasound in veterinary medicine as this imaging/Doppler technology continues to demonstrate its value in both institutional and private practices.

Significant advances in this technology have improved diagnostic capability, and a wide range of systems and features is available to the practitioner. Specialty ultrasound courses are now offered on a regular basis for those wanting to learn sonography and so incorporate it into their practice. The list of applications for medical ultrasound continues to grow each year, and although many of these uses are included in this book, this chapter provides an overview of growth trends, current status, and selected topics that will most likely impact the future of diagnostic and therapeutic ultrasound in veterinary medical practice.

MARKET STATUS

In 1993 and 1994, a survey was taken to establish the history and current status of ultrasound and its diagnostic use in veterinary medicine.[4] Completed survey questionnaires were received from 27 schools of veterinary medicine in North America as well as from 35 private practitioners that routinely use sonography in their practice. The results clearly indicate that ultrasound is an important diagnostic tool in veterinary medicine. During the period between 1979 and 1987, ultrasound imaging and Doppler techniques have been incorporated as a primary diagnostic method in all veterinary medicine teaching institutions (Fig. 16–1).

The diagnostic utility of sonography and the growing number of veterinary applications for ultrasound, particularly in the fields of abdominal, cardiovascular, and reproductive (obstetrical) examinations, have resulted in the use of multiple systems at many institutions. Currently, most teaching facilities have between three and six ultrasound systems located in various hospital departments or for field use in mobile vehicles.

In the private sector, 58% of practices have one ultrasound system and 42% have two or more systems (Fig. 16–2). As veterinarians become more familiar with the diagnostic advantages of sonography, more and more practitioners will use this technology in their practice.

In the United States, total annual sales revenues for veterinary ultrasound systems continue to grow at an impressive rate as this technology diffuses into all aspects, i.e., hos-

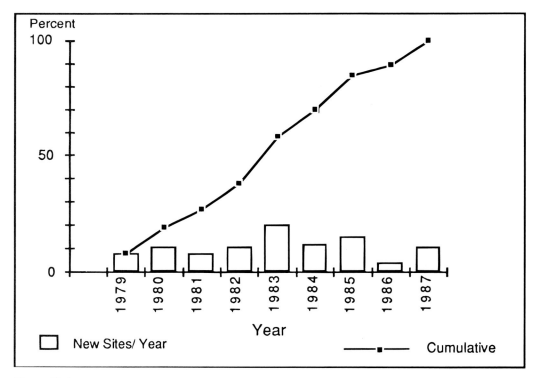

Figure 16–1

Institutional adoption of diagnostic sonography.

pital, office, and field settings for small and large animal use, as well as in the food animal industry. It is estimated that by the year 1996, over 1300 systems will be sold per year into veterinary environments (Table 16–1).

The ultrasound systems most often used in veterinary medicine tend to be those with a price in the low to middle range. These systems combine both linear and sector imaging, with some units providing integrated spectral Doppler capabilities. The survey results indicated that ultrasound imaging systems manufactured by Aloka, Corometrics, ATL, and Ausonics dominate the current installed base at veterinary teaching institutions (Fig. 16–3). With the advent of multiple probe configurations, quantitative Doppler, and color Doppler imaging, it is estimated that higher priced, high performance systems will be purchased in the future, particularly at teaching institutions. As of 1994, most veterinary teaching institutions were already using a variety of Doppler techniques (Fig. 16–4).

This growth appears to be fueled by an increased awareness of the diagnostic capabilities of sonography, appropriate budget allocations for ultrasound systems, and the availability of educational courses that ultimately stimulate interest and a decision regarding purchase. Approximately 75% of all schools of veterinary medicine surveyed offer

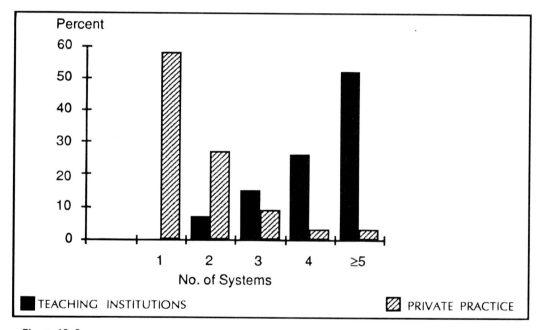

Figure 16–2

Number of installed ultrasound systems (1994).

TABLE 16–1
United States Veterinary Ultrasound Sales Revenues, 1986-1996

Year	Sales Revenues ($ Millon)	Annualized Growth Rate
1986	9.4	—
1989	13.5	14.5%
1992	17.4	9.6%
1996	26.6	13.2%

Source: Market Intelligence Research Corporation[5]

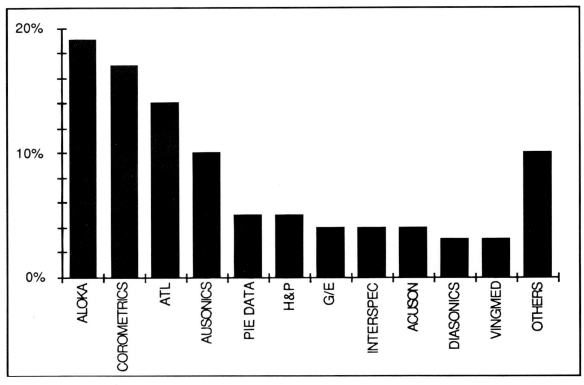

Figure 16–3

Ultrasound installations by manufacturer in teaching institutions.

courses in diagnostic ultrasound. In addition, the incorporation of veterinary sessions at major medical and scientific meetings has helped to stimulate interest and growth in diagnostic sonography.

With greater use of sonographic techniques to assist in the diagnosis of disease states in a wide variety of animals, the number of sonographic procedures done at teaching institutions and in private practice has significantly increased (Fig. 16–5). Approximately 85% of all veterinary teaching institutions conduct between 25 and 200 sonographic procedures per month, with 15% reporting monthly case loads greater than 200 procedures. As might be expected, the total number of sonographic procedures conducted by private practitioners is less than their institutional counterparts, although 24% reported doing more than 50 procedures per month.

Sonographic techniques are now being used in a wide variety of animals, as shown in Table 16–2. Even with different species, however, the diagnostic sonographic procedures for animals parallel those specific procedures used in human medicine. Abdominal, cardiac, and reproductive (obstetric) examinations dominate the procedures routinely conducted in veterinary practice (Fig. 16–6). In teaching institutions, ultrasound-guided biopsies and ocular examinations are among the most common applications. Other sonographic procedures being performed with increasing frequency include musculoskeletal (tendon/ligament) evaluations, noncardiac vascular blood flow studies, intraoperative ultrasound, and neurosonography. As the technology improves, this positive growth trend in the use of ultrasound in veterinary medicine, which has accelerated over the last 10 years, will undoubtedly continue.

In her article on health care for pets, Marguerite T. Smith stated that "Americans pay out $20.3 billion a year on their pets, about half of that on health care. . . . From 1987 to

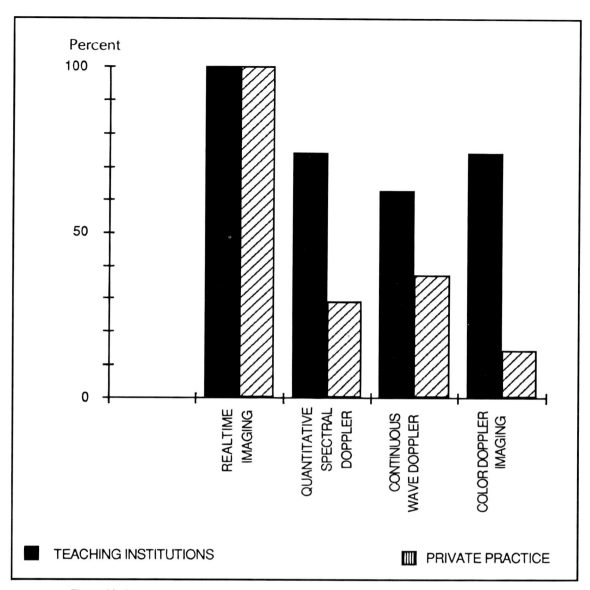

Figure 16–4

Ultrasound technology used in veterinary medicine (1994).

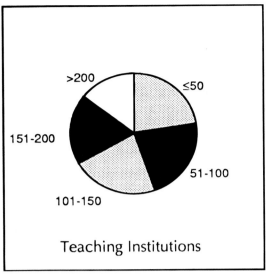
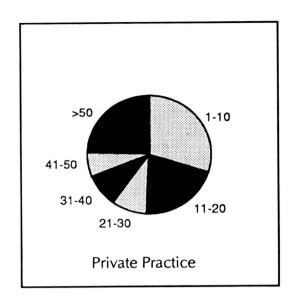

Figure 16–5

Diagnostic sonographic examinations per month (1994)

TABLE 16–2
Diagnostic Sonographic Procedures by Animal Species

Animal Species	Teaching Institution (%)	Private Practice (%)
Canine	18	40
Equine	18	10
Bovine	18	5
Avian	10	4
Other	18	1

1991, national expenditures for veterinary services climbed from $5 billion to $7.4 billion—a 49% jump."[6] Although the procedural fees of other imaging methods such as computed tomography (CT) and magnetic resonance (MR) imaging for animals is high (range: $250 to $1000),[6] diagnostic sonography is a cost-effective imaging tool that has the potential to generate significant annual revenues. Survey results showed that the overall range of prices charged for sonographic procedures, in both teaching institutions and private practice, is $20 to $165 (Table 16–3). These fees are consistent with the technical skill and time required for the examination as well as the cost of the equipment.

In conclusion, it is clear that diagnostic sonography has had a major impact on the practice of veterinary medicine. Developmentally, teaching institutions will continue to be the major influence in the positive growth of this specialty as more advanced technology is introduced into the educational and diagnostic environment. Clinically, combining real-time imaging with Doppler techniques will provide a practical approach to diagnostics in many animal species and in most parts of the body where there is acoustic access. Economically, diagnostic sonography remains cost effective and has the potential to increase institutional and private practice veterinary annual revenues. The future of diagnostic sonography in veterinary medicine is bright and holds promise for all those willing to learn this discipline.

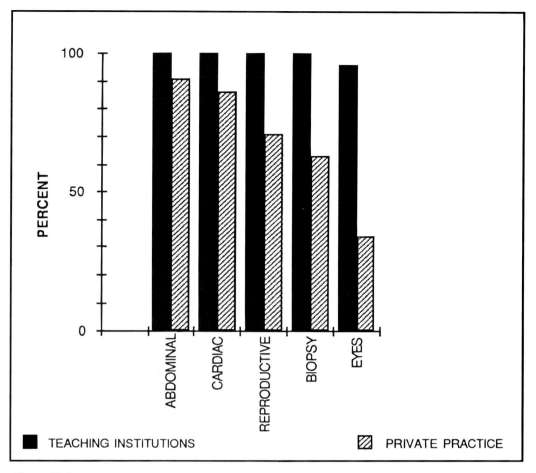

Figure 16–6

Veterinary sonographic procedures by application.

TABLE 16–3
Sonographic Procedure Fee by Application (1994)

Examination	Teaching Institution		Private Practice	
	Mean ($)	Range ($)	Mean ($)	Range ($)
Abdominal	54	30–110	93	50–165
Cardiac	59	35–165	100	35–165
Reproductive	40	20–75	56	29–120
Biopsy	70	35–90	71	60–85
Ocular	50	40–60	—	—
Musculoskeletal	46	30–75	82	75–90
Vascular	46	30–90	50	50–85
Intraoperative	52	30—90	68	35–130

FUTURE APPLICATIONS

Color Doppler Imaging

Color Doppler imaging (CDI), a recent extension of duplex ultrasound technology, has revolutionized its clinical utility. Duplex sonography combines the advantages of sonography providing morphologic information (anatomic data) with Doppler blood flow information (hemodynamic data) to assist in the detection of disease.[7] Color Doppler imaging adds an additional dimension that allows visualization of blood flow in the image, providing a powerful noninvasive tool to diagnose disease in almost every part of the body where acoustic access is possible. The addition of CDI promises to make the Doppler data more readily understandable when compared to conventional Doppler techniques of plotting complex spectral frequency and velocity displays. In fact, CDI will most likely supersede the use of continuous wave (CW) and pulsed waved (PW) Doppler techniques, because it rapidly allows vascular evaluation of the entire B-scan image field and facilitates more accurate placement of the discrete Doppler sample volume or range gate to study localized flow characteristics.

Color Doppler imaging, introduced in the middle 1980s, found initial acceptance in the areas of cardiac and peripheral vessel evaluation. Its use has since expanded to whole body vascular evaluation, and is limited only by the principles of Doppler physics and the skill level of the user. The technique provides noninvasive imaging of blood flow based on Doppler frequency shifts resulting from moving blood cells in vessels in the ultrasound field of view. The color-coded blood flow display (map) is simultaneously superimposed on the B mode image, thus providing a complete evaluation of both anatomy and blood flow dynamics over the entire two-dimensional fields of view. When using CDI, the color-coded image of flowing blood acts as a contrast agent that outlines the patent lumen of vessels and pinpoints areas of vascular pathologic change. Thus, the Doppler flow information is given spatial orientation, similar to angiography, which displays the spatial details of flow in relationship to anatomy and improves diagnostic capability.

The basic characteristics of blood flow displayed in the Doppler flow map are direction of flow, mean (relative) velocity, size and shape of vessels or chambers, and the extent of flow disturbances, which are visually displayed over the gray-scale image by means of color encoding of the Doppler-generated flow signal. The standard convention for color coding is to use red for flow toward the transducer and blue for flow away from the transducer, although most CDI systems allow the user to assign the color-code scheme regardless of vessel angle or direction of interrogation. In addition to direction, mean velocity information is displayed as varying hues of either red or blue. The brighter the hue, the faster the relative velocity and the duller the hue, the slower the velocity. Additional color maps (yellow, green) can also be used to distinguish disturbed flow or turbulence (an abnormal spread of frequencies around the mean frequency) and allows the user to discriminate between normal and abnormal flow states (Fig. 16–7). Color Doppler imaging has proven to be an exceedingly useful adjunct to conventional duplex sonography and, in fact, can shorten examination time, improve diagnostic confidence, and facilitate more reproducible quantitative spectral Doppler analysis.

Because CDI has the advantages of being noninvasive, portable, and relatively inexpensive when compared to angiographic equipment, it will find a unique role in diagnostic veterinary medicine. Its potential clinical applications are broad and will expand as users explore its diagnostic usefulness in a wide variety of animals. Some of the more common current applications of CDI include the following:

Echocardiography - For detection of valvular regurgitation, abnormal septal defects, flow through great vessels, and the presence of stenotic jets (Fig. 16–8).

Peripheral Vascular Disease - For detection of arterial stenoses, detection of venous thrombosis and venous flow patterns, development of aneurysms, and assessment of vessel patency postoperatively and after angioplasty.

Abdominal Region - For the evaluation of blood flow to critical organs (Fig. 16–9), flow characteristics in the portal and hepatic veins and hepatic artery, detection of renal artery stenosis, and detection of vascular abnormalities associated with organ-specific tumor growth.

Organ Function - As an adjunct to other imaging techniques to evaluate organ function and structure based on blood perfusion (Fig. 16–10).

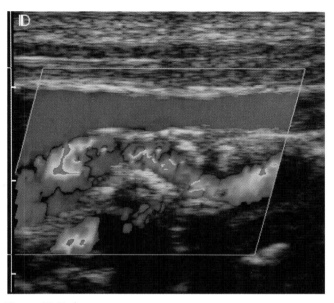

Figure 16–7

Color Doppler image displays blood flow in the internal jugular vein (blue) and disturbed flow patterns in the internal and external carotoid arteries (courtesy of Diasonics, Milpitas, CA).

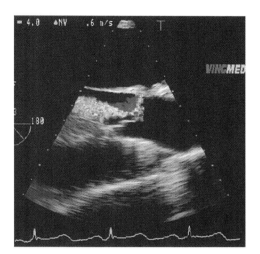

Figure 16–8

Color flow Doppler image reveals aortic insufficiency in this view of the left ventricular outflow tract (courtesy of Vingmed Sound, San Francisco, CA).

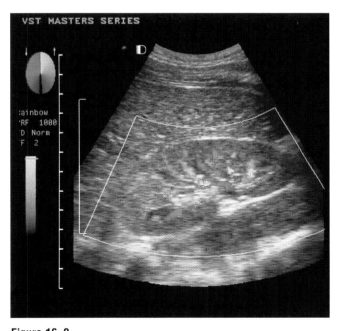

Figure 16–9

Improved sensitivity with Color Doppler clearly shows detailed blood flow patterns in the branching arcuate arteries in the kidney (courtesy of Diasonics, Milpitas, CA).

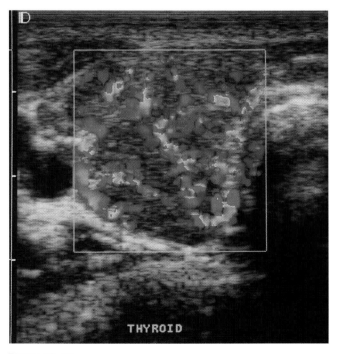

Figure 16–10

Color Doppler imaging demonstrates glandular tissue perfusion, as in this thyroid image, as it relates to tumor neovascularization or other flow abnormalities (courtesy of Diasonics, Milpitas, CA).

Oncology - Quantitative evaluation of tumor flow may provide a means of assessing tumor response to radiotherapy.

The diagnostic application of CDI continues to expand rapidly. Integration of color flow mapping with three-dimensional imaging has achieved promising results.[8] The ability to display the blood flow architecture and characteristics through tumor tissue three dimensionally may provide new criteria for more accurate detection and differential diagnosis of benign and malignant conditions.

Ultrasound Angiography

An important new enhancement to color Doppler imaging systems is the use of amplitude-based Doppler information to map blood vessels down to 1 mm in diameter. This new technology significantly improves sensitivity and spatial resolution, with the potential to allow the evaluation of tissue perfusion and blood flow found in vascular beds. Several manufacturers (Diasonics, ATL, Acuson) have developed this highly sensitive, real-time imaging technique that creates detailed vascular flow profiles similar to those seen with angiography.

Unlike CDI, "ultrasound angiography" uses amplitude rather than frequency shifts to identify blood presence or density of red blood cells within the volume sampled by the ultrasound beam rather than blood flow velocity. The resultant color flow display is independent of velocity, angle, and directional information and allows precise visualization of blood flow in all vessels, including small vessels, tortuous vasculature, and vessels at angles that are difficult to evaluate with conventional CDI. Because Doppler frequency shifts are not translated into images, the vasculature displayed is uniform in color, regardless of the blood flow direction.

A more recent innovation with ultrasound angiography takes advantage of its improved sensitivity and edge definition using blood/tissue discrimination algorithms. The discriminator amplifies the distinction between extremely small vessels and adjacent tissue in a manner similar to a topographic map. Thus, differentiation of microvasculature can be readily visualized by using a highly dimensional display that creates an embossed look at the edge of the vessels. As an example, the ultrasound topographic display of renal blood flow clearly delineates the presence of microvasculature (blood flow perfusion) at the edge of the renal cortex (Fig. 16–11).

Another interesting application of ultrasound angiography, leveraging on its increased dynamic range over conventional CDI, may be in detecting increased soft tissue perfusion; it might be possible to monitor the effects of therapy on tissue hyperemia resulting from musculoskeletal inflammatory and infectious diseases.[9]

Both ultrasound angiography and topographic mapping are complementary to CDI and promise to expand the horizons of potential applications of this dynamic Doppler technique in veterinary medicine.

Intracorporeal Sonography

Externally applied extracorporeal or transcutaneous sonography is the conventional technique used for many clinical applications. Over the last several decades, however, clinical researchers have attempted to place miniaturized ultrasound transducers in vessels and various body cavities. Technologic advances, coupled with miniaturization of transducers and custom-designed probes, have sparked the growth of what is now emerging as a new field of interest, "intracorporeal sonography." For the purposes of this discussion, intracorporeal sonography is presented with respect to three types of applications: endoluminal, intraoperative, and laparoscopic.

Endoluminal Sonography
The first attempts to visualize organs via a body cavity were with endorectal probes, fol-

lowed by transducers inside of endoscopes (both rigid and flexible) to evaluate the esophagus (Fig. 16–12), stomach, and heart. This endoscopic application was further adapted to a transvaginal technique used to evaluate the uterus and ovaries and transurethrally to evaluate the urinary bladder.[10,11]

With the development of miniaturized probes, with diameters in the millimeter range, a new set of endoluminal applications is evolving. Strong interest has been shown for the evaluation of peripheral blood vessels, coronary artieries, and aortic abnormalities (Fig. 16–13) using small, high-frequency (10 to 30-mHz), catheter-based transducers for high resolution visualization of vascular structures.[12] Endoluminal sonography has drawn great interest and will establish itself as an important diagnostic tool.

Intraoperative Sonography

Intraoperative ultrasound (IOUS) imaging has been slow in gaining acceptance. In human medicine, this slow evolution has resulted in part from nonoptimized equipment, the lack of third party reimbursement, and the unfamiliarity of the surgeon with sonography. In veterinary medicine, because reimbursement is not as important an issue, IOUS has the potential to become a valuable addition to surgical practice as more custom ultrasound probes are developed. Direct intraoperative sonographic examinations provide a practical method to identify anatomic relationships, recognize anomalies, detect pathologic lesions, and determine their resectability.[13]

Survey results show that close to 50% of all veterinary teaching institutions are using IOUS, whereas only 3% of private practice groups reported the use of intraoperative sonography.

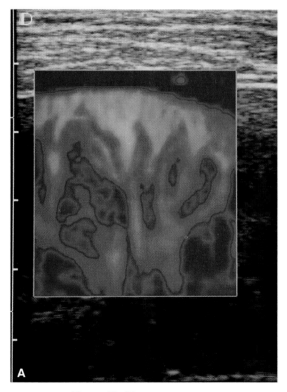 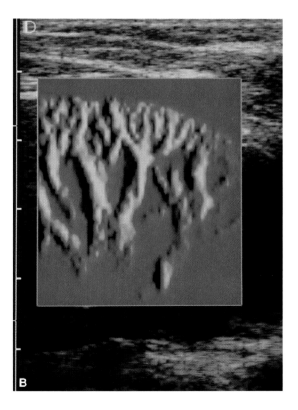

Figure 16–11

A, UltrasoundAngio vascular profiles of cortical blood flow perfusion in the kidney is similar to flow patterns seen with x-ray angiography. **B,** Discrete renal microvasculature is demonstrated using a sensitive blood/tissue discrimination algorithm that creates a topographic blood flow map (courtesy of Diasonics, Milpitas, CA).

Figure 16–12

Endoluminal 12.5-mHz sonogram displays the five layers of the esophagus (courtesy of Diasonics, Milpitas, CA).

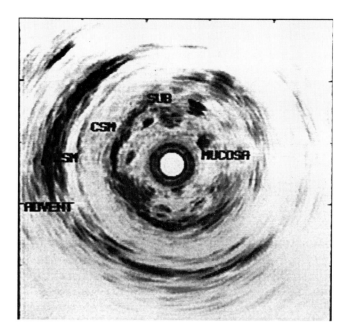

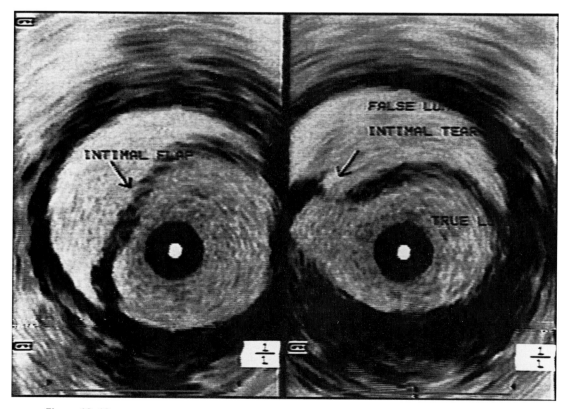

Figure 16–13

Endoluminal 12.5-mHz sonogram allowed detection of a dissecting aortic aneurysm showing an intimal tear with an expanding false lumen (courtesy of Diasonics, Milpitas, CA).

Historically, attempts to use A mode ultrasound in open surgery were first reported in the early 1960s for localization of renal stones[14] and common bile duct stones.[15] With the introduction of real-time B mode imaging in the late 1970s came a renewed interest in using ultrasound intraoperatively.

Real-time scanning has many advantages in the surgical environment and was quickly used to assist and expedite surgical treatment. With practice, IOUS was used to examine the common bile duct and accurately localize and characterize masses of all types. Since then, it has proven useful for biopsy guidance, cyst aspiration, and directed resection of tumors. Because lesions can be precisely localized, the need for exploration as well as blind and unnecessary dissection is reduced. With multiplane IOUS imaging, precise localization of normal anatomic structures reduces the potential for their injury during procedures, and no contrast materials or ionizing radiation are required.

Intraoperative sonography has several device requirements that, to this date, have not all been met in one probe, i.e., small size, variable frequency (3.0 to 7.5 mHz), suitable penetrability, and easy sterilizability. Even without the "ideal" probe, IOUS has great potential in veterinary surgery for a wide spectrum of applications.

In the abdomen, IOUS should prove to be an important imaging tool for the liver, bile ducts, pancreas, kidney, gallbladder, and extrahepatic biliary ductal system, and it appears to be an ideal method for delineating liver lesions, especially metastases. Several studies in man have determined that intraoperative sonography of the liver appears to be more accurate for the detection of common bile duct stones[16] and intrahepatic metastases than either CT or sonography performed preoperatively.[17] Intraoperative sonography can also help detect nonpalpable tumors, guide the direction of liver transection, assist biopsy of small nodules, and guide catheterization into the bile duct.

Although the pancreas is one of the most difficult organs to assess adequately with extracorporeal sonography, IOUS may influence the management of pancreatitis and pancreatic neoplasms. For pancreatitis, IOUS can be used to localize the pancreatic duct, detect nonpalpable intrapancreatic pseudocysts, and direct needle aspirations of fluid collections. For cancer surgery, IOUS can assist in selecting the optimal site for biopsy, as well as provide visualization of the tumor margin to aid intraoperative staging before resection.[18,19]

Intraoperative sonography is useful in the evaluation of the gallbladder and biliary tract. Visualization of gallstones as well as exploration of the common bile duct are possible without the use of ionizing radiation and contrast agents. Other applications include intraoperative renal sonography for the localization or sizing of renal stones, which can help to minimize the surgical nephrotomy. In the evaluation of the brain and spinal cord, IOUS has been used primarily to localize lesions and to direct dissectional or needle aspiration biopsies.

Although IOUS is in its infancy, its diagnostic and therapeutic applications in veterinary medicine promise to grow with increased usage, improved technology, and more exposure to its advantages, particularly in teaching institutions.

Laparoscopic Sonography

Laparoscopic sonography is the newest entry in the field of surgical sonography, and is a logical extension of IOUS. The concept of using ultrasound laparoscopically in the abdomen was first reported in 1964,[20] but not until 1982 were the first real-time two-dimensional imaging studies reported.[21]

The ability to examine the surface of organs and structures within the abdominal cavity from outside the body is now a reality with the use of a laparoscope. In comparison to open surgery, however, this technique has inherent limitations, including restricted fields of view with difficulty in hand-eye coordination, lack of binocular vision and depth perception, and lack of tactile sensory feedback, which is useful in the detection of palpable tumors. Laparoscopic sonography holds the potential to alleviate some of these limitations by providing the surgeon with another visual dimension, i.e., the ability to see into organs and structures.

Several manufacturers are developing custom ultrasound probes that are designed to fit through a 10-mm laparoscope trocar. Different imaging configurations providing end-on and side-looking transducers are currently available (Fig. 16–14). With the addition of Doppler, these devices promise additional utility in the detection of vascular structures, facilitating the process for selecting sites for incision and surgical procedures.

In 1986, the invention of the computer chip (CCD) video camera was a major breakthrough. This device allows transmission of the laparoscopic visual image to a television monitor, which provides an efficient method of viewing the operative field by the surgeon and the surgical assistants. The addition of picture-in-picture technology (Fig. 16–15) superimposed on the ultrasound image provides yet more utility for laparoscopic ultrasound evaluations.

Although laparoscopic sonography is still basically a research tool, the technique holds promise to provide information about a variety of structures not directly visualized during surgery. Initial studies have been directed to the liver, pancreas, and gallbladder, providing visualization of the intrahepatic biliary system, cystic duct, and common bile duct. In addition, laparoscopic sonography can be used to identify stones and to detect liver mestastases, and has the potential to guide needle aspiration or biopsy.

The current veterinary survey did not indicate use of laparoscopic sonography in veterinary applications. As this technology develops, it could offer significant advantages for use in animals for which a minimally invasive procedure is preferred and physical access is limited.

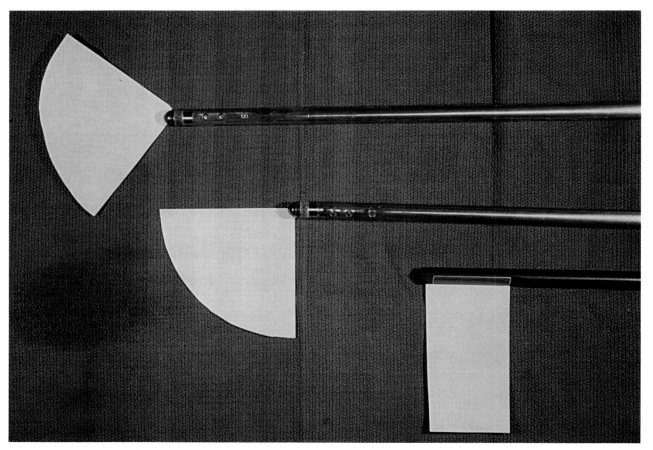

Figure 16–14

The current design of laparoscopic ultrasound probes provides forward viewing (mechanical sector), oblique viewing (mechanical sector), and side viewing (linear array) with a rectangular field of view (courtesy of W. McMullen, Endomedix).

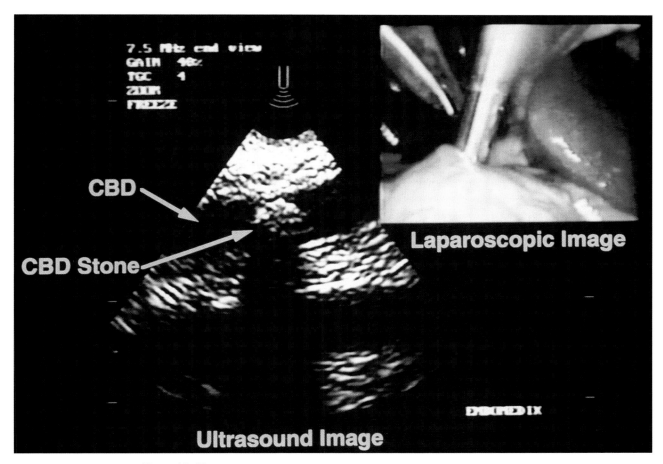

Figure 16–15

Picture-in-picture technology superimposes the laparoscopic image over the sonographic image. A stone is visible within the common bile duct (courtesy of W. McMullen, Endomedix).

Sonographically Guided Needle Procedures

Sonographic imaging is well suited for guidance of biopsy needles in that the real- time display allows visualization of the needle tip as it passes through tissues. With the use of smaller gauge needles, multiple biopsy samples can be easily taken, which often leads to a quick and accurate diagnosis. Ultrasound-guided percutaneous needle biopsy or aspiration is now a widely accepted technique that can be used for histologic diagnosis of malignancies and either drainage or aspiration of abscesses.[22,23] Improvements in sonographic image quality, biopsy devices, and reflectivity of needles hold promise to expand the utility of this technique in veterinary medicine without radiation hazard.

Sonographic guidance can be used for the biopsy of many organs and tissues in a large number of animal species, as long as an acoustic window is available through which to operate. Most sonographically guided biopsies are performed under continuous real-time visualization. If, however, the tissues visualized are not relatively homogeneous but produce bright echoes, the procedure is more difficult. Theoretically, any mass that is visible sonographically is amenable to needle biopsy.

Several approaches are used to guide aspiration or biopsy procedures. With the free-hand approach, ultrasound is used to simply locate the position of the anatomy of interest. The operator must then exercise a reasonable degree of manual dexterity to execute the procedure. The freehand approach is best applied for larger masses that are located more superficially. Another alternative is to use ultrasound probes that have incorporated needle channels that direct the insertion of the needle within the B-scan image plane. Other biopsy guides are fitted on the side of the probes to guide the needle at a predetermined angle to specific depths within the image field. These devices, combined with computer-generated graphics and grids, have greatly improved the ease of use and accuracy of sonography in facilitating the biopsy procedure (Fig. 16–16).

Sonographic visualization of the biopsy needle can be a frustrating aspect of biopsy procedures. The B-scan image plane (slice thickness) is only a few millimeters wide, and the needle must be in this plane to be visualized. Several techniques have been developed to enhance the visualization, and thus location, of the needle.[24] Larger caliber needles (16 to 19 gauge) are easier to see than smaller needles. Increased visibility of the needle has been achieved by scoring the needle surface to increase its reflectivity. Research is underway to develop a needle that contains a piezoelectric acoustic transponder on the tip (ATL). This transponder is activated by the ultrasound imaging frequency and transmits a signal (bright spot) that is mapped on the B mode image to show the location of the needle tip in the organ. This concept has also been used on a 2-mm catheter (Fig. 16–17) to show its location inside the body (Echo Locator, Diasonics, Milpitas, CA).

Figure 16–16

Soft tissue biopsy is facilitated by use of biopsy needle guides and visual guide lines superimposed on the real-time B mode image.

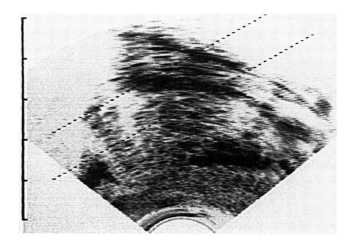

Figure 16–17

A 2-mm acoustic transponder mounted on the tip of a catheter was inserted into a phantom. When activated, it generates a signal that is superimposed on the sonogram and serves as a pointer for localization.

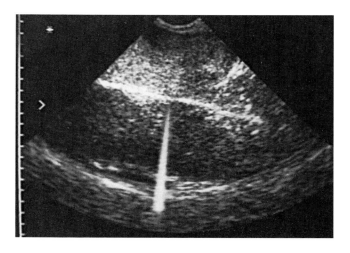

Ultrasound-guided biopsy and aspiration is currently used on a regular basis at all veterinary teaching hospitals and by approximately 75% of the private practitioners surveyed. Continued improvement in image quality and biopsy devices, along with the use of phantoms to help develop the hand-eye-screen coordination, will increase the interest and ability of practitioners to use this technique.

In the future, it is expected that other ultrasound-guided needle procedures will evolve. Alcohol ablation for the treatment of tumors involves direct percutaneous needle injection of alcohol under ultrasound guidance.[25] Other applications may include the deposition of chemotherapeutic and radioactive agents to selected sites for focal or localized treatment of tumors.

Contrast Agents

The use of radiopaque contrast agents for radiologic techniques to delineate vascular structures is well established. Using contrast agents with sonographic imaging, however, presents a new set of challenges that have been under investigation for over 25 years. This concept was first introduced in the late 1960s to increase the reflectivity of blood during echocardiographic recording.[26] The basic principle involves injecting a solution containing entrapped gas-filled microbubbles into a vein or artery to enhance both Doppler signals and visualization of vascular beds in solid tissues. The increased acoustic backscattering (echogenicity) observed is directly related to the presence of the echo contrast microbubbles.

Researchers have sought different methods of producing microbubbles, with the most promising agents involving either a sugar or albumin matrix. Current investigations are directed toward agents that use encapsulated gas bubbles,[27] colloidal suspensions,[28] emulsions,[29] and carbon dioxide.[30] The ideal echo contrast agent should be nontoxic and provide microbubbles that are of relatively uniform size (1 to 8 μm in diameter), are small enough to pass through the capillaries, and remain intact for 1 to 5 minutes. Two sonographic agents that appear to meet these criteria are Albunex, air-filled human albumin microspheres (Molecular Biosystems, San Diego, CA) and Levovist, a monosaccharide agent (Schering AG, Berlin, Germany).

Most research to date with such contrast agents has been directed to studies of the heart and the cardiovascular system.[30] More recently, investigators are focusing on using sonographic contrast agents to help differentiate areas of normal vascularity from areas of reduced flow caused by the presence of tumor necrosis or areas of ischemia or occlusion. In addition, these agents are being used to evaluate the effectiveness of enhanced detection of slow blood flow in the microvasculature, particularly flow related to vascular architecture within tumors. The potential to study microvascular flow may result in significant tissue enhancement (echogenicity), allowing characterization of organ perfusion in both normal and pathologic conditions.[31] Using color flow imaging combined with sonographic contrast enhancement could result in more rapid and accurate methods of diagnosing malignant tumors based on their neovascular and perfusion patterns.

An alternative to encapsulated gas-filled microbubbles is direct injection of carbon dioxide gas into the hepatic artery to enhance the visualization of tumors. Although evaluation of this technique is in its early stages, studies to date indicate that carbon dioxide-enhanced sonography may be a useful tool in detecting small liver tumors as well as in differentiating various hepatic disorders.[32]

In addition to intravenously administered agents, cellulose-based oral sonographic contrast agents are being investigated with the intent of improving sonographic visualization of abdominal anatomy.[33] SonoRx (Squibb Diagnostics, Princeton, NJ), one of the first products specifically formulated for acoustic enhancement, has significantly improved pancreatic visualization, bowel marking, and bowel wall detail with reduced gas artifacts.

The utility of diagnostic sonography in veterinary medicine will certainly expand further given the clinical potential of their use in such ways as increasing the reflectivity of blood (thus Dopplers signals) or enhancing visualization of organ- or tumor-specific tissues to allow improved detection and differentiation of disease.

Three-Dimensional Imaging

Three-dimensional (3-D) imaging techniques are well established for CT and MR visualization of anatomic structures, 3-D sonographic imaging presents a special set of challenges. When 3-D sonography becomes a reality, a new visual data will become available to aid diagnosis, volume calculations, and surgical/therapeutic planning.

Advanced sonographic imaging techniques, combined with faster and more powerful computer technology, continue to motivate investigators in the quest to develop 3-D sonography. Much early research has been directed toward 3-D visualization of the heart and major vessels.[34,35] Echocardiology is still the primary target for many of the research and clinical programs directed to 3-D imaging.[36,37] More recent applications include obtaining image of the fetus (Fig. 16–18), breast, liver, prostate, and eye, and in combination with color Doppler may provide a unique assessment of the neovascular architecture associated with tumors.[38–40]

The basic scanning technique for 3-D reconstruction using ultrasound requires the acquisition of multiple two-dimensional images (tomographic planes) with known spatial orientation. Major technical challenges relating to 3-D sonography are currently under investigation at numerous research sites and involve a host of interrelated topics that include:

—Probe/transducer registration in reference to anatomy
—Limited acoustic windows and organ movement
—Methods for on-line, high speed multiplane data acquisition

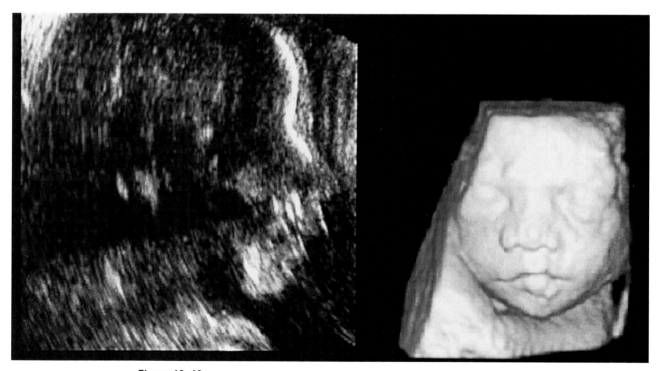

Figure 16–18

A normal two-dimensional (2D) sonogram of a 25-week fetal face (left) and the three-dimensional (3D) reconstruction (right). The 2D image is one slice that was acquired to build the 3D reconstruction (courtesy of Tomtec Imaging Systems, Inc. and Kretztechnick, Denver, CO).

—High capacity digital storage and processing
—High speed image processing for multiplanar reformatting
—Display format for 3-D presentation to user

Several unique approaches for probe registration and multiplane image acquisition are being developed. Custom-designed transducer housings incorporate electromechanical devices to sweep the probe and images are obtained through a predefined angle. Two-dimensional phased arrays have been developed that allow visualization of different tomographic planes by electronic steering of the ultrasound beam in any direction in 3-D space.[41] Although different approaches are being evaluated, many practical limitations dealing with frame rates, data acquisition time, number of scan lines, and spatial resolution still exist and present a formidable challenge.

Determining the probe position and orientation in relation to anatomy is yet another challenge. Methods of determining the probe orientation in three dimensions as well as how to scan serial B-mode planes at known incremental distances are under development. Probe position and orientation can be determined using either electromechanical, acoustic, or electromagnetic sensing devices, all of which have inherent advantages and disadvantages. It is interesting to note that the now defunct static B scanner used a probe interfaced with a 3-axis mechanical scanning arm, now a requirement for 3-D imaging. Serial planes of image data can be obtained by mounting the probe on a translation stage that contains precise stepper motors to control the probe position. Sonographic image data can thus be collected from different planes that are incrementally separated by 0.5 to 2.0 mm. Individual image plane RF data from various tissue orientations (sections) is then digitized and sorted for subsequent analysis.

In addition to the transducer locating system customized for 3-D data acquisition, the reconstruction of 3-D images from multiple two-dimensional tomographic planes requires the use of a digital scan converter to obtain volumetric image data in Cartesian coordinates.

Current RF data acquisition and digitization can be done on-line (real time), although 3-D image reconstruction is a timely process that requires a large digital memory, high speed processing capability, and between 5 and 30 minutes to complete. The image reconstruction time depends on the complexity of the anatomic presentations, spatial resolution requirement, and the time required for multiplaner reformatting in any arbitrary plane.

Undoubtedly, 3-D sonography will be an integral part of diagnostic imaging in the future. This unique capability will, however, come at a cost that may limit its utility for at least another decade.

Combined Sonographic Imaging and Therapy

Several unique technologies are evolving that combine the use of ultrasound energy for both diagnostic imaging and therapy. Because ultrasound can be focused, it can be delivered to remote sites inside the body. Used in the pulse echo mode at low intensities (SPTA < 100 mw/cm^2), B-mode images can be produced. If high intensity ultrasound is focused inside the body, selected tissue can be destroyed, resulting from localized thermal effects, cavitation, and mechanical stress. These principles are incorporated into the design of a new generation of devices that are used to break stones (lithotripters) and to selectively kill tissue (acoustic ablation).

EXTRACORPOREAL PIEZOELECTRIC LITHOTRIPSY

Lithotripsy or the breaking of stones with shock waves had its birth in Germany in the early 1970s.[42] The first generation of lithotripters used spark-induced focused shock waves that were targeted inside the body using x-ray techniques to localize the renal stones. More recently developed lithotripters use ultrasound-induced shock waves coupled with sonography for accurate targeting of the focused energy into the calculi (Fig. 16–19). Several companies are developing piezoelectric lithotripters, each with a slightly different shock wave generator configuration (EDAP, France; Wolf, Germany; Diasonics, USA).

An ultrasound-based lithotripsy system has several clinical advantages: the procedure is painless, it affords real-time monitoring during treatment, and it imposes no radiation hazard. Most therapeutic applications for extracorporeal shock wave lithotripsy have been directed to the noninvasive fragmentation of renal or biliary calculi (Fig. 16–20). As this technology matures and equipment costs are reduced, it is possible that lithotripsy may be used in veterinary medicine.

Figure 16–19

The B-mode imaging transducer is coaxial, with the shock wave focus providing accurate targeting of the calculi and real-time monitoring during treatment (courtesy of Diasonics, Milpitas, CA).

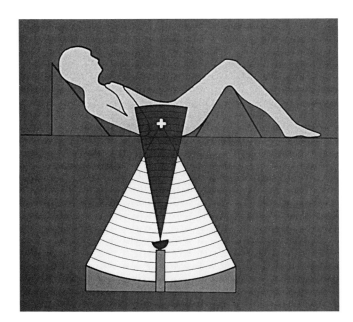

Figure 16–20

Sonogram of the gallbladder shows sand-like debris from a 2.5-cm calculus after piezoelectric lithotripsy treatment.

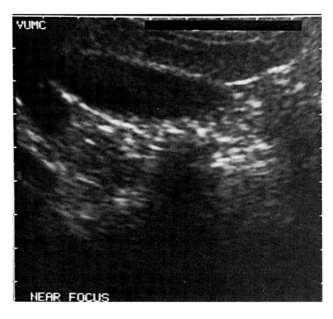

In addition to fragmenting kidney stones and gallstones,[43,44] one must consider the lithotripter as a unique method to deliver high energy, short duration acoustic pulses (microseconds) to various internal tissues and organs. The typical piezoelectric beam characteristics and energy levels result in the deposition of high pressure sound waves in a focal area of several centimeters in diameter. When considered as a focal energy source, the benefit of the lithotripter has the potential to expand beyond that of just fragmenting calculi. Researchers have indicated the applicability of lithotripsy to the stimulation of bone growth and fracture repair. In veterinary medicine, another potential application might be the use of lithotripsy for the noninvasive removal of bone spurs. Although the use of shock wave lithotripsy has become widespread only over the last 10 years, researchers are no doubt challenged by this technology and will apply it to new and yet unexplored ends.

Acoustic Ablation

Another exciting new imaging/therapeutic application is the use of high-intensity focused ultrasound (HIFU) to destroy selected tissues and tumors.[45–47] The high energy ultrasound is focused to a small zone (millimeters in size) to generate high levels of heat ($>70°C$), resulting in tissue death produced by coagulation necrosis. A unique characteristic of HIFU technology is the fact that the ultrasound energy can be focused on tissues within the body without injuring intervening tissues. Thus, this type of tool could be considered an acoustic (or invisible) knife that can be used to perform noninvasive surgery.[48]

Several companies are developing HIFU technology (FOCUS Surgery, Milpitas, CA.; EDAP, Marne-la-Vallee, France), and have coupled it with sonography to provide accurate targeting of the focal zone in the organ of interest. To date, the only commercial system available for HIFU surgery is the Sonablate (FOCUS) (Fig. 16–21), which incorporates an endocavity probe. The piezoelectric crystal in the probe is concave and focuses the high energy sound at a fixed distance from the probe tip, creating a focal lesion approximately 2 mm in diameter by 10 mm long. Under computer control, the crystal is mechanically moved to different positions, creating many overlapping focal lesions to ensure that the entire targeted tissue volume has necrosed (Fig. 16–22).

In the research environment, HIFU has been used experimentally for in vitro and in vivo animal research to study the ablative effects on normal tissue and implanted tumors.[49–51] In 1985, Heimberger reported the use of HIFU for the treatment of malignant brain tumors in man.[52] Since then, image-guided HIFU ablation has been reported to be clinically useful in the treatment of glaucoma[53] and benign prostatic hyperplasia.[54] Acoustic ablation treatments take between 15 to 60 minutes and can be done using local anesthesia, thus making this technique an attractive alternative to conventional surgery.

Although HIFU technology has not yet entered the arena of veterinary medicine, its noninvasive surgical potential is great and it is just a matter of time until the "invisible knife" is part of veterinary surgical instrumentation.

Figure 16–21

The Sonablate acoustic ablation system incorporates a 4-mHz endocavity probe that provides both B mode imaging for targeting and high-intensity focused ultrasound to ablate selected internal tissues without damaging intervening tissues (courtesy of FOCUS Surgery, Fremont, CA).

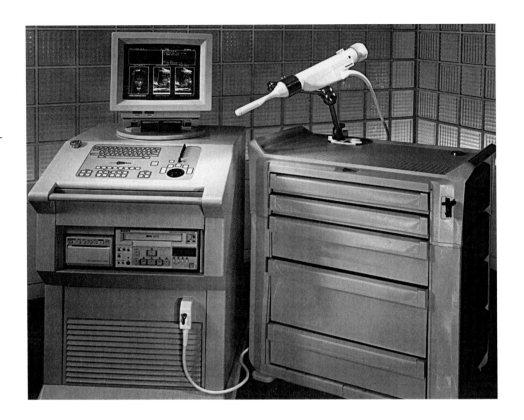

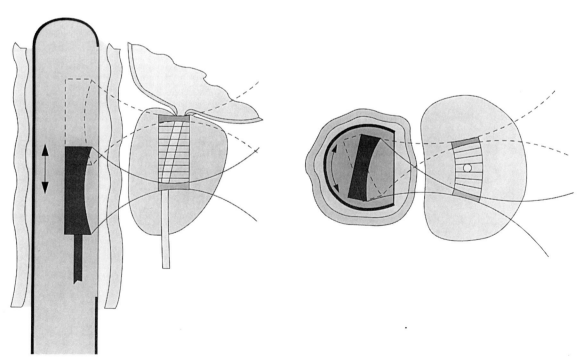

Figure 16–22

For thermal ablation of prostate tissue, the endocavity probe is positioned in the rectum, the high-energy ultrasound is focused on the targeted tissue, and overlapping focal lesions are created, resulting in coagulation necrosis (70° to 90°C).

ACKNOWLEDGEMENT

The author is greatly indebted to Karen Morgan for her efficient and skilled assistance in the manuscript preparation of this chapter.

REFERENCES

1. Howry DH, Bliss NR: Ultrasonic visualization of soft tissue structures of the body. J Lab Clin Med *40:*579, 1952.
2. Goldberg BB, Gramiak R, Freimanis AK: Early history of diagnostic ultrasound: The role of American radiologists. AJR Am J Roentgenol *160:*189, 1993.
3. Beach KW: 1975–2000: A quarter century of ultrasound technology. Ultrasound Med Biol *18:*4:377, 1992.
4. Showise Strategies, Veterinary Medicine Survey, 3844 Suncrest Ave., San Jose, CA. 95132.
5. Market Intelligence Research Corp., 2525 Charleston Road, Mountain View, CA. 94043.
6. Smith MT: The wild new world of health care for your pet. Money *47:*April, 1994.
7. Salles-Cunha SX, Andros G: Atlas of Duplex Ultrasonography, Pasadena: Appleton Davies, 1988.
8. Picot PA, et al: Three-dimensional true velocity colour Doppler imaging. J Ultrasound Med *11:*S-9, 1992.
9. Newman JS, et al: Power Doppler sonography: Applications in musculoskeletal inflammatory disease. J Ultrasound Med *13:*S-5, 1994.
10. Goldberg BB, et al: Endoluminal laparoscopic ultrasound. J Ultrasound Med *11:*S-16, 1992.
11. Schiller VL, et al: Interoperative ultrasound guidance of hepatic cryosurgery: Techniques, pitfalls and complications. J Ultrasound Med *13:*S-56, 1994.
12. Goldberg BB, Liu JB: Endoluminal ultrasound: Vascular and nonvascular. Ultrasound Q *9:*245, 1992.
13. Sigel B: *Operative Ultrasonography.* Philadelphia: Lea & Febiger, 1982.
14. Schlegel JU, Diggdon P, Cuellar J: The use of ultrasound for localizing renal calculi. J Urol *86:*367, 1961.
15. Eiseman B, Greenlaw RH, Gallagher JQ: Localization of common bile duct stones by ultrasound. Arch Surg *91:*195, 1965.
16. Sigel B, et al: Comparative accuracy of operative ultrasonography and cholangiography in detecting common bile duct calculi. Surgery *94:*715, 1983.
17. Makuuchi M, et al: The use of operative ultrasound as an aid to liver resection in patients with hepatocellular carcinoma. World J Surg *11:*615, 1987.
18. Plainfosse MC, et al: The use of operative sonography in carcinoma of the pancreas. World J Surg *1:*654, 1987.
19. Klotter HK, et al: The use of intraoperative sonography in endocrine tumors of the pancreas. World J Surg *11:*635, 1987.
20. Yamakawa K, et al: Laparoechography—An ultrasonic diagnosis under the laparoscopic observation. Jpn Med Ultrasonics *2:*26, 1962.
21. Fukuda M, Mima F, Nakano Y: Studies in echolaparoscopy. Scand J Gastroenterol *17:*186, 1982.
22. Holm HH, et al: Ultrasonically guided percutaneous puncture. Radiol Clin North Am *13:*493, 1975.
23. Reading CC, et al: Sonographically guided percutaneous biopsy of small (3 cm or less) masses. AJR Am J Roentgenol *151:*189, 1988.
24. McDicken WN: *Needle guidance techniques.* In *Advances in Ultrasound Techniques and Instrumentation.* Edited by PNT Wells. New York: Churchill Livingstone, 1993.
25. Shiina S, et al: Percutaneous ethanol injection therapy for the treatment of hepatocellular carcinoma. AJR Am J Roentgenol *154:*947, 1990.
26. Gramiak R, Shah P, Kramer D: Ultrasound cardiography: Contrast study in anatomy and function. Radiology *92:*939, 1968.
27. Hilpert PL, et al: IV injection of airfilled human albumin microspheres to enhance arterial Doppler signal: A preliminary study in rabbits. AJR Am J Roentgenol *153:*613, 1989.
28. Parker KJ, et al: A particulate contrast agent with potential for ultrasound imaging of liver. Ultrasound Med Biol *13:*555, 1987.
29. Fink IF, Miller DJ, Shawker TH: Lipid emulsions as contrast agents for hepatic sonography: An experimental study in rabbits. Ultrasonic Imaging *7:*191, 1985.
30. Feinstein SB, et al: Two-dimensional contrast echocardiography. In vitro development and quantitative analysis of echo contrast agents. J Am Coll Cardiol *3:*14, 1984.
31. Chen RC, et al: Carbon dioxide-enhanced ultrasonography of liver tumors. J Ultrasound Med *13:*81, 1994.
32. Dittrich HC, et al: Multiple organ tissue perfusion by intravenously (IV) administered novel ultrasound contrast agents in dogs. J Ultrasound Med *13:*S-9, 1994.
33. Lev-Toaff AS, et al: Evaluation of an oral contrast agent to improve ultrasonic visualization of abdominal anatomy: A phase I trial. J Ultrasound Med *13:*S-8, 1994.
34. Howry DH, et al: Three-dimensional and stereoscopic observation of body structures by ultrasound. J Appl Physiol *9:*304, 1956.

35. Geiser EA, et al: A mechanical arm for mechanical registration of two-dimensional echocardiographic sections. Cathet Cardiovasc Diagn 8:89, 1982.
36. Itoh M, Yokoi H: A computer-aided three-dimensional display system for ultrasonic diagnosis of a breast tumor. Ultrasonics 17:261, 1979.
37. Levaillant JM, et al: Three-dimensional ultrasound imaging of the female breast and human fetus in utero: Preliminary results. Ultrasonic Imaging 11:149, 1989.
38. Brown TG: Visualization of soft tissues in two and three dimensions, limitation and development. Ultrasonics 5:118, 1967.
39. von Ramm OT, Smith SW, Pavy HG: High speed ultrasound volumetric imaging system. Parts I and II. IEEE Trans Ultrason Ferroelect Freq Contr 38:100, 1991.
40. King DL, et al: 3-D echocardiographic techniques for quantitation of ventricular volume and function: Clinical validation. J Ultrasound Med 13:S-65, 1994.
41. Hottier F, Collet-Billon A: 3-D echocardiography: Status and perspective. In 3-D Imaging in Medicine. Edited by KH Hohne, H Fuchs, SM Pizer. Berlin: Springer, 1990.
42. Chaussy C, et al: Contact-free renal stone destruction by means of shock waves. Eur Surg Res 11:36, 1979.
43. Martin X: Ultrasonic stone localization for ESWL. In State of the Art Extracorporeal Shock Wave Lithotripsy. Edited by LB Kandel, LH Harrison, DL McCullough. Mt. Kisco: Futura Publishing, 1987.
44. Marich KW, et al: Ultrasonic reflex transmission imaging improves stone localization and characterization for biliary lithotripsy. In Lithotripsy and Related Techniques for Gallstone Treatment. Edited by G Paumgartner, et al. St. Louis: Mosby-Year Book, 1991.
45. Fry WJ, et al: Production of focal destructive lesions in the central nervous system with ultrasound. J Neurosurg 11:471, 1954.
46. Oka M: Application of intense focused ultrasound in brain surgery and other fields. Clin All-Round 13:1514, 1974.
47. Linke CA, et al: Localized tissue destruction by high-intensity focused ultrasound. Arch Surg 107:887, 1973.
48. Catalano P: Gamma knives and ultrasound microcookers. In The World & I. Vol. 9. New York, News World Communications, May 1994, p. 192.
49. ter Haar GR, et al: High-intensity focused ultrasound for the treatment of rat tumours. Phys Med Biol 36:1495, 1991.
50. Sanghvi NT, et al: Ultrasound system for noninvasive focal lesioning in organs and tissue. J Ultrasound Med 3:S-30, 1984.
51. Vallencien G, et al: Focused extracorporeal pyrotherapy: Feasibility study in man. J Endourol 6:173, 1992.
52. Heimberger RF: Ultrasound augmentation of central nervous system tumor therapy. Indiana Med 78:469, 1985.
53. Lizzi FL, et al: Thermal model for ultrasonic treatment of glaucoma. Ultrasound Med Biol 10:289, 1984.
54. Bihrle R, et al: High-intensity focused ultrasound for the treatment of benign prostatic hyperplasia: Early United States clinical experience. J Urol 151:1271, 1994.

GUIDE TO THE SONOGRAPHIC DIAGNOSIS OF DISEASE IN ANIMALS APPENDIX

Normal brain general	Need persistent fontanelle or craniotomy to see in adult. Can image puppies until 3 to 4 weeks old. The appearance of the lateral and third ventricles varies depending on the relative amounts of cerebrospinal fluid (CSF) (anechoic) or choroid plexus (hyperechoic). May see pulsations in choroid plexus.
Head of caudate nucleus	Transverse images: hyperechoic superficially
Sulci	Transverse: The falx cerebri, splenial sulci, and callosal sulci comprise a hyperechoic umbrella-like structure, respectively forming the stem, roof, and handle of an umbrella. Parasagittal: Splenial and callosal sulci appear as hyperechoic lines.
Lateral ventricles	Transverse: Rostrally, appear as anechoic, slit-like areas medial to the respective head of the caudate nucleus. More caudally, can see choroid plexus (hyperechoic) and/or CSF (anechoic) in dorsal and ventral horns of the lateral ventricles. Parasagittal: Appears as a C-shaped structure. Mean height measured at or immediately caudal to the level of the interthalamic adhesion was 0.15 mm (0.04 to 0.35 mm). Cerebral mantle ratio = height of the lateral ventricle/ thickness of cerebral mantle (brain parenchyma dorsal to the lateral ventricle) was 0.08 (range: 0.05 to 0.18). Ventricle hemisphere ratio = height of the lateral ventricle/ hemispheric width was 0.07 (range: 0.04 to 0.17). Percent of brain occupied by the dorsoventral dimension of the lateral ventricle was 0.14%.
Hippocampus	Transverse: Dorsally, shows as a hypoechoic structure on either side of the midline, medial to the lateral ventricles, in the diencephalon. May see ventrally, medial to hyperechoic choroid plexus in the ventral horns of the lateral ventricles.
Mesencephalon	Transverse: Dome-shaped hypoechoic structure outlined dorsally and laterally by interfaces between CSF, vessels, and trabeculae in the subarachnoid space.
Cerebellum	Transverse: Vermis presents as a stack of horizontal hyperechoic lines in caudal images. The cerebellar hemispheres are hypoechoic and are located laterally.
Osseous tentorium	Transverse: In the adult, this structure resembled an upside-down "V." Blocked visualization of deeper structures.
Thalamus	Parasagittal: Thalamic adhesion is hypoechoic but is outlined by hyperechoic choroid plexus in the lateral ventricle.
Hydrocephalus	Lateral ventricular height measured at the level of the interthalamic adhesion >3.5 mm. Ventricle mantle ratio >0.25.

Ventricle hemisphere ratio >0.19.
Moderate enlargement if the percent of brain occupied by the dorsoventral dimension of the lateral ventricle was 15 to 25%.
Severe dilatation was indicated by a percentage greater than 25%.

Brain neoplasia	Most (not all) are hyperechoic
Brain abscess	Center with variable echogenicity
Brain hemorrhage	Initially hypoechoic but rapidly becomes hyperechoic
Normal spinal cord	Need laminectomy or osseous defect to see. Sagittal images: Dura mater and adjacent thin arachnoid = linear horizontal echo. Subarachnoid space = May not see or anechoic because of CSF. Pia mater = second hyperechoic linear echo on the surface of the spinal cord. Spinal cord parenchyma = variable echogenicity with no distinction between gray and white matter. Central canal = 1 to 2 hyperechoic lines located centrally. Fat and connective tissue in the ventral epidural space = lobular echoes. Surrounding bone = Bright hyperechoic surface but absorbs sound, causing distal acoustic shadowing. Transverse: Central canal appears as a circular echogenicity surrounded by a relatively hypoechoic spinal cord parenchyma.
Trauma	The spinal cord is hyperechoic after trauma, possibly because of hemorrhage
Disk disease	Hyperechoic disk material can be seen compressing the spinal cord after laminectomy. Doppler sonography may help evaluate vascularity.
Syringomyelia	Multiple cystic (anechoic) areas that may not be interconnected
Arteriovenous malformations	Usually appear as multiple, cystic masses, although echogenic masses have been reported. Doppler sonography may aid in resection.
Tethered cord syndrome	Caudal displacement of the spinal cord
Meningocele	Hypoechoic tract
Extramedullary intradural lipoma	Appeared as a hyperechoic mass in cat with tethered cord syndrome
Neoplasia	Intramedullary spinal neoplasms in people and dogs usually are more hyperechoic than the normal spinal cord. May be expansion of the cord with disruption or loss of the central canal echo complex.
Edema	Diffusely expanded, echogenic spinal cord. Must consider neoplasia.
Normal spinal cord	Sagittal images: Hyperechoic near and deep surfaces with multiple linear echodensities internally. (Hudson JA, Steiss JE, unpublished research.)
Transection	Follow normal section of nerve to area of possible transection. Nerve undergoes Wallerian degeneration distally and is difficult to identify. Be careful where nerve changes course. Must know normal anatomy. Look for muscle atrophy.
Wallerian degeneration	Nerve distal to transection appears slightly smaller than normal. The borders are less hyperechoic and become slightly irregular. Confusion with blood vessels or muscle or tendon fibers is more likely to occur. Look for muscle atrophy.

CHAPTER 5: THE EYE

DISEASE	SONOGRAPHIC APPEARANCE
Hypopyon	Increased anterior chamber echoes
Iris/ciliary melanoma	Echogenic mass extending into anterior chamber or vitreous originating at the iris or ciliary body
Cataract	Thick echogenic anterior and posterior lens surface
Blood clot in vitreous Fungal granuloma Purulent panophthalmitis	Echogenic mass in vitreous
Asteroid hyalosis	Small echogenic specks in vitreous
Retinal detachment	Thin echogenic lines in vitreous; "V" shaped
Metallic foreign body	Highly echogenic focus with shadows or reverberations
Retrobulbar mass	Often echogenic and mass-like; may deform shape of the globe

CHAPTER 6: THE SALIVARY, THYROID, AND ADRENAL GLANDS, THE PANCREAS, AND LYMPH NODES

DISEASE	SONOGRAPHIC APPEARANCE
Benign salivary mass	Hypoechoic—sharply marginated
Malignant salivary mass (abscess)	Hypoechoic—irregular margin
Sialoadenitis	Inhomogeneous, hypoechoic
Salivary hemangioma	Anechoic
Thyroiditis, hyperthyroid, abscess	Decreased echogenicity
Pancreatitis—mild	Hypoechoic with hypoechoic foci, anechoic finger-like projections
Pancreatitis—severe	Irregular areas of increased and decreased echogenicity, displaced duodenum
Pancreatic cyst	Anechoic area
Neoplasia of pancreas	Discrete hypoechoic nodule
Adrenal enlargement (tumor)	Diameter to length measurement of >30%
Adrenal cyst	Anechoic area within adrenal
Metastatic lymph node	Transverse to length ratio of > 2:1
Lymphadenitis	Hyperechoic center
Benign lesions	Linear pattern
Malignant lymphoma	Spotty—linear pattern

CHAPTER 7: THE HEART AND VESSELS

Definition of Terms

Left ventricle diameter diastolic (LVDd)—Diameter of the lumen of the left ventricle during diastole. Usually made from M-mode image (MM).

Left ventricle diameter systolic (LVDs)—Diameter of the lumen of the left ventricle during systole. M mode usually (MM).

Left ventricle ejection time (LVET)—Time from opening of the aortic valve until its closing. M mode.

Shortening fraction (%) (SF)—The percent change in the diameter of the left ventricle from diastole to systole. Calculated.

Aortic root dimension (Ao)—Diameter of aortic root. M mode or B mode. End of diastole.

Interventricular septal wall thickness diastole (IVSd)—Thickness of IVS end diastole. M mode or B mode.

Interventricular septal wall thickness systole (IVSs)—Thickness of IVS end systole. M mode or B mode.

Left ventricular posterior wall thickness diastole (PWd)—Self explanatory. M mode or B mode.

Left ventricular posterior wall thickness systole (PWs)—Self explanatory. M mode or B mode.

Left atrial diameter (diastole LAd, systole LAs)—Self explanatory. M mode or B mode.

Heart rate (HR)

Cardiac output (CO)—Amount of blood ejected from left ventricle at end of systole or for one minute.

Left atrium diameter aortic ratio (LAD/AO)—Divide LA diameter by aortic diameter. M mode or B mode.

Ejection fraction (EF)—The fractional volume of blood pumped out of the left ventricle during systole.

Left ventricle stroke volume (LVSV)—Volume of blood pumped from the left ventricle during systole.

Left ventricle posterior wall thickening fraction (LVPWTF) (%)—Percent change of wall thickness from diastole to systole. Calculated from M mode.

$$\frac{LVPWs - LVPWd}{LVPWs} \times 100$$

Left ventricle wall excursion (LVWE)—Initial excursion to peak excursion. M mode.

Interventricular septal thickness fraction (IVSTF) (%)—Percent change of thickness from diastole to systole.

Right ventricle diameter diastole (RVDd)—see above

Right ventricle diameter systole (RVDs)—see above

Right ventricle free wall diastole (RVFWd)—see above

Right ventricle free wall systole (RVFWs)—see above

Right ventricle free wall thickening fraction (RVFWTF)—see above

Pericardial effusion (PE)—Distance between pericardium and heart

Heart Disease

Atrial septal defect (ostium secundum)
1. Dilatation of hyperdynamic right ventricle, right atrium, and pulmonary artery
2. Paradoxical motion of IVS
3. Visual defect
4. One–third of cases have mitral valve prolapse

Atrial septal defect (ostium primum)
1. Dilatation of left ventricle
2. Defects of left and right AV valves
3. Defects of both IVS, IAS
4. Pulmonary artery hypertension

Patent ductus arteriosus
1. Dilatation of left atrium and ventricle
2. Hyperdynamic left ventricle or IVS
3. Possible visualization of ductus
4. Reduced fractional shortening

Coarctation of aorta
1. Left ventricular hypertrophy

Pulmonary valve stenosis
1. "a" dip on M mode
2. Thickened, more prominent valve on B mode
3. Dilatation of right ventricle and atrium
4. Right ventricular hypertrophy, IVS, hypertrophy

Tetralogy of Fallot
1. Visualize VSD (B mode)
2. Overriding aorta visualization (B mode)
3. Right ventricular enlargement
4. Right ventricular outflow obstruction
5. Septal hypertrophy with paradoxiae motion

Pulmonary hypertension
1. Right ventricular hypertrophy (M mode, B mode)

Aortic stenosis
1. Thickened/calcified aortic valve leaflets (B mode)
2. Left ventricular hypertrophy (B mode, M mode)
3. LA/AV ratio increased

Aortic regurgitation
1. Aortic valve vegetation or dysfunction
2. Diastolic fluttering of mitral valve
3. Premature mitral closure
4. Left ventricular dilatation

Mitral stenosis
1. Valve thickened (EF slope decreased on M mode)
2. Posterior leaflet drawn ventrally during diastole (B mode, M mode)
3. Mitral calcification possible (B mode)
4. Left atrial enlargement (B mode, M mode)
5. Pulmonary trunk enlargement (B mode, M mode)

Mitral regurgitation
1. Hyperactive IVS
2. Left atrial dilatation
3. Prolapse valve (B mode)

Tricuspid stenosis
1. Dilated right atrium
2. Hypertrophy of right ventricle

Tricuspid regurgitation
1. Dilated right atrium and ventricle
2. Abnormal Doppler flow or valve motion

Pulmonary regurgitation
1. Dilatation of right ventricle

Endocarditis
1. Vegetation B mode (90% sensitive)

Myocarditis
1. May be normal
2. May see atrial and ventricular dilatation (B mode, M mode)
3. Ventricular hypokinesis (B mode, M mode)
4. Mitral and/or tricuspid regurgitation (B mode, M mode)
5. Pericardial effusion (B mode, M mode)

Dilatory cardiomyopathy
1. Dilatation of ventricles and atria (B mode, M mode)
2. Ventricular systolic and diastolic dysfunction (B mode, M mode)
3. Hypokinesis, especially in left ventricle (B mode, M mode)

Hypertrophic cardiomyopathy
1. Disproportionate thickening of IVS and/or left ventricular free wall
2. End systolic diameter of left ventricle lumen is decreased
3. Left atrium enlarged

Restrictive cardiomyopathy
1. Hyperechoic endocardium
2. Some pericardial effusion
3. Ventricular wall thrombus (echogenic focus)
4. Myocardial "sparkle" with amyloidosis

Pericardial effusion
1. Echo-free space around left and/or right ventricle

Cardiac tamponade
1. Diastolic collapse of right atrium and right ventricle
2. Swinging of heart in pericardial sac

Constrictive pericarditis
1. Thickened pericardium
2. Abnormal motion of IVS
3. Short, steep E to F slope of anterior leaflet of mitral valve

CHAPTER 8: THE LIVER AND GALLBLADDER

DISEASE	SONOGRAPHIC APPEARANCE
Hepatic lipidosis	Diffuse increase in echogenicity. Decreased visualization of portal vein wall echogenicity. Liver margins smooth.
Nodular hyperplasia	Variable. Hyperechoic nodules. Hypoechoic nodules.
Cirrhosis	Diffuse increase in echogenicity with irregular liver margins.
Abscesses	May see echogenic focus (gas) with reverberation artifact. Early = small hyperechoic focal area with variable wall thickness. Late = hypoechoic to anechoic with variable wall thickness.
Cysts	Focal to multifocal anechoic foci, often demonstrate posterior enhancement.
Hepatocellular carcinoma	Solitary hyperechoic mass. Can be multifocal with mixed echogenicity.
Cholangiocellular carcinoma	Usually multifocal, hyper- or hypoechoic.
Lymphosarcoma	Highly variable. Diffuse to multifocal, hyper- or hypoechoic.
Metastatic neoplasia	Focal or multifocal. Hyper- or hypoechoic masses. Mixed patterns possible.
Portasystemic shunt	Often small hypovascular liver. May see communication between portal vein and liver. Acquired shunts may show dilated tortuous portal vasculature.
Cholelithiasis	Hyperechoic foci in gallbladder. Posterior shadowing.
Biliary obstruction	Dilated intrahepatic ducts. Tortuous branching pattern, irregular wall. Too many hepatic tubular structures.
Benign hyperplasia/ hypertrophy	Normal to increased size. Often symmetric, uniform, and slightly hyperechoic. Cystic lesions can be seen.
Prostatic cyst	Anechoic with posterior enhancement. Smooth to slightly irregular margins. Some may have internal echoes.
Prostatic abscess	Hypo- to anechoic, solitary or multiple lesions. Prostate often asymmetric, inner margins often irregular.
Paraprostatic cyst	Large anechoic structure adjacent to prostate. Smooth margins with thin or thick walls. May demonstrate posterior enhancement or contain low-level internal echoes.
Chronic prostatitis	Variable appearance. Diffuse or multifocal. Hypo- to hyperechoic.
Prostatic adenocarcinoma	Mixed nonuniform echogenicity. May contain mineralized foci.

CHAPTER 9: THE ESOPHAGUS AND GASTROINTESTINAL TRACT

CONDITION OR DISEASE	APPEARANCE/SIZE/SHAPE
Normal esophagus	Seen inconsistently; poorly defined structure with a hyperechoic, star-shaped center representing intraluminal mucus and air; identify by watching swallowing or move esophageal stethoscope in anesthetized animal
Normal stomach	Five layers alternating hyperechoic and hypoechoic echoes 1. Inner hyperechoic layer, mucosal surface 2. Inner hypoechoic layer, mucosa 3. Central hyperechoic layer, submucosa 4. Outer hypoechoic layer, muscularis propria 5. Outer hyperechoic layer, subserosa and serosa Thickness, 3.0 to 5.0 mm; abnormal: >6.0 to 7.0 mm

Small intestine	Five layers; thickness, 2.0 to 3.0 mm; abnormal: >5.0 mm; mucosa noticeably thickest layer
Large intestine	Usually hyperechoic with no through transmission because of large amount of gas. Five layers but harder to measure. Thickness, 2.0 to 3.0 mm. Mucosa not as thick as that of stomach and small intestine. Contractions may not be seen in the descending colon.
Foreign body	May transmit or attenuate sound. Reflective near interface, hyperechoic near border with deep acoustic shadowing (e.g., rocks, sewing needle, acorn, some rubber balls). Shape of near interface can help identify. Attenuation with minimal reflection, acoustic shadowing but no hyperechoic near border. Transmission of sound, shape can be identified. Surrounding fluid may help identify shape. "Clean" or crisp, complete shadow is more likely to occur with a soft tissue-bone interface or a soft tissue-foreign body interface. "Dirty" shadow may be caused by reverberations between the transducer and intraluminal gas.
Linear foreign body	Hyperperistalsis and intestinal plication has been reported with linear foreign bodies.
Obstruction	May see distension of GI tract with decreased or absent motility proximal to obstruction. May be seen with pancreatitis with enlargement of the pancreas, free peritoneal fluid, and enlarged mesenteric lymph nodes.
Neoplasia	Symmetric or asymmetric, localized or generalized wall thickening. Disruption of wall layers common. Masses can be present. Wall mineralization, mesenteric lymphadenopathy, or ileus can occur. Ulceration in neoplasia and inflammation. Ulcers hyperechoic because of trapped gas.
Ileus	Decreased motility often with increased intraluminal fluid and mucus. Seen with foreign body, neoplasia, pancreatitis, and parvovirus enteritis.
Intussusception	Multiple concentric rings surrounding an echogenic core in transverse images. May be a target-like pattern. Multiple layers in longitudinal images. Pattern varies with degree of edema, luminal fluid content, scanning location, and invaginated contents.
Parvovirus enteritis	Normal wall thickness, fluid distension, and a lack of motility.
Nonfungal inflammation	Normal or increased wall thickness. Normal wall layers generally preserved with nonfungal inflammation unlike with neoplasia (see Fig. 9–23).
Exocrine pancreatic insufficiency	May be thickening of intestinal wall with preservation of normal wall layers, corrugation (spasticity) or increased echogenicity.
Acute hemorrhagic pancreatitis	May be hemorrhage in adjacent intestine with loss of the normal layered appearance.
Fungal enteritis (e.g., Candida albicans, Histoplasma capsulatum, Aspergilla, and phycomycetes)	Involves mucosa or all layers, specific segments or entire bowel. May cause dramatic thickening of wall or cause disruption of wall layers. Lymph nodes may be enlarged. Phycomycetes can cause mass requiring differentiation from intussusception or foreign body obstruction.
Feline infectious peritonitis	Pyogranulomatous disease. Similar appearance to fungal enteritis. May be concurrent increased echogenicity of the kidney and renal capsule.
Bowel adhesions	Diagnosed in horses suffering from intermittent bouts of colic. Examination for a significant length of time showed no independent movement of involved segments of the intestine. Ileus not always present.
Mesenteric vascular disease	Can use transrectal sonography to evaluate the cranial mesenteric artery in horses with verminous arteritis. Can use color flow Doppler imaging and Doppler spectral analysis to evaluate gastrointestinal vascularity.
Displacement of bowel	Cranial or caudal displacement with small or large liver, respectively. Diaphragmatic herniations can be recognized by following the cranial edge of the liver and diaphragm from side to side. Inguinal hernias have a "tornado" appearance. Observation of a beating heart adjacent to the cranial aspect of the liver and diaphragmatic discontinuity is diagnostic of congenital peritoneopericardial herniation.
Enteric duplication	Rare. Cyst-like formation is adjacent to a bowel segment with a common wall and muscular layer. Cyst may contain hypoechoic fluid.

CHAPTER 10: THE SPLEEN

DISEASE OR CONDITION	SIZE/SHAPE/APPEARANCE
Normal	Smooth borders; fine echogenic line represents splenic capsule when visualized incident to the beam. Has uniform echo pattern slightly hyperechoic to liver. Venous branches seen near hilus. Cannot see intraparenchymal splenic arteries without Doppler. Echogenic flow seen in large normal vessels. Volume averaging can cause fat adjacent to vessels and hilus to appear artifactually like a hyperechoic mass.
Hemangiosarcoma	Usually causes a complex mass with echogenicity ranging from anechoic to hyperechoic. Anechoic to hypoechoic areas usually have well-defined borders but no capsule.
Lymphosarcoma	"Swiss cheese" appearance. Nonhomogenous echo patterns with poorly marginated hypoechoic to anechoic nodules (4 mm to 3 cm). Usually no acoustic shadowing or enhancement of the underlying tissues. Complex masses or nodules reported in horses. Check for lymphadenopathy.

Mast cell tumor	Splenomegaly or spleen may appear normal in spite of splenic metastases. Decreased echogenicity, generalized or patchy.
Carcinomatosis	Hyperechoic nodules (3 to 20 mm) reported on serosal surfaces in a mare.
Hemangioma	Cannot differentiate from hemangiosarcoma or hematoma sonographically. Absence of other organ involvement help differentiate. Need histopathologic analysis for definitive diagnosis.
Passive congestion	Splenomegaly. Normal or decreased echogenicity. (Chronic congestion can lead to increased echogenicity in people.)
Myeloproliferative disease	Hypoechoic mass in one cat. Enlarged spleen with normal or increased echogenicity in people.
Extramedullary hematopoiesis	Splenomegaly or non-neoplastic splenic mass. Can appear as a hypoechoic, ill-defined lesion.
Hematoma—general	Cannot differentiate from hemangiosarcoma with ultrasound. Difficult to differentiate on fine needle aspiration.
Hematoma—acute	Initially anechoic-hypoechoic but becomes hyperechoic with clotting.
Hematoma—96 hrs	Hypoechoic or anechoic as clot hemolysis occurs.
Hematoma—chronic	Hyperechoic with reorganization and eventual calcification of the hematoma.
Splenitis	Can appear similar to neoplasia. The spleen of one dog was enlarged with multiple hypoechoic nodules that varied in size. Diffusely hypoechoic spleen in people.
Abscess	Usually hypoechoic, occasionally complex. Variable encapsulation. Mild to no through transmission.
Nodular hyperplasia	Common in old dogs. Nodules usually project from the surface and vary up to 2 cm or more in diameter. Can appear similar to hemangiosarcoma if necrosis or hemorrhage occurs. Peritoneal effusion more commonly accompanies hemangiosarcoma.
Infarction/necrosis	Anechoic (occasionally cystlike) or hypoechoic round lesions in acute infarcts. Hyperechoic wedge-shaped lesions with the apex toward the hilus in chronic infarcts. Round, hypoechoic or isoechoic, well-marginated nodules may deform the splenic border. A heteroechoic or hypoechoic, diffuse coarse/"lacy" appearance in the affected area of the spleen without deformation of the splenic border may represent splenic necrosis secondary to infarction.
Splenic torsion	Usually affects large or giant breed dogs. Frequently associated with gastric dilatation-volvulus. Splenomegaly and distension of the splenic veins. Subsequent splenic infarction and necrosis may cause a diffusely hypoechoic spleen with linear echodensities separating large, anechoic areas (coarse/lacy heteroechoic pattern). Doppler sonography may aid in diagnosis.
Splenic rupture	May see hematoma formation or free peritoneal fluid. Possible parenchymal splenic lesions. Possible rupture of a neoplasm.

CHAPTER 11: THE KIDNEYS

DISEASE	CATEGORY	APPEARANCE
Calculi	Focal/multifocal	Hyperechoic focus, ± shadow
Cysts	Focal/multifocal	Circular, anechoic, through transmission
Neoplasia	Focal/multifocal	Altered shape, heteroechoic, cats-hypoechoic
Infarcts	Focal/multifocal	Initially hypoechoic with bulging margins, later hyperechoic and depressed surface
Abscess	Focal/multifocal rare	Anechoic to echogenic focus, ± through transmission
Hematomas	Focal/multifocal	Early hypoechoic, subacute-echogenic (fibrin), late-complex
Perirenal pseudocyst	Regional	Encapsulated, anechoic fluid around kidney
Hypercalcemic nephropathy	Regional	Thin, continuous hyperechoic band at corticomedullary junction (medullary rim sign)
Ethylene glycol toxicity	Regional	Dramatic increase in cortex, later medulla, medullary rim sign
Pyelonephritis and hydronephrosis	Regional	Anechoic renal pelvis (pyelectasia), ureter ± anechoic tube
Advanced hydronephrosis	Regional	Marked anechoic dilatation of renal pelvis, rim of cortex, ± septa
Nephrocalcinosis	Regional or diffuse	Continuous hyperechoic inner cortex or diffusely hyperechoic
FIP, infiltrative LSA, early amyloidosis	Diffuse	Diffusely hyperechoic, enlarged, poor corticomedullary definition
Glomerulonephritis, CIN, nephrosclerosis, late amyloidosis, end-stage kidneys	Diffuse	Hyperechoic, small, irregular, poor internal definition
Early infiltrative renal disease	Diffuse	May be normal

CHAPTER 12: THE URINARY BLADDER

DISEASE	CATEGORY	APPEARANCE
Crystals, "sand"	Intraluminal	Mobile bright echoes, gravitate down, shadow when accumulate
Cellular debris	Intraluminal	Mobile low level echoes, mimic tissue when accumulate
Calculi	Intraluminal	Bright curvilinear foci, shadow if large, gravitate, appearance unaffected by composition
Gas	Intraluminal	Mobile bright echoes, float upward, reverberate near top
Blood clots	Intraluminal	Mobile mass-like, gravitate, no shadow
Foreign body	Intraluminal	Parallel-lined catheters, bright shadowing BBs, branching grass awns
Ureterocele	Mural	"Small bladder within bladder," anechoic, thin-walled, trigone
Ectopic ureter	Mural-congenital	Anechoic tube with low flow, continue caudal to trigone
Diverticula	Mural-congenital or traumatic	Persistent conical thinning of wall at vertex
Rupture	Mural	Partial-subserosal anechoic halo around bladder; complete-free fluid, adherent tissue, wall defect
Hematoma	Mural	Fixed mural mass effect, echogenicity "age" related, usually hypoechoic
Herniation	Mura	Absent normal bladder, smooth-walled anechoic structure in hernial sac
Acute cystitis	Mural	Thick irregular hypoechoic wall, loss of layers, intraluminal debris, angular shape, ± nodules
Chronic cystitis	Mural	Thick wall, irregular bright "heaping up" of mucosa, intraluminal debris, ± nodules
Emphysematous cystitis	Mural	Thick irregular wall, bright reverberating intramural gas, intraluminal gas
Neoplasia	Mural	Papillary, polypoid, or sessile, complex hypoechoic, abrupt transition to normal wall unless infiltrative ± mineralization

CHAPTER 13: THE REPRODUCTIVE SYSTEM

DISEASE	SONOGRAPHIC APPEARANCE
The Ovaries and Uterus	
Ovarian cyst	Thin-walled anechoic with distal enhancement >2.5 cm
Ovarian neoplasms	Bilateral, mostly solid with small cysts, irregular margins
Uterus proestrus	Increased diameter—hypoechoic tubular structure
Uterus estrus	Hyperechoic lines radiating outward, fluid in lumen sometimes
Uterus post partum	Multiple alternating hyperechoic and hypoechoic layers
Pregnancy	17 to 20 days following LH surge, mass appears on day 25
Pyometra	Uniform hypoechoic tube with enhancement
Uterine neoplasia	
Benign	Homogenous isoechoic to uterine wall
Malignant	Mixed echogenic mass
The Prostate	
Benign prostate	Normal to increased size. Symmetric. Uniformly hyperechoic cysts possible.
Prostatic cysts	Anechoic with posterior enhancement. Smooth to slightly irregular margins. Some may have internal echoes.
Prostatic abscess	Anechoic solitary or multiple. Inner margins are asymmetric, may have posterior enhancement.
Paraprostatic cyst	Large, anechoic, adjacent to prostate. Smooth margin with thin or thick walls.
Chronic prostatitis	Diffuse or focal hyperechogenicity, patchy with granulomatous prostatitis.
Neoplasia adenocarcinoma, transitional cell carcinoma	Mixed pattern, possible mineralized foci—capsule irregular.

The Testicles

Seminoma intestinal cell tumor	Mixed echogenic pattern
Sertoli cell tumor	Hypoechoic focal area
Hydroceles	Anechoic area around testicle
Orchitis	Mixed patterns
Testicular torsion	Vascular flow reduced. Diffuse decrease in echogenicity.

CHAPTER 14: THE INTEGUMENT, MUSCLES, TENDONS, JOINTS, AND BONES

DISEASE	SONOGRAPHIC APPEARANCE
Integument	
Dermatitis (humans) (animals?)	Subepidermal band of hypoechogenicity
Scleroderma (humans) (animals?)	Skin thickened and subcutaneous fat echogenic
Tumors (humans) (animals?)	Hypoechoic mass
Cysts (humans) (animals?)	Anechoic area
Muscles	
Trauma—tear	Loss of regular pattern. Hypoechoic area.
Hemorrhage	Anechoic or hyperechoic area
Lipoma	Echogenic mass
Rhabdomyolysis	Patchy areas of decreased echogenicity
Sequestrum	Hyperechoic area with shadows
Tendons	
Tears	Hypoechoic area
Synovitis	Anechoic area around tendon
Fibrosis	Hyperechoic area
Joints	
Synovial fluid increase	Increase anechoic area in joint capsule
Septic synovitis	Echogenic foci in increased anechoic joint capsule
Bones	
Osteomyelitis	Anechoic layer superficial to bone

Index

Note: Page numbers in *italics* indicate figures; page numbers followed by t indicate tables.